New Rules

· ·

12/22/95

Maureen –

Happy Holidays.
We are looking for
great things in your
new job! Congratulations

Troy

Troyen A. Brennan
Donald M. Berwick

New Rules

Regulation, Markets, and the Quality of American Health Care

Jossey-Bass Publishers
San Francisco

Substantial discounts on bulk quantities of Jossey-Bass books are available to corporations, professional associations, and other organizations. For details and discount information, contact the special sales department at Jossey-Bass Inc., Publishers. (415) 433–1740; Fax (800) 605–2665.

For sales outside the United States, please contact your local Simon & Schuster International Office.

 Manufactured in the United States of America on Lyons Falls Pathfinder Tradebook. This paper is acid-free and 100 percent totally chlorine-free.

Library of Congress Cataloging-in-Publication Data

Brennan, Troyen A., date.
    New rules : regulation, markets, and the quality of American
health care / Troyen A. Brennan, Donald M. Berwick.
      p.   cm.—(The Jossey-Bass health series)
    Includes bibliographical references and index.
    ISBN 0-7879-0149-0 (alk. paper)
    1. Medical care—United States—Quality control.   2. Medical care—
Law and legislation—United States.   3. Medical care—United
States—Cost control.   I. Berwick, Donald M. (Donald Mark), date.
II. Title.   III. Series.
RA399.A3B74   1996
362.1'0973—dc20
                                                            95-30487
                                                             CIP

HB Printing   10 9 8 7 6 5 4 3 2 1   FIRST EDITION

Contents

Acknowledgments

The authors would like to thank a number of people who were very helpful in the development and writing of this book. Oliver Sangha, M.D., contributed greatly to the information and interviews in Chapter Three. We are also indebted to Robert Brook, John Williamson, Avedis Donabedian, Kerr White, and Paul Sanazaro for spending a good deal of time with us during interviews. Erik Ramanathan and Christine Solt both provided a great deal of help in researching legal issues. Their work was critical in Chapters Two, Four, and Five. Kathryn Guare did a good deal of the word processing for Chapter Three. Ann Marie Hultmark typed much of the rest of the manuscript and uncomplainingly did revision after revision. Carlisle Knowlton Rex-Waller skillfully edited our first draft. Tim Jost carefully read an early draft and gave us many great suggestions. These and a number of our other colleagues were extraordinarily helpful to us in writing this book.

To George and Vivian Brennan,
my parents

To Dr. Philip Berwick,
my father

The Authors

. . . .

TROYEN A. BRENNAN is professor of law and public health at the Harvard School of Public Health, and professor of medicine at Harvard Medical School. He practices internal medicine at the Brigham and Women's Hospital, where he is executive director of the Brigham and Women's Physician Hospital Organization. He holds a B.S. degree from Southern Methodist University, a master's of art degree from Oxford University, an M.D. and a master's of public health degree from Yale Medical School, and a Juris Doctor degree from Yale Law School.

DONALD M. BERWICK is president and CEO of the Institute for Healthcare Improvement, a nonprofit organization dedicated to accelerating the pace of improvement of the health care systems in the United States and Canada. He is also associate professor of pediatrics at the Harvard Medical School, and adjunct associate professor of health policy and management at the Harvard School of Public Health. He holds an A.B. degree summa cum laude from Harvard College, a master's of public policy degree from the John F. Kennedy School of Government, and an M.D. degree from Harvard Medical School.

The Role of Regulation

Describing a recent visit to his hospital by a survey team from the Joint Commission for Accreditation of Health Care Organizations (JCAHO), the physician administrator began to grow animated, even passionate. The JCAHO, or the "Joint" as it is known in the hospital industry, inspects hospitals every three years and accredits them if they have met a variety of standards. In most states, this accreditation is critical because hospital licensure is contingent on accreditation. Moreover, Medicare and in some cases, Medicaid funding is available only to accredited institutions. The survey is a serious business.

The administrator had every reason to be pleased with the way his institution was being run. He and his colleagues had undertaken a series of exciting measures to improve the quality of care at the hospital. Among these innovations was a tracking system for nosocomial infections. Using definitions of infections set forth in a program administered by the Centers for Disease Control, the hospital was able to monitor the incidence and treatment of infections and compare its results to those of other institutions. With this information, the hospital could identify its areas of weakness and address them directly. The infectious disease team was justifiably proud of its work thus far.

But the surveyors from the JCAHO were unimpressed. They focused upon structural measures of attention to nosocomial

infections, such as minutes from meetings held by the hospital's epi-
demiologists. They were not interested in the hospital's endorsement of cutting-edge methods like "outcome measures" and
"benchmarking." The JCAHO's failure to notice a serious investment in quality improvement had infuriated the hospital's leaders,
including the physician administrator. "What good," he asked, "was
regulation if the regulators ignored quality improvement efforts?"
Overall, in this hospital, the visit from the surveying team of the
JCAHO had become mostly a big headache, absorbing energies that
otherwise could have gone into quality improvement.

The hospital administrator's experience was not unique. Indeed,
it reflected a pattern we have witnessed frequently in the past two
years as we have tried to understand how to improve health care
regulation. The frustration with traditional regulation is apparent
throughout the industry, even in the regulatory community itself.
But there are subtleties behind the sharp points this story makes
about regulation.

First, although the physician administrator was completely focused
on the issues of hospital quality and regulation when speaking about
the accreditation survey, in other parts of our interview, he was quite
articulate about the need to expand and integrate his organization
and also about the virtues of managed care. His hospital is part of a
large network of health care institutions, including several hospitals,
a number of very large group practices, a fledgling health maintenance
organization, and affiliated nursing homes and rehabilitation centers.
The administrator confined his concerns about regulation to the
traditional hospital context, yet acknowledged only minutes later
that health care has moved well beyond the traditional physician/
hospital/third-party insurer arrangements that for the past twenty-five
years have dominated thinking about medical care. In doing so, he
demonstrated how anachronistic most conceptions of regulation have
become as health care has evolved. Views on regulation, whether positive or negative, are years behind the facts and circumstances of the
rapidly changing health care environment.

Second, the shape of the institutions is not the only thing that is changing in medical care. The market in which this physician practices medicine is one of the most advanced in the United States, with increasing reliance on capitated payment. Cost competition is extraordinarily severe. Yet in our interview with this leader, he never mentioned the potentially troubling issues raised by the cost/quality trade-offs that must come as health care institutions are forced to take below-cost payment in order to guarantee sufficient patient volume.

Our interview with this physician in many ways crystallizes the problems we face in trying to improve regulation. We want to consider how to convert health care regulation from a meaningless waste of resources into something that can really help practitioners provide better care, but this agenda is complicated by the rapid changes in health care institutions and by the increasing cost competition in the health care market that can negatively affect quality. We need to understand not just how to modify regulation, but how to do so in a reformed and dynamic health care system that faces significant cost pressures.

The task is a difficult one for a number of reasons. First, too little scientific attention has been given to technologies that can be used in regulating the quality of medical care. Many good books and articles are written every year on regulation, but most avoid discussing medical care, and almost none address the quality of medical care in particular. The student of regulation learns from sophisticated models in areas such as risk regulation undertaken by the Food and Drug Administration or the Occupational Safety and Health Administration. But regulatory experts have not provided models directly applicable to the concern of this study—regulation of health care quality—so we have few paths of analysis to follow.

Another obstacle to redesigning health care regulation is the lack of agreement on key terms, an issue that has troubled commentary on regulation generally. Justice Stephen Breyer, writing in 1981 about regulatory reform, acknowledged at the outset of his important book *Regulation and Its Reform* that he would make no serious effort to define regulation.[1] We might define *regulation* as any set of influences exterior to the practice or administration of medical care that imposes some rules of behavior.[2] In the law, we would include in regulation both traditional agency-developed rules as well as rules issuing from common law litigation. Of course, some prescriptions created by a market in medical care might fit well within this definition of regulation, yet the distinction between markets and regulation is central to most analyses of the regulatory state.

Even if we agree on a working definition of regulation, we are left with the thorny issue of what we mean by "quality of medical care." The difficulty of this definition is one of the main reasons that legal scholars have avoided using quality of medical care as an illustration of the problems with regulation. Indeed, the law—in particular, common law courts—has largely left the definition of quality of medical care up to the profession itself, and the profession has historically been little interested in bold searches for new definitions. The negligence standard in medical malpractice litigation, for example, is defined by medical custom—that is, by the testimony of expert physicians. In essence, the practitioner has tended to say, "Quality, by definition, is what we do."

We have a slightly more critical understanding of high-quality care. For our purposes, *quality* is the optimal match between work and need. It will also be efficient, for more work than is necessary to meet need is, by definition, of poor quality. Throughout our book, we will return to this definition of quality, and we will spend more time specifying its meaning in health care, especially in Chapter Three.

Yet another difficulty in thinking about regulation of health care is the relative lack of structural regulation in this section of the economy. Quality has traditionally been regarded as a matter primarily of the physician's ethical commitment to the patient. No other field has been as highly dominated by a sense of professional paternalism. Both the profession and society have long seen the individual doctor's devotion to the patient and conscientiousness in providing appropriate care as sufficient. Insofar as there has been regulation, it has been self-regulation. The profession has policed both itself and the institutions like hospitals in which care occurs. Although external inspections, like those of the JCAHO, have been tolerated (and in many ways have actually been a form of self-regulation, as we will discuss), regulation has largely been viewed as a meaningless sideshow compared with the physician's altruistic commitment to the patient.[3] This approach to assuring the quality of medical care has persisted through this century, even as the modern medical industry has grown far beyond traditional structures.

The evolution of the medical industry has been continuous, although the pace has increased recently. At the turn of the century, hospitals were still emerging from their past as almshouses and were largely dominated by their lay philanthropic boards. Over the course of the next thirty years, however, they transformed into more sophisticated institutions of medical care, and control passed from the board to the organized medical staff.[4] Hospital administrators had to be especially responsive to their own medical staffs. The organized physicians retained their independence, in great part because of the belief that patients chose a doctor, not a hospital. The hospital was thus a passive service provider for the physician. Young administrators in training learned that it was critical to the success of the hospital to keep referring physicians happy.

This model was reinforced by the nature of private insurance. Insurance began as Blue Cross/Blue Shield plans that were often created by statute and were closely supervised by the medical profession. After World War II, large commercial insurers emerged, but they did little to diminish the professionals' influence on health insurance. Physicians continued to charge customary rates of reimbursement, and insurers rarely questioned the costs or nature of the care provided. In 1964, the government endorsed this arrangement by imitating in Medicare and Medicaid the existing insurance relationships.[5] Thus, twenty-five years ago, the triad of passive hospitals, unquestioning insurers, and dominant physicians was well still secure.

By 1970, change was under way. Health care costs were rising at a rate that alarmed both private and public payers. Efforts at cost containment began, involving both review of appropriateness and oversight of technology. Moreover, models of managed care, initially developed by health maintenance organizations (then a very small industry), slowly emerged. However, the underlying shape of medical practice still involved the individual physician committed to the individual patient, supported by fee-for-service financing and utilizing compliant hospitals.

Perhaps the most salient feature of the traditional health care system was its insulation from market forces. Although it is an exaggeration to suggest that market forces did not affect health care at all, physician control of the knowledge that lay behind medical care allowed practitioners to shape both the demand for medical technology and its supply, inhibiting the development of an active role of the patient as a consumer. In the half-century between 1925 and 1975, the profession persisted in its efforts to limit exterior influence on health care—including market incentives. One motivation for doing so (suggested by Paul Starr and Eliot Friedson, among others[6]) may have been that the monopoly of knowledge and the inhibition of the patient's role as consumer furthered the profession's own economic interests. Another (and in many ways more probable) explanation is that the espoused ethic of medicine required the reduction of market incentives so as to eliminate all influences on the healing relationship except the physician's commitment to the patient. According to this view, fee-for-service payment provided by passive insurance companies allowed the doctor to concentrate on the good of the patient. Similar arguments obstructed any hospital oversight or managerial intervention in the relationship between doctor and patient.

Today, the isolation of this relationship is no longer tenable or possible. Health care has become a true industry, with numerous loci of authority well beyond the doctor's office. The care of the patient is increasingly understood to depend on the precise functioning of a complicated organization. Though the physician still acts as the patient's advocate, practitioners are more and more economically integrated into the structure of health care, either as employees, as members of physician-hospital organizations, or as participants in managed care plans. In many ways, the relationship of the patient to the doctor is of less importance than is the role of the patient as consumer in a health care system. Patient choice and patient discrimination are the hallmarks of intrinsic health care reform. Of course, this means that market incentives are more sharply felt in health care today. In addition, traditional medical ethics, based on the doctor-patient dyad, must be reformulated to fit the new mold of the delivery of health care. The roles of physicians and their patients change with the changes in structure and financing.

The evolving health care system and the changing role of the doctor provide the context for our main subject in this book: the quality of health care and its regulation. Modern advocates of quality improvement recognized much earlier than most that sound health care delivery in the future will require the precise functioning not only of individuals but of complicated organizations—high-performance systems. No longer can the emphasis be simply on the doctor's commitment to the patient; rather, the system of care must be improved, through rational measurement and carefully planned, continual change. As we discuss in Chapter Three, health care quality improvement is undergoing a revolution.

We believe regulation of quality improvement must also undergo a revolution. The traditional and still dominant methods of quality oversight come from an era characterized by passive institutions, "hands-off" financing, and physician hegemony. That era has passed, and regulation must evolve. Moreover, regulation must take note of the influence of the market in medical care. Most of the competition in health care today emphasizes cost, but we have every reason to believe that quality competition will develop quickly as well.

Regulators in medicine, long unused to noticing market incentives, must now come to understand how competition affects quality.

Quality regulators must also be aware of the trade-offs between cost and quality that could come with an environment focused too exclusively on control of expenditures. Unrelenting pressure to reduce costs in medical care, especially the demands emanating from sources uninformed in modern methods of process improvement, can easily lead to deficiencies and errors. Regulation must take this into account and adapt appropriately.

Most important, however, regulators must understand the theory and practice of modern quality improvement, lest they inadvertently impede such improvement. Techniques learned from other industries are taking root at hospitals like the one our physician administrator represents. Surveyors, certifiers, and other regulators must be open to innovative approaches to improving care and must have clear opportunities to enhance and disperse such techniques.

Reform of regulation must then address three key issues. First, regulators and regulated must understand how today's rules obstruct integration of innovative methods of quality improvement into health care. Regulation should enable and promote, not discourage, continuous improvement. Second, new rules must take account of both the virtues and the drawbacks of the burgeoning market in health care. Especially insofar as the market promotes cost restraint at the expense of quality, regulation must be deployed to benefit the patient. Third, regulators themselves should be prepared to adopt new methods, based on modern notions of quality improvement. Responsive and cooperative new rules based on regard for patient welfare must be the goal.

The Regulatory State

What sort of regulatory philosophy should guide the formulation of new rules? As our goal is to describe a better system of regulating the quality of health care, we cannot afford the luxury of simply taking the definition of regulation for granted. We must spend some effort, at the outset, to understand what regulation is, how it has developed, and what function it is intended to serve in our society.

As we have already discussed, no less an authority than Justice Breyer has stated that he will not adequately define regulation. A different sort of authority, *Merriam-Webster's Collegiate Dictionary*, defines regulation as "an authoritative rule dealing with details of procedure." To regulate is to "govern or direct according to rule . . . to bring under the control of law or constituted authority."[7] Regulations are rules provided by an authority. Regulating for improved medical care thus involves designing appropriate rules invested with authority.

Not all rules are the same. Regulation involves prescriptive, not descriptive, rules. As Frederick Schauer points out in his fascinating book *Playing by the Rules*, descriptive rules are a matter of regularity, whether mathematical or empirical. They are not intended to change or channel behavior. They reflect the world as it is. On the other hand, "prescriptive rules are employed, not to reflect the world, but to apply pressure to it."[8]

This definition of prescriptive rules is still quite general. Indeed, some might note that it can accommodate the notion of "principles." But rules imply specificity. Ronald Dworkin argues, for instance, that rules are dispositive if applicable, whereas principles can be applicable without being controlling.[9] Yet as Schauer counters, this distinction may not capture all the dimensions of rules that Dworkin has in mind.

The linguistic and philosophical analysis that would be required to sort these issues further goes well beyond the scope of this book, but the nuances are helpful. Regulation implies prescriptive rules that are legitimate and specific for certain kinds of activities. We treat regulation as consciously formulated and intended by a source of authority. Hence although the market may have a certain rationality and coherence, giving rise to behavior that appears to follow certain rules, we see these rules as descriptive. Our attention is focused not on the rules of the marketplace, the economic facts of life created by the market, but rather on prescriptive rules of behavior that can be enforced by exterior authority. We will advocate the use of rules to correct the market when necessary.

This understanding of regulation as prescriptive is reflected in the history of American regulation.[10] Though the roots of the regulatory state in this country can be traced to legislation passed in the middle and latter parts of the nineteenth century, regulation assumed its modern aspect in the years of the New Deal. The reformers who gave birth to the modern administrative state were convinced that existing regulation, enshrined primarily in the common law of contracts, torts, and property, failed to protect its intended beneficiaries. As a result, a great deal of activity that had been considered part of the private sphere, issues of personal liberty, became subject to public attention and public rules. Property rights were curtailed so that a whole new set of rights could be created— rights to what Rawls would call "primary goods"[11] Primary goods are those things necessary to take advantage of the opportunities of liberalism: food, shelter, some education, and self-respect.

To enforce the new rules that created these rights, a superstructure of new administrative agencies was constructed in Washington, and to some extent in the state governments. The creation and enforcement of rules required a great deal of human capital. For example, between 1933 and 1939, the number of civil service employees grew from 572,000 to 920,000.[12] Among the new agencies created were the Works Progress Administration, the Civil Conservation Corps, the Tennessee Valley Authority, the Farm Security Administration, the Social Security Administration, the Federal Deposit Insurance Corporation, the Securities and Exchange Commission, and the Food and Drug Commission. In a very short time, social regulation far more extensive than that possible through the common law courts became widely accepted. Notably, however, little of this new regulation affected the medical care industry.

Although not quite on the scale of the New Deal revolution, the redistributive programs enacted thirty years later during the Johnson administration's Great Society initiatives again set forth a series of rights and an oversight structure. The Democratic Congress passed the Food Stamp Act and began Head Start, enacted a series of historic antidiscrimination statutes, and initiated Medicare and Medicaid. Though the latter programs were essentially passive insurers at the outset, they laid the foundation for regulatory activity in health care financing.

Remarkable growth of the administrative state occurred again in the late 1960s and early 1970s, especially in the sphere of human welfare and health protection. (Many have previously noted that economic regulation preceded social regulation.) In a short period of time, and largely under the Ford and Nixon administrations, the Environmental Protection Agency, the Occupational Safety and Health Administration, the Mine Safety and Health Administration, the Nuclear Regulatory Commission, and the National Highway Traffic Safety Administration were created. These authorities had a host of new statutes to enforce, especially in the environmental area. Much of this regulatory activity reflects a sense of urgency about the need to protect the environment and create a safe workplace. Concurrently, especially at the state level, as we shall see, some regulation began to touch health care as well.

This brief history suggests that at times, public consensus creates a context for government intervention in the private sphere. We are not arguing, however, that there is an unwavering historical progression toward greater regulation, for at other times the social consensus favors limits on government, and deregulation occurs. The role of deregulation is the subject of Richard Vietor's perceptive book *Contrived Competition: Regulation and Deregulation in America*.[13] In Vietor's view, the Depression created an overwhelming pessimism regarding the critical institutions of capitalism, including but not limited to the stock market and banks. This explains the turn of Roosevelt's Brain Trusters to national planning and economic regulation, leading in a space of five years to the passage of the Banking Act, the Securities Exchange Act of 1934, the Communications Act of 1934, the Motor Carrier Act of 1935, the Civil Aeronautics Act of 1938, the Public Utility Holding Company Act of 1935, the Natural Gas Act of 1938, and the Robinson-Pattman Act. These regulations remained in effect over the next forty years, as Keynesian economics ushered in an era of annual growth in real GNP that averaged 4.3 percent from 1938 to 1968.

Vietor is unwilling to infer any causal relationship between economic regulation and economic prosperity. On the contrary, he sees economic regulation as the root of the economic slowdown from 1968 through 1974. He argues that inflationary recession that proved so immune to the regulatory efforts of the Nixon administration was "as fundamental a structural change as the great Depression."[14] The best thinking in economics could not solve the problem of stagflation in the 1970s, just as in the Depression, non-Keynesian economists were unable to find methods of stimulus.

By the mid-1970s, academics, stimulated by Alfred Kahn's work on the economics of regulation, were advocating deregulation and use of market incentives.[15] In the late Ford and early Carter administrations, these ideas took hold. No less a liberal than Senator Edward Kennedy organized congressional hearings on deregulation. At the same time, the presidential candidates, Jimmy Carter and Gerald Ford, both ran on platforms emphasizing limited government. Once in office, the Carter administration engaged in economic deregulation with a vengeance.

More surprisingly, Vietor argues that the major economic deregulation was complete by 1980. The Reagan administration passed only three deregulatory laws after 1980: the Bus Regulatory Reform Act of 1982, the Cable Television Act of 1984, and the Garn-St. Germaine Banking Act of 1982, which created the conditions for the savings and loan crisis.[16] Although Reagan paid ideological lip service to reducing the regulatory burden on industry, after a few years of effort, the deregulation campaign waned. In the first two years of the Reagan administration, expenditures on regulation decreased by 3 percent and personnel involved in regulation at the federal level declined by 20 percent. Major health and welfare programs in the Environmental Protection Agency, the Consumer Product Safety Commission, and the Occupational Safety and Health Administration were reduced. But by 1984, the antiregulation ammunition had largely been spent.

Perhaps even more surprising, there was an impressive rebound in regulation in the mid- to late 1980s. As Ayres and Braithwaite argue, by 1982, enforcement actions under the Clean Water Act had dropped to 27 percent of the 1977 level, but 1984 enforcement expenditures exceeded the 1977 level.[17] Enforcement of a variety of federal environmental claims increased dramatically in the late Reagan and early Bush administrations. OSHA civil penalties had dipped in the early Reagan years, but by 1987, there were record numbers of enforcements, and the average size of penalties had increased dramatically. Many of these programs at the Department of Energy increased by more than 100 percent from 1985 through 1989. However, in 1995, during a Democratic administration, the Republican Party's Contract with America intended to sweep away much existing social regulation.

These numbers challenge the conventional wisdom. Deregulatory rhetoric is not always backed by deregulation. Nor are presumably pro-social-regulation administrations (Carter's, for example) necessarily strong advocates of new rules. Thus one must be careful not to assume that widespread deregulation occurs in an era in which antiregulatory rhetoric dominates. Moreover, a wave of regulation will not swamp every industry simultaneously or homogeneously. Consider health care. Insulated by a commitment to the individual and to professional decision making, medical care saw regulatory intent arrive only very slowly. One might expect regulatory or deregulatory tendencies in health care to follow slightly behind those occurring in other social sectors. But the New Deal's economic regulation barely brushed the health care sphere of the economy, and the new welfare regulation of the Great Society left the structure of medicine untouched—except that new payers were added. Significant new regulations were to take shape early in the 1970s. All this suggests that an understanding of the history of the government's use of prescriptive rules and a grasp of their relation to market-based, private activity will be critical to the design of new rules for health care quality.

The Functions and Forms of Regulation

Prescriptive rules are recognized as legitimate when they are embedded in widely held beliefs about the way a government should act. Their general function is to restrict the satisfaction of individual, private choices and desires in the interests of the community. Regulation allows coordination and collective action to thwart some private choices. It places certain public values before certain private ones. Some would even suggest that prescriptive rules help individuals to better understand their private preferences and to adapt and evolve in their choices.[18]

Any generic classification of government rules reveals these abstract functions of regulation. For example, Breyer has produced a somewhat economically oriented list of the functions of regulation.[19] First, he suggests, regulation is intended to compensate for spillover costs, or externalities. Breyer relies on important cases in the common law of torts to illustrate externalities. Steam engine sparks can ignite fires on crop lands near the railway. Regulation of sparks reduces the risk of such a fire. Prevalent social beliefs about the appropriate bearer of the costs of accidents can be translated into prescriptive rules by the legislature. The railroad can be forced to "internalize" the costs of the fires.

Another function of regulation is to compensate for inadequate consumer information. Technically, a market should provide sufficient information for consumers on a routine basis, because customers prefer to buy products they understand. However, when buyers have inadequate bargaining power, producers have less incentive to supply appropriate information. An obvious example may be the doctor-patient relationship, in which the patient's desire for information has often subordinated itself to the provider's paternalistic commitment to patient welfare: "Trust me," says the doctor. "Whatever you say," responds the patient. Trust replaces the exchange of information.

Closely related is the notion of so-called *moral hazard,* which occurs when a third-party buyer purchases on behalf of another. The primary buyer (patient) is bound by none of the economic restraints experienced by the financing buyer (insurer) and hence has no economic reason not to overpurchase. In situations of moral hazard, the sellers' ethical code is often relied on to moderate spending. But commitment to codes can easily break down, and some see spiraling medical care costs as an excellent example of such a breakdown.

Governments may also regulate to combat scarcity. Scarcity occurs when the markets deteriorate in some way. Without a market, even widely held beliefs that certain kinds of commodities *should* be more widely available may be insufficiently strong to create appropriate supply. This is especially true with regard to certain publicly valued services or goods. In such cases, the government must step forward to alleviate the scarcity, usually through regulation. The relative lack of primary care doctors in the United States is a good example of scarcity due to breakdown of market forces. It has had to be addressed through regulation of physician training and distribution.

Each of these various forms of regulation can in some way be understood as countering market failures. Even stronger oversight of market failures occurs when governments address monopolies. Inefficiency of monopolies can in some cases drive up costs of services and also diminish product quality. Here it is not so much that the market has failed to function appropriately, but that the market has been deformed. The point of antitrust law, for instance, is to modify monopolistic relationships in such a way as to increase competition. Though the antitrust laws, at least in the United States, were founded on the populist sense that monopolies are by definition harmful to the economy, recent insights suggest that monopolies may sometimes be efficient.[20]

Closely related to regulation of monopolies is regulation of rent. As referred to by economists, rent is the profit that occurs when one firm is able to produce a good at a price cheaper than that currently existing in the market, such as when the firm holds the patent to a breakthrough process. Rent is a target of public regulation when it is seen to influence legislatures. Well-disciplined and well-organized interest groups are able to provide information to legislators at much lower costs than those charged by their competitors and so are able to bring about changes in legislation (prescriptive rules) that serve those groups. Such *interest group transfers*, or *rent seeking*, offend the public interest.

Rent-seeking behavior can be a target of regulation such as limits on lobbying activities, but it can also be a shaper of the process by which certain kinds of regulation are created. In their most extreme form, interest group transfers lead to *industry capture or regulation*, which permits the regulated industry to dictate the sort of rules that it will follow.[21] Although further attention to these public choice models is beyond the scope of this book, we think the understanding of health care regulation must include an awareness that regulation of the regulatory process itself may sometimes be necessary and appropriate.

An entirely different set of functions for regulation aims at increasing equality in society, as opposed to repairing the market or extending market efficiencies into areas in which the market is very weak. Examples are regulations that attempt to redistribute income or wealth; those that support pluralism and diversity, such as regulation of public broadcasting; and those that overcome inequality of opportunity, such as various antidiscrimination statutes. In health care, this sort of regulation typically involves efforts to increase access to health care.[22]

Some of these rationales for regulation have special importance for health care. As the health care market evolves, rules intended to make the market more efficient, to bring efficiencies to areas in which the market has been retarded, or to correct the market's emphasis on a single dimension (such as cost) may be especially important. In addition, because decision making in health care has traditionally been decentralized and uncoordinated, collective values may have suffered and may need correction through regulation. In this light, we suggest the following as a reasonable list of the primary functions of regulation in health care, especially as they affect the quality of medical care:

1. To constrain decentralized, individual decision making so as to achieve the efficiencies of a more coordinated, cohesive approach
2. To control elements of monopoly power
3. To provide consumers with adequate information so as to facilitate effective bargaining
4. To curb moral hazard in insurance arrangements
5. To weigh public welfare against the choices of private consumers

We can gain further insights into health care regulation by reviewing its failures. We have already mentioned one way that regulations fail: specific interest groups can transfer their own desires and agendas into public policy by capturing regulators or legislators. It is of course highly desirable to have the ears of those who make the laws, for if the original statutory rules can be written to benefit one group, those selective benefits become foundational to subsequent legislation. However, given the public nature of lawmaking, such interest group transfers cannot always be accomplished. It is often easier, if less efficient, to influence the regulators who design the specific measures through which laws are given effect. We now refer to influence on regulators, as opposed to influence on legislators, as *agency capture*.

Each of these approaches has a similar outcome: the paradigm of regulations as prescriptive rules reflecting public sentiment that certain kinds of activities are inappropriate or inefficient is undermined. Legal enactments are created that favor a specific portion of society, often at the cost of the majority, or well-intended rules are foiled by inappropriate application and enforcement.

This characterization of interest group transfer and agency capture may suggest too strongly that the failure of regulation is due to corruption. Much more common is that good intentions reap poor outcomes. To use a medical metaphor, well-motivated legislators and regulators must diagnose a specific problem and develop innovative therapy. The more complex the system, the more difficult the diagnosis is and the more uncertain the treatment. In many cases, statutes or regulations fail simply because they are based on a poor understanding of a complicated system. They represent not failed intent but failed prediction. Policy analysis is in many ways much more difficult than health care's diagnostics and therapeutics. The legislature must play hunches, surrounded always by the uncertain dynamics of policy science.

A corollary involves unanticipated consequences. Regulation does not only fail by not bringing about an intended outcome. It can also create unforeseen outcomes or consequences that produce greater harm or inefficiencies. Market-reverent antagonists of regulation usually cite retarded innovation as the critical unanticipated consequence of regulation. The important point for regulators is that a certain modesty and humility are appropriate to their enterprise. Policy making is a double-edged sword.

Coordination is also critical to the success of prescriptive rules. Many regulated industries are pushed and then pulled by the successive activities of their regulators. This can be the result of insufficient strategic planning by an agency, but it can come also from the complexity of government. A variety of regulatory agencies may have their attention focused on a single industry. This is certainly the case in health care. Yet these regulators may pay insufficient attention to each other's goals and activities, consequently producing discordant signals. Coordination failures are rampant, as we will see, and they can be especially telling in health care. A cost-conscious federal agency—the Health Care Financing Administration, for example—may be encouraging the elimination of hospital beds in an oversupplied area, yet the affected hospitals are prevented by the threat of federal antitrust actions from engaging in the cooperative planning most likely to achieve that result.

Finally, a common concern, perhaps more frequently found among students of policy making than in regulated industries, is that regulatory agencies will favor technocratic expertise over political judgment. To succeed, regulation must be founded on legitimate political choices that reflect the good of the public. Yet such choices can sometimes recede if technical expertise suggests other courses. This is not a matter of capture; the technocratic expertise may be that of the regulatory agency. Rather, it is a substitution of goals resulting from an overemphasis on the technical or scientific problems that arise in the regulatory process. The technical decision is easier to make than the political one, so regulators choose the former. One good example is the decision by the Environmental Protection Agency to insist on use of scrubbers for smokestack emissions in the mid-1970s. As documented by Bruce Ackerman, Congress chose to allow the continued use of "dirty" coal from Appalachia and "fixed" this by insisting on use of a technology: scrubbers.[23] This strategy led to greater costs and greater pollution—all because an easy technical fix was available.

These insights into the functions of regulation and the ways in which regulations fail are not new. They have been grist for the academic mill for more than two decades. Unfortunately, understanding regulatory failure has led to relatively little innovation in the design and operation of regulations. In fact, we still employ the same two generic methods of regulation that have been in place since the New Deal upheaval: standard setting and culling.

First, regulatory agencies set standards, the true prescriptive rules. They are usually designed in a highly stylized administrative rulemaking procedure that allows appropriate due process for regulated parties. Standards are difficult to write. As Breyer notes, their degree of specificity, their extensive technological content, their characteristics as performance or design standards, and the need for coherence in their messages all provide ample opportunity for debate by the participants (adversaries) in the rulemaking.[24] Understandably, the result is all too often an imperfect set of compromises.

The second fundamental method of regulating is culling, which involves, for example, distribution of permits or screening of applicants. *Permitting standards* set criteria for regulators to apply when deciding who will be allowed to carry on certain activities and who will not. An example from environmental regulation is illustrative. Regulations deriving from the Clean Water Act of 1972 are largely based on a system of permits for potential sources of pollution. The Environmental Protection Agency (EPA) must identify any significant source of discharge of effluents into surface water and apply (usually) technological controls for various classes of sources through permits. The regulation identifies and screens particular contributors to the overall problem of water pollution. By contrast, the Clean Air Act of 1970 relies more fundamentally on standards. The agency sets certain standards for levels of so-called criteria pollutants in the environment and then leaves enforcement to the regional air pollution councils. The latter may choose to focus on specific major sources of pollution, but the EPA's enforcement criteria dictate levels of pollution, not distribution of permits.

Standard setting relies on rulemaking; culling or screening depends more on adjudication. This coherent distinction is embodied in the federal Administrative Procedure Act.[25] In health care, regulation has relied on screening. Perhaps, as we shall argue, it is time to use standards.

No matter what their historical contexts, function, or format (standards versus permits), the shape of regulations will often depend on the intent of regulators. The dominant philosophy of regulators, the degree of their adversarial commitment, and their view of the true intentions of the regulated entities may all be more influential in determining the impact of their rules than are the forms of the rules themselves. It is therefore critical to understand not only the design and intellectual foundation of regulatory prescriptions but also the manner in which they are enforced.

Others have recognized the importance of enforcement, but perhaps none so perceptively as John Braithwaite, whose research spans a variety of regulatory domains and countries.[26] As he points out, much of the academic debate about enforcement revolves around the distinction between deterrence and compliance. The deterrence model is founded on the belief that the regulated concerns must be given firm rules, not advice. Advocates of compliance, on the other hand, take the gentler view that regulation should largely be a matter of persuasion. The former belief leads to tough inspectors with strong sanctioning authority. The latter leads to a major role for regulators as consultants. Self-regulation is a possibility in the compliance model; it is ruled out in a deterrence model. Neither the nature of regulation nor its format necessarily determines which model prevails. Even within the same industry, some regulators will be focused on deterrence whereas others will be compliance seekers.

Braithwaite has explored these issues through empirical research in a number of industries. His study of coal mine safety is especially revealing.[27] Reviewing coal mining disasters, he finds a mix of regulatory responses ranging between, in his terms, *persuasion* and *punishment*. In this analysis, he makes a good case that corporations are rational and concerned about their reputations, and that these characteristics create the possibility of persuasive regulations. Corporations can be rehabilitated through persuasion.

Of course, the danger with the persuasive (compliance) method is that the persuasive regulator may be co-opted by the regulated entity. Braithwaite argues, however, that a persuasive regulator can rely on negotiation as long as it is backed up by the power to punish, which is a safeguard against regulatory capture. Moreover, he argues that punishment based on violations of codes simply cannot work in a complicated undertaking like a coal mine, in which it is impossible to monitor every possible safety threat. Hence some mixture of the two enforcement methods is better than either alone.[28]

Braithwaite also maintains that self-regulation is a viable alternative to government command and control. Self-regulating companies have a better understanding of their own processes and functions and can therefore be expected to identify sources of problems more readily. More important, both sanctioning and persuasion authority are much greater in the private sphere than in the public, as the former is much less padded by due process protections. Braithwaite would argue that any time new regulation is considered, self-regulation should be the first option.

An alternative to simple self-regulation is what Braithwaite calls *enforced self-regulation*. Enforced self-regulation requires the regulated industry to write its own set of rules that address a problem area. The rules are submitted to the regulatory agency, which either ratifies them or returns them to the regulated industry for modification. This approach is much less costly than command-and-control regulation because most of the costs of enforcement can be internalized by the company itself. Moreover, writing one's own rules and regulations allows companies to avoid compliance with inappropriate or unnecessary regulations. The regulations can also be adjusted to fit changing industry structure. Of course, the risks remain of co-optation or clever dodging of the regulatory intent.

Another important point Braithwaite makes is that regulatory regimes must be evaluated empirically. His book on coal mine safety goes into great detail on safety records and accident reports. Like any other intervention, the effects of regulation must be measurable. Most regulatory innovations are simply hypotheses; outcomes must be specified and followed. We see this evaluative process all too infrequently in the establishment of new government rules.

Braithwaite's proposals are food for thought as we begin our analysis of regulating the quality of health care. Both punishment and persuasion are likely to figure in our exploration of regulation for improvement. It will therefore be important to understand the mixture of enforcement models currently utilized in the United States to regulate health care quality.

In summary, all regulations share a common definition, a set of functions, and similar enforcement modalities. They are also embedded in a common history. Health care regulation is no different, except that it has lagged far behind other areas of regulation since the time of the New Deal. Even the major federal health and welfare regulatory initiatives of the late 1960s and early 1970s affected health care much less than a number of other public health fields. As we have discussed, much of the retarded progress of health care regulation may be attributable to the dominance of health care providers and the emphasis on their ethical commitment to the patient. This commitment has been viewed as obviating the need to assert the public interest through prescriptive rules. Yet the insulation of medical care has clearly ended, and the industry is now rapidly developing into a much more open target for regulators, albeit a difficult one to understand.

The lesson of this review of regulatory functions is that regulation can sometimes obstruct what it is designed to promote, as a result of capture by those regulated, insufficient specification of goals, or poor implementation of good ideas. An analysis of regulation of health care quality must distinguish these issues, understanding both how regulatory intent is foiled and how implementation falls short. As suggested earlier, both strategy and tactics are critical to formulation of new rules for health care.

The Right Time to Study Regulation of Quality

The regulation mandate ebbs and flows in our country. Certain periods are primarily deregulatory, whereas others produce a variety of new regulatory initiatives. Within sectors of the economy, regulatory imperatives depend on the public's perception of how well the unregulated market functions and how cohesive the structures that compose that sector are. Some sectors remain quite untouched by a period of deregulation or reregulation until a sense of crisis develops.

In health care, prescriptive rules enforced by those outside the doctor-patient relationship have traditionally been rare and quite lenient. The regulation that has occurred has often been feeble if not dysfunctional. Now the traditional structures of health care are changing rapidly, especially as many aspects of a market economy begin to show signs of growth. Competition is sharper than ever. At a time like this, one might think, existing regulation should be replaced altogether by market incentives.

But we doubt this will be a period of deregulation. The ideological insulation created by the profession is being peeled away. No longer is the physician, paternalistically committed to the patient, the driving force in medical care. Health care is being rationalized through critical pathways and guidelines, and integrated business structures can increasingly define the care they want to buy. In these circumstances, the espoused central guarantee of quality of care, the ethical commitment of doctors, may weaken. Hence as the market develops, we may find a greater need for regulation, not a lesser one. The time thus seems right to seek to understand how the quality of care is regulated today and how it might be better regulated in the future.

The subject has not been completely ignored. Nursing home regulation has attracted some scholars interested in the general subject of regulation, including Braithwaite. A handful of health law scholars, most notably Timothy Jost, have tried to understand regulation in general and regulation of quality of care in particular.[29] But more notable is the absence of research in this field. Throughout administrative law, authors such as Breyer, Ayres, Sunstein, and others illustrate their views of regulation with examples from a kaleidoscope of regulatory initiatives, including antitrust, civil aeronautics, health and safety, and environmental protection, yet almost never do they delve into medical care. Hence our undertaking here is motivated in part by the relative lack of scholarship in this area.

Our project is imbued with a sense of urgency, because we perceive a lack of cohesion in the rather wildly changing health care environment of the mid-1990's. Much of the regulation of quality in the past was oriented toward the traditional pillars of medical care: the physicians, the hospitals, and to some extent, the insurers. As horizontal and vertical integration remake the organization of medical care, traditional rules become inapplicable. The reordering of the delivery of medical care has to be accompanied by a reordering of regulatory initiatives.

Even more important, we fear that the quality of care could suffer severely during this reconstruction. Already, it is clear that the country lacks sufficient redistributive impulse to guarantee access to care for the poor. Competition among networks of care, downsizing in major institutions, deflation in incomes for key players, including doctors, and increasing insistence on efficiency could all contribute to erosion in quality of care, at least for some populations.

For the past decade, a number of authors have been concerned about the risk of poor trade-offs between cost and quality in a market-dominated medical care system.[30] Many vulnerable populations at first, and perhaps the majority of those seeking medical care eventually, could face situations in which provider interests are at odds with the best standards of patient care. Though the high levels of inappropriate and excessive care that have driven an ever-spiraling inflationary trend in costs are nothing to be nostalgic about, we may be poorly prepared for a system that creates strong incentives to reduce benefits and resources. We may therefore need oversight of quality more badly than ever.

If so, the good news is that we now have some tools and methods to use to improve care. As we will discuss, over the past two decades, researchers have formulated useful approaches to evaluating quality of care. No longer is it necessary to rely simply on structural measures, such as the number of times the safety committee meets during a twelve-month period. The outcomes movement, though still young, has produced a series of patient-centered measures of quality to track satisfaction, problem scores, health status, and other dimensions of output from the system of care. Moreover, there are now greatly improved methods of determining compliance with appropriate processes of care and of specifying appropriate patterns of care through guidelines and critical pathways. This is a boon for those interested in bringing market forces more thoroughly into medical care, because reasonable knowledge about quality can help make the patient a better consumer. The same tools are also available to regulators.

Furthermore, notions of quality improvement are gradually supplementing more traditional notions of quality assurance. Quality improvement, based on ideas from modern industry, emphasizes the need for changes that will produce better functioning of the system and better results. Total Quality Management, Continuous Quality Improvement, or a variety of other names and aliases under which modern quality methods travel in medical care, can empower improvement efforts throughout health care institutions. Now more than ever, there are leaders ready to react to regulatory requirements and to work closely with regulators to develop new forms of cooperation. Rather than being trapped in the role of meddling outsiders, regulators need to understand how to cooperate with and encourage those who do pay attention to maintaining and improving quality within medical care.

Our goal in this book is ambitious: to offer a framework for a redesign of regulation governing medical care quality that

Recognizes the market-based changes in the structure of medical care

Takes into account the evolution of prescriptive rules in health care

Is cognizant of the context of regulation in the present political world

Draws upon the best possible scientific research on development
of tools and methods for measurement and improvement

Helps to prioritize and address the key quality problems that
may arise over the next decade

We approach these problems without a great deal of ideological
baggage (or at least, so we tell ourselves). The war between those
who favor regulatory solutions and others who want more market
incentives has gone on long enough. Most of the proponents on
either side have rehearsed the various arguments well, and the more
honest of them recognize that they have reached an intellectual
stalemate. Therefore we do not start with any extreme *a priori* beliefs
about the virtuous market or the wise administrative state.

We do, however, believe that regulation should be context-
specific. Each industry is slightly different, and understanding the
interrelationships between market incentives and prescriptive rules
within any given field is challenging.[31] We are drawn especially to
Ayres and Braithwaite's idea of *responsive regulation*. They note that
regulation should be "responsive to industry structure in that different structures will be conducive to different degrees and forms of
regulation."[32] In short, we think it is appropriate to start with the
assumption that medical care is an industry different from many
others and that regulatory solutions in medical care will have to be
tailored to its peculiarities and values.

We also rely on what we see as another treasure in the culture of
medical care: cooperation. Because a commitment to high-quality
care is really part of the commitment to an individual patient, we
see little need for or benefit in antagonistic relationships between
the various professionals who work on behalf of the patient, be it the
health care provider at the bedside or the regulator who is attempting to bring about the best possible incentives for good care. Patient

care at its best is team-oriented, and we believe this should transcend the boundaries of the profession at the bedside. Our vision of the new rules of health care, though not fixed as we begin this enterprise, is nonetheless one of cohesion and cooperation, not acrimony and divisiveness. The regulator is a member of the team that will determine how the system of care will serve its beneficiaries.

Our thesis then is really threefold. First, regulation in health care must be carefully evaluated to identify areas in which capture, anachronistic theories, or misguided initiatives are obstructing the development of better care. Second, regulators must be responsive, and the first steps in that direction may be to develop tactics that dovetail with new tools for quality improvement. Third, we recognize a place for regulation as the health care market rapidly evolves, possibly in the direction of inadequate attention to quality of care.

With all this in mind, our approach will be deliberate. We believe it is important to understand the historical evolution, both of quality thinking in medical care and of regulation of the quality of care. Therefore we begin in Chapter Two with a more complete review of the foundations of quality regulation in health care. As we have suggested, the regulation of health care quality has been relatively sparse in the United States until recently. Physician oversight has been accomplished through state licensing authorities, many of which are still controlled directly or indirectly by the profession's medical societies. Hospital oversight has been the province of the Joint Commission for Accreditation of Health Care Organizations, which grew out of the Hospital Standardization Program of the American College of Surgeons. The JCAHO, as will be shown, represents a form of self-regulation, although since the late 1960s, it has had sufficient autonomy to be viewed as external, and its relationships with hospitals have become primarily adversarial.

The only other major source of quality influence on medical care has been the medical malpractice system. Malpractice law, like the rest of tort law, is intended to deter substandard or negligent behavior. In most analyses of regulation, tort law is marginalized. Indeed,

regulation is usually seen as remedying the inefficiencies or inade-
quacies of the common law. However, in medical care, malpractice
has such a central role that we examine it as a key regulatory influence and will include its reform as part of a full framework of regulating for improvement.

We will examine the emergence of the modern medical malpractice system from a series of doctrinal changes that occurred from
the 1920s through the 1960s. Though malpractice litigation did not
become a major source of concern for physicians until the mid-
1970s, the ground had been prepared for increased claims rates and
more and higher settlements well before then.

In Chapter Three, in parallel fashion, we review the scientific
foundations of quality assurance and improvement in medical care.
We find that much of what is helpful today in progressive thinking
about health care quality was well established thirty to forty years ago.
Many important ideas, such as the need to link quality improvement
to professional education, the role of statistics and data analysis in
providing a basis for quality improvement, and the critical institutional focus for quality improvement projects, were carefully developed by a few outstanding thinkers, but were never widely pursued.
We offer some explanations for why such critical advice was not
heeded and also describe the importance of this intellectual inheri-
tance for a later generation of academics. We end our exploration of
the intellectual foundations of quality improvement by looking at the
involvement of several leading reform proponents in the efforts of the
Department of Health, Education, and Welfare to integrate quality
regulation into the Medicare program, primarily through the Experimental Medical Care Review Organizations (EMCROs).

We then pick up the contemporary story of the conceptualization
and measurement of quality of care, especially by academics. The last
quarter-century is most notable for consolidation of the ideas developed since 1920, as well as the rationalization of a variety of measures
of quality of care. The work of researchers, especially those associated
with the Rand Corporation's Health Insurance Experiment, has been

nothing short of revolutionary.[33] Those interested in understanding quality are superbly well equipped today with methodologically sound measurements. This more than anything else has changed the enterprise of quality improvement.

But equally important, especially in the past ten years, has been the rapid influx of Total Quality Management, or Continuous Quality Improvement, methods in medical care. Modern quality thinking, established in the writings of such visionaries as Deming and Juran, long paused at the doorway of medicine, but has now entered.[34] Nearly every hospital administrator responsible for quality of care today must at least attempt to understand and integrate modern industrial notions of quality improvement. The story of the development of quality measurement and the integration of Total Quality Management will bring us to the present state of the quality enterprise in health care. Designing responsive regulation will depend on understanding these theories.

Chapters Four and Five explore the current structure of health care, specifically as it relates to regulation of clinical quality. The structure of medical care has changed rapidly in the past twenty-five years. We see 1970 as roughly the pinnacle of the traditional architecture emphasizing private physicians, fee-for-service practice, passive hospitals, and cost-unconscious insurers. This architecture, at least superficially, changed little through the 1970s, although cost inflation had already made it clear that passivity was no longer possible. Since that time, the framework of medicine has undergone a metamorphosis. In retrospect, the brief fling with structural health care reform led by the federal government in the mid-1990s shows how quickly the structure of health care is changing. As we approach the year 2000, the house of medicine has been completely redesigned, and the locus of power has shifted from independent physicians to integrated institutions. Understanding this evolution, as well as the complex interplay of existing quality of care regulation, at both the state and federal levels, is central to our task of designing responsive regulation.

In Chapter Six, we put these intellectual musings in perspective by probing the real world of health care, relying on interviews conducted in 1993 and 1994 with health care executives interested in the quality of medical care. These interviews provide insights into quality of regulation that would not otherwise be attainable. What we find, somewhat disturbingly, is the impossibility of developing a broad perspective. Attitudes toward regulation are based on the patterns of the past and fail to reflect the rationalization of the present health care system. Our interviews also reveal the few strengths and many weaknesses of the current methods of regulating quality. Finally, it appears that competitive pressures are making it ever more difficult to invent and actualize new strategies of improvement.

Our interviews, and our understanding of the evolution of regulation with respect to the quality of medical care, lead to our conclusion in Chapter Seven that some radical restructuring must occur, consistent with the dominant paradigm of competing integrated delivery structures. Both regulators and regulated must come to understand that they share a common goal, and in many cases a common vision. Cooperation and emphasis on identifying and sharing superior methods of improving the quality of care should be the goals of regulation, in keeping with Ayres and Braithwaite's notion of responsiveness. Regulators must also help the health care providers learn about and create new methods for improving the quality of care. The older goals of surveillance and punishment must be left behind without compromising the public safety they were meant to ensure. The challenge of the next century must be to design new rules that do not obstruct quality but enable it; that do not reduce competition but ensure that the market does not harm quality; and that allow regulators to incorporate the new theories of quality improvement into their own work.

Notes

1. S. Breyer, *Regulation and Its Reform* (Cambridge, Mass.: Harvard University Press, 1982), 7.

2. We will not delve into the philosophical notions of rule-based behavior. Those interested in this subject should see F. Schauer's excellent book *Playing by the Rules: A Philosophical Examination of Rule Based Decision-Making in Law and in Life* (New York: Oxford University Press, 1991).

3. See T. A. Brennan, *Just Doctoring: Medical Ethics in the Liberal State* (Berkeley: University of California Press, 1991), chaps. 1–3.

4. See generally, C. E. Rosenburg, *The Care of Strangers: The Rise of America's Hospital System* (New York: Basic Books, 1987).

5. See Brennan, *Just Doctoring,* chap. 4.

6. See Brennan, chap. 2.

7. *Merriam-Webster's Collegiate Dictionary* (10th ed.)

8. See Schauer, 2.

9. See R. Dworkin, *Taking Rights Seriously* (Cambridge, Mass.: Harvard University Press, 1977), 22–28, 72–80.

10. Here we follow a number of authors, but primarily C. R. Sunstein, *After the Rights Revolution: Reconceiving the Regulatory State* (Cambridge, Mass.: Harvard University Press, 1990), 20–30.

11. See J. Rawls, *A Theory of Justice* (Cambridge, Mass.: Harvard University Press, 1971).

12. See Sunstein, 22–23.

13. R. Vietor, *Contrived Competition: Regulation and Deregulation in America* (Cambridge, Mass.: Harvard University Press, 1994), 6–12.

14. Vietor, 24.

15. A. E. Kahn, *The Economics of Regulation: Principles and Institutions* (New York: Wiley, 1970).

16. Vietor, 15.

17. See I. Ayres and J. Braithwaite, *Responsive Regulation: Transcending the Deregulation Debate* (New York: Oxford University Press, 1992).

18. See, for example, Sunstein, 25–40.

19. See Breyer, 23–35.

20. See R. H. Bork, *Antitrust: A Policy at War with Itself* (New York: Basic Books, 1978).

21. The large literature on public choice, especially in the political science and legal fields, suggests that all that occurs in the operation of legislatures is a series of interest group transfers. Existing entitlements are treated as simply exogenous variables. See generally, R. A. Epstein, *Takings: Private Property and the Power of Eminent Domain* (Cambridge, Mass.: Harvard University Press, 1985). We are convinced that this process essentially removes the civic nature of government and regulation and should be resisted through regulations that, for instance, curb lobbying and contributions to political action committees.

22. A whole other set of functions of the regulatory state has to do with endogenous preferences. See Sunstein, 64–66. Advocates believe that many people have poorly formed preferences and that regulation can be used to correct them, or more pointedly, to allow their true preferences to rise to the surface. This kind of regulation is most worrisome to the classic liberal, who is concerned about the state's use of positive freedom to reduce negative freedom. See Isaiah Berlin, *Four Essays on Liberty* (London: Oxford University Press, 1969). Regulation oriented toward endogenous preference development is increasingly questioned in the United States.

23. See T. A. Brennan, "Environmental Torts," *Vanderbilt Law Review* 46 (1993):1.

24. Brennan, 23.

25. See Breyer, 12–15.

26. See, for example, J. Braithwaite, *Corporate Crime in the Pharmaceutical Industry* (Boston: Routledge, 1984); J. Braithwaite, *To Punish or Persuade: Enforcement of Coal Mine Safety* (Albany: State University of New York Press, 1985); J. Braithwaite, T. Makkai, V. Braithwaite, D. Gibson, and D. Ermann, *The Contribution of the Standards Monitoring Process to the Quality of Nursing Home Life: A Preliminary Report* (Canberra, Australia: Department of Community Services and Health, 1990); J. Braithwaite and P. Pettit, *Not Just Deserts: A Republican Theory of Criminal Justice* (Oxford, England: Oxford University Press, 1990).

27. Braithwaite, *To Punish or Persuade*.

28. As Braithwaite notes, "The trick of successful regulation then becomes that of imposing punishment when needed without undermining the capacity of inspectors to persuade" (*To Punish or Persuade*, 117).

29. See Braithwaite and others, *The Contribution of the Standards Monitoring Process to the Quality of Nursing Home Life*; T. S. Jost, "The Joint Commission on Accreditation of Hospitals: Private Regulation of Health Care and the Public Interest," *Boston College Law Review* 24 (1983):835–923; T. S. Jost, "The Necessary and Proper Role of Regulation to Assure the Quality of Health Care," *Houston Law Review* 25 (1988): 525–598.

30. For one of the earliest discussions of this topic, see E. H. Morreim, *University of California Law Review* 75 (1987):1719.

31. See S. R. Ackerman, "Progressive Law and Economics—and the New Administrative Law," *Yale Law Journal* 98 (1988): 341–368.

32. Ayres and Braithwaite, 4.

33. J. Newhouse and the Insurance Experiment Group, *Free for All: Lessons from the Rand Health Insurance Experiment* (Cambridge, Mass.: Harvard University Press, 1993).

34. See W. E. Deming, *Out of Crisis* (Cambridge, Mass.: Institute of Technology, Center for Advance Engineering Study, 1992).

2

• •

The Regulatory Landscape
Through the Early 1970s

The first step in our endeavor to define new rules for health care quality is to explore the basis for our assertion that current regulation obstructs efforts to improve quality. We suggested in Chapter One that physicians have long idealized the image of the isolated practitioner doing what is best for the patient according to professional judgment. Allowing quality regulation to remain the purview of the medical profession has been consistent with this ethic of individual provider responsibility. But although self-regulation recognizes the traditional commitment of the medical profession and reinforces its self-image, it also fosters a perception of external regulation as intrusive, unwanted, and unnecessary. Rather than being seen as helpful and collegial, regulators are viewed as meddlers.

Furthermore, we have suggested that capture can be an important issue when regulation is viewed as hostile, especially when the regulated entity is as dominant in its sphere as the medical profession has been in health care. We have hypothesized that rational regulation could be frustrated by professional concerns about prerogative and resulting efforts to dominate regulators.

Unfortunately, we find that the history of health care regulation is inextricably linked with these themes. A review of this history, as it relates both to quality and to other areas of oversight, builds our case that misconceptions and antagonisms have created the context for obstructive rather than enabling rules, and for hostility rather than cooperation.

For those who do have access to care, the major point of contention has been not how to improve quality but how to maintain the high levels of care that already exist in the face of rapid reorganization of health care costs. The American public widely perceives our health care system as providing excellent technological care.[1] Studies that suggest widespread deficiencies in the quality of care even for those with insurance have had little influence on the policy debate until very recently.[2] But now, new quality initiatives are being proposed by the public and by providers to preserve what both believe we already have.

In this chapter, we survey health care regulation through the early 1970s. (In some cases, we actually follow the regulatory history through to the 1990s.)

The Recent Past of Quality Assurance: Self-Regulation of Hospitals and Doctors

The traditional practice of medicine reached its zenith in the late 1960s and early 1970s.[3] With the passage of Medicare and Medicaid in 1964, the medical profession had ensured that the tenets of private practice, including fee-for-service practice, passive insurance companies, and hospitals controlled to a large extent by their medical staff would remain in place. After 1964, federal subsidies, administered by the same insurance companies that provided private insurance, began to flow to hospitals and doctors. Despite nearly two decades of pressure for greater governmental influence over financing of medical care, physician ascendance in a largely private system remained virtually unchallenged.[4] The evolution of the structure of medical practice through the early 1970s deserves some scrutiny before we address quality.

Organized medicine has struggled continuously through the twentieth century to maintain political control over the practice of medicine and to keep the doctor-patient relationship free from external influences. The reasons for this struggle have been characterized in sociological, economic, and ethical terms, but there is little disagreement that government regulation and business influences were anathema to physicians.[5] Medical care was viewed by most physicians as too important to be subject to outside control.

Indeed, doctors preferred and cultivated the passive role of indemnity insurers who provided first-dollar insurance and performed little if any oversight of the practice of medicine. First the Blue Cross/Blue Shield plans, then the commercial insurers, and finally the federal payers were integrated into the financing of medical care in a manner that erased the usual principles of economics. With passive insurance financing and patient ignorance about health care needs, physicians could decide about both supply and demand of health care goods. Unfortunately—and likely unexpectedly—with federal funding in hand and continued importation of expensive technology into a variety of specialties, the stage was set for unabated health care inflation.[6]

Nor did hospitals offer any countervailing influences. They were the only other structural element in health care (the nursing home industry never rising in prestige or power and the managed care industry not yet reaping the benefits of the Health Maintenance Organization Act of 1973), but they rarely had administrations that were independent of the professional staff.[7] They operated primarily as accommodations for the patients admitted by physicians and tried hard to please the doctors, who could usually take their business elsewhere. An overwhelming majority retained a nonprofit status, but the lay boards rarely exercised strong influence after the early part of the century. The peculiar financing arrangements inhibited any rational cost-accounting systems. Instead, most hospitals charged what the insurer could afford, and a rough system of cross-subsidization developed that effectively financed the care of the poor in separate wards, often by the house physicians.

None of this is to suggest malevolent or even monopolistic

tendencies on the part of the medical profession. Many of the activities of the organized medical profession were undertaken in the belief that they were critical to excellent patient care. Private practice was understood as the best culture for the altruistic commitment of physician to patient that was central to medical ethics and also critical to high-quality medical care. Benign intentions created the structure of medical practice that many of us grew up with. Indeed, as medical care rapidly changes today, many may find the arrangements of twenty-five years ago to be preferable.

Up through the early 1970s then, there were few external influences on the health care industry. Hospitals were overseen to some extent by state public health authorities, but they in turn generally deferred to the inspection and accreditation process of the Joint Commission for Accreditation of Hospitals (and later of Health Care Organizations). Physicians were licensed by state boards. Physicians and to some extent hospitals were also subject to tort litigation. But accreditation, boards, and tort law were only nominal regulatory methods and were subject to capture, as will be seen.

Joint Commission for Accreditation of Health Care Organizations (JCAHO)

Incorporated in 1951, the JCAHO was the product of doctors' efforts—particularly those of the American College of Surgeons—to standardize practices at hospitals so that professionals could easily move from one institution to another.[8] The JCAHO was and is dominated by the major professional organizations of providers, including the American Medical Association, the American College of Physicians, the American College of Surgeons, and the American Hospital Association, each of which has institutional seats on the governing board. Though it has taken on a life of its own, the JCAHO was for many years a form of pure self-regulation.

As outlined by the JCAHO in the 1970s, the purposes of the organization were largely unchanged since its incorporation twenty years earlier: to establish standards for hospitals and other health care organizations and to conduct audits (surveys) that would promote high-quality care, applying certain basic principles of physical plant safety, and maintaining essential services in the facilities through the coordinated efforts of the organized staffs and the governing bodies. In particular, the JCAHO manual states, "A primary step in the accreditation process is to identify the basic supporting elements of hospital life for which standards can be set."[9]

The details of the accreditation process evolved somewhat from 1951 to 1971, but the general form remained much the same until very recently. Hospitals were accredited every three years and paid a fee to the JCAHO for the survey. They received a fairly constant flow of information from the JCAHO concerning the criteria or "standards" on which they were judged. New standards were added as the accreditation manual was revised. Hospitals had to comply with the standards in order to pass the inspection. The outcome of the survey was either accreditation for three years, accreditation for one year for those manifesting certain shortcomings, or nonaccreditation.[10] It is notable that the detailed results of the accreditation visit were confidential, to be shared only between the hospital and the "Joint."

Slowly, however, the relationship between the JCAHO and the hospitals changed. The JCAHO came to be viewed as an outside regulator, and relationships became more adversarial. Though hospitals still paid for accreditation, many began to perceive the JCAHO in much the same light as they would official state inspectors.

The JCAHO expected the same approach to quality of medical care in every hospital. The hospital governance was to be split along traditional lines, with the hospital administration generally responsible for the "hotel" aspects of the institution and the medical staff largely responsible for the quality of patient care. The methods of ensuring high-quality care were fairly simple. First, only well-qualified physicians were to be allowed on the staff. Second, if a physician proved deficient, his or her privileges for admission of patients would be restricted or revoked. Third, staff committees were to undertake quality assurance oversight of medical practice.[11]

The first two tasks fell to the credentialing committee. Typically composed of the leading members of each clinical department, the credentials committee would review applications of potential new staff members and recommend acceptance or denial. They would also review questionable practices by staff members and consider suspension or revocation of privileges. Their control was basically unchallenged. Most hospitals assumed, and the few courts that reviewed the issue agreed, that the hospital administration could not overrule the determinations of the medical staff.[12] According to the JCAHO, the medical staff bylaws governing these matters were to be approved by the governing body of the hospital, but such approval was not to be unreasonably withheld. Nor in most cases were courts able to review decisions by medical staff.[13]

Although there are few good sources of statistics on revocation of privileges by hospitals, it appears from anecdotal evidence that such actions were quite infrequent through the 1960s. Most actions taken by peer review bodies such as credentials committees are cloaked in confidentiality by state law; the collection of data on credentialing decisions is thus all but impossible. Over the past four years, however, we have had discussions on this subject with top administrators at more than 150 hospitals, and only one reports more than one action by a credentialing committee to revoke privileges during the 1960s and 1970s. Since that time, the rise of corporate negligence theories in tort law and nations of economic credentialing have led to greater oversight, topics reviewed later.[14]

The JCAHO standards themselves indicated the formal manner in which the regulatory process reinforced the physician-dominated quality assurance process. The standards required that there be a single medical staff responsible for the quality of all professional services.[15] This staff was to be organized into a committee structure to meet its quality assurance responsibilities, with several layers of membership including active staff and courtesy staff. The process of selection and oversight of staff members had to be set forth in detailed bylaws. The integrity of the appointment/

reappointment process was also monitored by the review of minutes from selected meetings.[16]

The leadership of the JCAHO realized that most of the measures of quality were primarily "input-oriented," or focused on the structure of the institution—not just staff credentialing but all aspects of the institution. This was so because of the belief that "there is a very high correlation between, on the one hand, a safe and functionally efficient physical plant, effectively qualified personnel, and properly developed procedures, and, on the other hand, the quality of care provided to patients."[17] Nonetheless, as set forth in various chapters in the accreditation manual, the criteria were vague and ineffective. Over the years, therefore, the JCAHO moved toward more explicit criteria.[18]

The specifics of ensuring clinical quality in hospitals fell to a number of committees on which staff members were required to serve. These included pharmacy and therapeutics, medical records, infection control, and utilization review. Otherwise, medical staff were given a good deal of flexibility in clinical quality assessment, although tissue and necropsy reports were mentioned explicitly.[19] Again, the committees were required only to show formal compliance with meeting and record-keeping requirements. Departments of surgery were typically quite rigorous in their review of cases; however, there was rarely any real disciplinary action.[20] Though committee activities resulted in some feedback to physicians, the relationship of such activities to quality improvement is unclear.[21]

The inspection team (or as the JCAHO prefers, surveyors) usually consisted of several professional members, including doctors, nurses, and an administrative expert. Specialists in laboratory medicine rounded out the group. They visited for a five-to-seven-day period, roaming the hospital to interview physicians, nurses, and other staff. They observed practices, looked over administrative documents ranging from credentialing files to fire plans, checked calibrations of laboratory equipment and other technology, and generally scrutinized practice and records of practice.

The survey was typically coordinated on the hospital side by a senior administrator who spent a majority of his or her time on the process for the three to six months leading up to the visit. (Hospital administrators' views of the JCAHO process will be discussed in Chapter Six.) Assisted by nurse-managers in the quality assurance department, the administrator's role was to ensure that the compliance with structural measures on the medical staff/clinical side and the various outcome measures on the hotel side were in order. Rarely did this preparation provide the opportunity for quality improvement.

Although, as Chapter Four will detail, the JCAHO is attempting some dramatic changes in its approach, throughout the 1960s and much of the next two decades, the emphasis was on the structures of care and the documentation of meetings rather than on evidence regarding the quality of care itself.[22] Moreover, important areas of care were largely left out of the evaluation. For example, accreditation manuals had no specific reviews of surgical care, although they did typically cover anesthesia in a separate section. The only detailed requirements were for such easily quantified issues as the control of specimens in hematology laboratories.[23]

The salutary effects of this regulatory effort are uncertain. The JCAHO measures of quality have never been carefully compared with other measures. In one of the few research efforts to determine the effectiveness of the standards, investigators found that in New York in 1984, hospitals with high numbers of JCAHO variances did not have higher standardized mortality rates or higher rates of negligent adverse events.[24] In fact, there was very little statistical correlation between the JCAHO ratings and other quality indicators. Studies such as this raise significant questions about the JCAHO's quality definitions. Nonetheless, the JCAHO has endured, largely because it has not disturbed medical practice.

This is not to say that hospitals have always scored well in the JCAHO's somewhat complex scoring system. As noted earlier, the survey process allows for some gradations in scores, ranging from full accreditation to nonaccreditation. In the American College of Surgeon's first Hospital Standardization Survey in 1917, only 89 out of 692 hospitals with more than 100 beds met the standard for full accreditation. Today, approximately 1 to 2 percent of those who seek accreditation do not achieve full status.[25] Nevertheless, there are very few examples of JCAHO accreditation failures and subsequent closure of facilities. So although surveys do cause much anxiety at hospitals, there is little real threat of loss of accreditation.

Federal regulators endorse JCAHO accreditation, a reasonable move given the lack of alternatives and the costs of developing an independent survey process.[26] The federal government has always considered JCAHO accreditation as sufficient to qualify for Medicare certification.[27] Just as the federal government has accepted the role of third-party administrators in Medicare financing, so too has it been willing to go along with the traditional method of overseeing hospital quality. Given the importance of Medicare funds, most hospitals have opted for JCAHO accreditation.[28]

States, too, have endorsed the JCAHO; an overwhelming majority have relied on accreditation status when they license hospitals. However, there has been some variation from state to state. A few states offer hospitals a choice of state inspection or JCAHO oversight. For example, in Georgia, the Department of Human Resources can inspect a hospital if it does not wish to seek JCAHO accreditation. Most Georgia hospitals choose the JCAHO (although a 1990 court ruling that accreditation records are public and not protected by peer review immunity may drive hospitals to rethink their commitment to the JCAHO).[29] Other states simply require a hospital to create a medical advisory committee responsible for adopting rules governing the hospital's performance.[30]

New York State has pursued a different strategy, empowering the Department of Health to survey hospitals every three years. Unlike the JCAHO, the state surveyors give hospitals as little as five days' notice of an impending visit. The surveys are similar to those undertaken by the JCAHO, involving a physician, a senior nurse, nurse surveyor, and survey coordinator. They review medical records, interview patients, evaluate quality assurance committee documents, visit nursing units, and confer with administrators.[31] A hospital receives a report card listing deficiencies within six weeks. It can then either address these shortcomings directly or, as most hospitals do for the majority of deficiencies, appeal their validity. As might be expected, the New York hospital industry has chafed under this additional oversight, persistently lobbying the legislature to accept JCAHO accreditation. Indeed, there are indications that New York may be interested in rejoining the JCAHO fold.[32]

The JCAHO history captures the spirit of regulation in health care. First, it was dominated by an ascendant profession and in many ways reinforced the primacy of the physician's role in determining quality. Second, and as a result, JCAHO rules did not evince an external rationality. Instead, the organization fell into a rather meaningless mode of external inspection that suited most parties. It was set on a course that could not lead to the ideal of cooperative interaction between regulator and regulated envisioned in Braithwaite's responsive regulation model. Indeed, one could predict that if the JCAHO were to demonstrate independence, the hospital industry and medical profession would probably interpret this as antagonism.

Medical Licensure Boards

The same set of lessons may be drawn from a review of oversight boards. However scanty the oversight of hospitals in the 1960s, it was independent and overbearing compared with the oversight of physicians. As part of the medical profession's consolidation of control over the practice of medicine in the late nineteenth and early twentieth centuries, the state medical societies came to dominate licensure functions at about the same time that the county and state medical societies forged an alliance with the American Medical Association.[33] For much of the first half of the twentieth century, the medical profession set forth the requirements for gaining a license and policed any professional deviations from the rules of conduct.

In most states, the licensure board was little more than an extension of the medical society itself. As Robert Derbyshire's history of licensure boards reveals, in 1969, it was clear that the boards were beholden to the medical societies because "without the support of the medical societies it is all but impossible to persuade the legislatures to act." In sixteen states, governors appointed members to the board from a nominating list provided by the state medical society. California was unique in that one of its board members had to be a nonphysician.[34] Even today, the boards are typically dominated by physicians; for example, the Michigan board consists of ten physicians, one physician's assistant, and three public members.[35]

While medical societies exerted significant independent control of medical practice, the relationship with disciplinary boards reinforced the power of the societies. But a trend toward judicial oversight of the state societies began in 1961 with the case of *Falcone* v. *Middlesex County Medical Society*. The New Jersey medical society had an unwritten ethics requirement that a physician spend four years at an AMA-accredited medical school. Though the plaintiff in this case had graduated from such a school, he had not spent four years in residence. The New Jersey Supreme Court, in compelling the medical society to admit Falcone into membership, ruled that the society's power was too great and that judicial scrutiny was necessary. The court's decision emphasized that the medical society is more than a private voluntary association; rather, it is an organization having an important and prominent public role. This public authority should not be unbridled, the court wrote.[36]

Oversight of medical societies led in turn to greater oversight of disciplinary boards. Over the course of the next two decades, a number of court decisions reduced medical society control over professional disciplinary activities. A good example is the decision of *Rogers* v. *Medical Association of Georgia et al.*[37] Here, the Supreme Court of Georgia found that allowing medical societies to screen and recommend candidates for membership on the state board, and by those recommendations limiting the Georgia governor's choice of candidates, represented an unconstitutional delegation of public authority to a private organization. Similar determinations were made in a variety of other states.[38]

Perhaps more important, boards with lay members were able to convince the courts that the board's expertise was sufficient to revoke licenses and that there was no need for the board to produce expert testimony regarding revocation.[39] This meant that the profession itself did not set the standard for licensure through expert testimony. Rather, licensure became a function of the state authority through the board. Other decisions reinforced the importance of lay membership on licensure boards.[40]

Although the profession's grip on the licensure boards through the societies loosened, the boards did not step forward to exert authority. Quality oversight was generally limited to granting licenses to those who had graduated from medical school and completed an appropriate postgraduate medical training program, and to removing licenses of (or more frequently, placing on probation) those physicians who had transgressed the professional definition of good behavior. Such actions were very infrequent. From 1963 to 1967, licensure boards across the country undertook only 938 actions, of which only 161 were suspensions (or less than one suspension per state per year).[41]

Many would say that little has changed through the mid-1990s. Boards are generally empowered to order a range of sanctions, including a "letter of admonition, private censure, public censure, suspensions for a definite or indefinite period, or revocation of a license to practice."[42] Physicians who are investigated by the board are permitted to provide answers or explain their behavior within a certain period of time. Physicians have a right to counsel, and any board hearing typically is governed by relatively formal rules of evidence. Much of the emphasis on procedure has been the result of litigation by physicians on due process grounds.

The jurisdiction of medical boards varies from state to state. Some have chosen to define professional oversight almost exclusively in terms of identification of impairment, either by drugs or alcohol. In Indiana, for instance, the medical licensure board must determine if the physician is endangering the public as a result of substance abuse.[43] Other state boards will investigate any infraction of professional codes, broadly defined. For instance, in Massachusetts, the Board of Registration in Medicine will discipline for lack of "good moral character" or for "conduct that undermines the confidence in the integrity of the profession."[44] Courts tend to defer to these professional determinations.[45] Clearly, this was the case before 1970. One study revealed that between 1963 and 1967, boards were overruled by courts only fifteen times, and this was a remarkable increase over the five-year period from 1957 through 1961, during which there had been only three reversals.[46]

Boards were not traditionally active in seeking out cases of unprofessional behavior. Their approach was more passive, waiting for complaints to arise from patients or others concerned about the behavior of a physician.[47] Those that came to the boards' attention were predominantly matters of substance abuse.[48] Although it is unassailable that there is an association between drug or alcohol abuse and poor care, the emphasis on such violations by state boards suggested that only rarely would one find a consistent provider of poor care, and only under extraordinary circumstances such as drug abuse.

Thus the chief target of the state boards seemed to be the occasional outlier. The average, non-substance-abusing physician who avoided sexual relationships with patients had little to fear from the licensure boards and probably perceived little oversight pressure with regard to quality of care. Quality regulation was essentially not a part of the board's function. In fact, board regulation of physicians probably had less impact on the practice of medicine than did the JCAHO's inspection on hospital practices.

In the mid-1980s, many boards were burdened with new responsibilities as a result of malpractice reform. The medical malpractice crisis of 1984–1986, which is discussed in detail in Chapter Four, had given rise to new provider cries for tort reform. Many state legislatures responded with measures designed to make it more difficult for patients to sue. To counterbalance these proposals, which theoretically weakened the deterrent (quality-inducing) effect of tort litigation, the legislatures created new requirements for hospitals and medical societies to report any quality problems or malpractice claims to medical boards. Typical was the Colorado requirement that any action taken by the governing board of a hospital to suspend, revoke, or limit the admitting privileges of a licensed physician or podiatrist must be reported to the state board of medical examiners.[49]

These new measures have not necessarily strengthened the function of state boards. Massachusetts is a case in point. A malpractice reform statute passed in 1986 empowered the Board of Registration in Medicine to review quality assurance information from hospitals. The following year, the board adopted regulations governing its Qualified Patient Care Assessment Program, which were challenged unsuccessfully by the hospital industry.[50] The regulations required that all credentialing information, as well as any complaints or disciplinary proceedings against physicians, be transmitted to the board. In addition, physicians were to report any patient injuries to the hospital's coordinator of patient care assessment, who in turn was to transmit any major incident reports to the state.[51]

With this amount of information in hand, there was at least the possibility that the Massachusetts board might mount a statistically based oversight system. But many predicted that the state would not commit sufficient resources to allow the board to process all of this data, and this prediction has proved correct. Funding for the Board of Registration continues to be inadequate. As a result, Massachusetts ranked forty-ninth in 1990, forty-eighth in 1991, and fiftieth in 1992 in Public Citizen Research Group's ranking of state disciplinary action.[52]

Massachusetts is not an isolated example. In New Jersey, only half of the malpractice claims transmitted to the Board of Medical

Examiners underwent any review.[53] Michigan's new reporting requirements were not funded, and in 1991, as part of budget cutting, the office that reviewed reports on lawsuits was eliminated.[54] In California, an investigation by the California Highway Patrol revealed that a backlog of three hundred cases had simply been dumped, most never pursued.[55]

New York is again an outlier. The New York legislature created an extensive incident-reporting program in 1986. Hospitals were required to inform the Office of Health Systems Management of any "emergencies or situations which might threaten the safety or well-being of patients or staff," including any "patient deaths or impairments in circumstances other than those related to the natural course of illness, fires, equipment failures, poisoning, strikes by facility staff, disasters or termination of any services vital to the continued safe operation of the health facility."[56] Reporting had to occur within twenty-four hours, with written notification to follow in five days and evaluation by the hospital within forty-five days.

The New York hospital industry has long wanted to eliminate these provisions, or at the very least require the state to specify exactly what kind of incidents should be reported.[57] Some large teaching hospitals have been sending out as many as thirty reports per month, each averaging five to seven pages.[58] It appears that the New York Department of Health follows up most of the reporting. Other boards are not as likely to follow up with complainants. In Ohio, for instance, of two hundred public complaints studied by Timothy Jost and colleagues, only 7 received individualized letters. Twenty-six percent of complainants received no reply at all.[59]

Nationwide, there is relatively little provider discipline. Public Citizen Research Group's monitoring of reports from the fifty states and the District of Columbia suggests that there are only about three thousand disciplinary actions each year (among the 584,900 medical doctors), and fewer than 10 percent of those may be for negligent or poor-quality care.[60]

One potentially salutary development among disciplinary boards has been a new emphasis on continuing medical education for doctors. At the time of license renewal, many states now ask physicians to demonstrate that they have participated in appropriate course work. In Michigan, the board requires 150 hours of continuing education courses or programs approved by the board.[61] Other states have similar provisions. Research has not yet confirmed the effectiveness of these reforms.

In short, if we take 1970 as our watershed, quality regulation in health care—whether represented by the JCAHO surveyors or by state licensing boards, or even by the rare threat of malpractice litigation—focused largely on structural details and on the discipline of defective hospitals and physicians. Consumers lacked appropriate information to avoid poor-quality providers, and the available evidence suggests that the medical industry controlled a good deal of its own regulation. The intrusiveness of the JCAHO surveys notwithstanding, quality regulation was generally ineffective and not particularly burdensome. More important, any independent rationality developed by regulators was likely to be seen as needless meddling. The stage was set for antagonistic rather than responsive regulation.

The Beginnings of Outside Regulation: Cost Control

Because quality regulation remained largely in the hands of providers or private organizations through the 1960s (and to a considerable extent through the 1980s), there was until recently no perception of a crisis in quality of care and hence no rethinking of the role of regulation. But contentment with the status quo was not a property of health care financing; it is therefore helpful for us to review regulation in this area. By 1970, the Medicare and Medicaid programs were expanding faster than expected, and government regulators began to step in with a variety of initiatives. The most important of these by far were 1) certificate-of-need programs to limit hospital expansion and spread of expensive technology, and 2) hospital rate setting, adopted by a few states as a form of budget control.

Reviewing these methods of regulating finance can provide some perspective for understanding the regulation of the quality of care generally. The assumptions that underlie the choice of programs, and the vagaries of the programs themselves, indicate the broader theme in health care oversight that we are exploring: the perception of obstruction. Tracing the evolution of health care financing reform can therefore shed further light on the quality reforms that developed somewhat later.

Certificate of Need

Certificate-of-need (CON) programs have the longest and perhaps the most interesting history of any issue in health law. The federal government has long been in the business of providing support for capital improvement at hospitals while simultaneously attempting to engage in some health planning. For example, the Hill-Burton Act of 1946 was fundamentally a mechanism for providing hospital construction grants.[62] The legislation did, however, require states to prepare medical facility plans that would help target construction in the most needy sites. This was accomplished through state agencies that reviewed construction applications from hospitals.[63] The regulation underlying the Hill-Burton enactments aimed primarily at promoting access. The same is true of the Comprehensive Health Planning and Public Health Services Amendments of 1966, which authorized funding for state and local health planning activities, particularly the assessment of the future needs of communities.[64]

However, the next round of planning regulations was influenced by theories of medical care costs. Milton Roemer had begun to make a strong case in the early 1960s that health care expenditures were directly linked to the number of hospital beds in any given region.[65] In many ways, his work foreshadowed the much more frequently discussed research of Jack Wennberg and others, which suggested that variations in rates of medical procedures could be explained by differences in the numbers of available physicians and

differences in practice styles among physicians.[66] The key point
made by both Roemer and Wennberg was that demand for medical
services would rise to fill supply—in this case, hospital beds. This
proposition would be quite questionable in a normal market, but as
we have seen, the health care market was one in which physicians
exerted substantial control over both supply and demand.

By 1972, with increasing inflation in the federal reimbursement
programs, the government began to integrate restrictions into
health planning. The Social Security Act amendments of 1972 created the so-called Section 1122 programs. Section 1122 empowered
the Department of Health, Education, and Welfare (HEW) to work
directly with states to conduct oversight of any major capital
improvement.[67] Those states that refused to participate would forgo
some federal funding; projects that failed to comply with Section
1122 could not take advantage of relatively generous capital funding available from Medicare and Medicaid.

Section 1122 gave impetus to the already emerging trend of state
oversight of hospital construction. Beginning with New York in
1964, states had required certificates of need from hospitals and
nursing homes for construction exceeding a certain threshold. In
1966, twenty-three states had such laws.[68] By 1973, as a result of the
federal funding incentives, all but West Virginia had CON programs
or Section 1122 functions in place, most adopting the federal
threshold of $100,000.

Even at this early stage, some lessons in health care regulation
emerge. The early certificate-of-need efforts were tangential to the
real issue—that is, the lack of market incentives and the resulting
provider-induced demand that operated as the inflationary engine
in health care. Hospital construction was essentially a symptom of
this critical problem. One can sense that regulators chose to avoid
a fight with the industry and the profession. Regulators did not
have, and probably did not want, the public support to get involved
in the kind of oversight of the clinical relationship that would have
been necessary for significant cost containment. Nor were their rela-

tionships with the regulated concerns of the kind that would be necessary to conduct cooperative, responsive regulation. The government did not force states to develop programs or hospitals to comply with regulations. It only threatened cut-off of very favorable federal funds.

One might draw the conclusion that the federal government was wary about undertaking thoroughgoing regulation in the health care industry, and not simply because the states were already engaged in appropriate oversight. Indeed, whereas Congress was showing a great deal of enthusiasm for comprehensive regulation in other areas of social welfare, such as environmental protection and occupational health, it was treating medicine very carefully and very conservatively. But concerns about health care costs would start to change this hands-off attitude. In 1974, Congress passed the National Health Planning and Resources Development Act (NHPRDA) in an effort to bring rising costs under control.[69] As with previous reform efforts, the NHPRDA did not employ a federal-led, frontal strategy but was primarily local in its focus, creating Health System Agencies (HSAs) in the states that were to promulgate health system plans (HSPs). The HSAs were also to develop implementation plans in concert with state CON authorities.[70]

As one commentator has observed, the NHPRDA was widely viewed as regulation "intended to achieve a more efficient and equitable allocation of resources than the competitive market managed to produce."[71] The government clearly recognized that the health care market was not a true market, and that regulation was required to improve it, though not necessarily by making it into a true market. The NHPRDA also implicitly recognized the need for non-provider influence in the health care system. Unlike the JCAHO and the licensure boards, the HSAs were not dominated by providers; HSA membership included consumer representatives and others. Not unexpectedly, however, most hospitals and physician groups resisted empowering the HSAs. In addition, the emerging managed care industry was able to garner an exemption from

NHPRDA requirements, setting a trend of special treatment for health maintenance organizations (HMOs) that was to continue.[72]

The CON effort generally and the NHPRDA structure in particular did not treat health care problems—in this case, cost inflation—as a matter that could be solved by addressing the behavior of physicians directly. Nor were the efforts at cooperation, through the HSAs, accepted by the regulated entities. The regulation of financing did not enter the clinical arena (in the way that managed care and prospective payment eventually would), but relied on systematic reforms based on economic incentives for states and for hospitals. Nevertheless, even though these somewhat tangential strategies had relatively little effect and were perhaps insufficiently oriented toward influencing physician decisions, they did reflect a significant departure from previous regulatory efforts. Cost reform treated health care as a modern industry, not as a guild, and treated hospitals as independent factors in an equation, not as doctor workshops.

One would have suspected that these efforts would fail, and by the early 1980s, some empirical research had begun to suggest that the CON programs were having minimal impact or none on health care costs. Moreover, state courts had raised questions about the planning function of state agencies.[73] Perhaps most important, the Reagan administration had little interest in regulation generally and no interest in command-and-control regulation that would cure the defects of the health care market administratively. As a result, the funding for the HSAs and State Health Planning and Development Agencies (SHPDAs) was allowed to expire in 1982, and general funding for the NHPRDA fell from $119.4 million in 1980 to $35.5 million in 1983, and was eventually repealed by Congress in 1987. In the absence of federal incentives, eleven states dropped their CON programs between 1983 and 1988.[74]

The evolution of the CON programs in the 1980s also provides insight into our thesis concerning the relative roles of regulation and market incentives.[75] This will be spelled out more clearly in Chapter Four, where we examine the ways medical practice is shifting from a physician-centric to an industry model,[76] but here we should note that the history of CON programs since the mid-1980s provides a good example of how government oscillates between regulatory and market incentive systems. One of the major reasons for the failure of regulation had been that hospitals had found ways to place certain capital investments slightly off-site to avoid state oversight. The 1979 amendment to the NHPRDA attempted to outflank this move by bringing under the scope of regulation any expenditures intended for inpatients, but this simply led to development of facilities that were completely independent of hospitals, undermining hospital finances as lucrative services, such as radiological imaging and minor surgery, moved off campus.

Once states dropped their CON programs completely, construction accelerated massively. For instance, in Virginia, the number of MRI scanners went from 38 to 72 in two years.[77] In Arizona, the state licensed twenty times as much capital construction in the six months after CON repeal in 1985 ($135 million) as it did in the comparable six months of 1984. These kinds of experiences have now led some states back to CON regulation. Other states have moved to extend the regulation to all health services, not just hospitals.[78]

As might be expected, New York has a strong certificate-of-need program buttressed by administrative regulations from the Department of Public Health. In deciding whether to issue a certificate of need, the Department of Health considers factors such as population characteristics of a designated area, age- and gender-specific utilization rates, standards for facility and service utilization, patient preferences, extent of access for the medically underserved, and current utilization.[79] New York maintains the certificate of need for a broad array of services, including ambulatory care units, inpatient beds, and particular technologies such as transplantation.

On the other side of the spectrum, Indiana's CON regulation expired in July 1994.[80] The current Georgia legislation is an example of a middle-of-the-road approach. Any investors must have a certificate of need from the State Health Planning Agency before they can buy or operate medical equipment worth more than $500,000.[81] State law lists specific criteria that the agency must consider before granting the certificate of need. However, the general objectives of state health planning may also be considered. Moreover, the State Health Planning Agency may require that any applicant for a certificate of need provide a specified amount of clinical health services to indigent patients as a condition of the grant of the certificate.[82]

Today, managed care organizations are often exempt from CON requirements. For example, in Massachusetts, an HMO or combination of HMOs does not need a certificate of need if 1) it has at least fifty thousand enrollees, 2) the facility is geographically located so that its services are reasonably accessible, and 3) at least 75 percent of patients receiving inpatient services are enrollees of the HMOs.[83] In Massachusetts, as elsewhere, the shift toward market-based approaches to health care has raised questions about the utility of certificates of need.[84] In the meantime, facilities once regulated by the CON law in Massachusetts, such as those for outpatient care, have been removed from review. Certain applications were exempted from full review and are now subject to much more lax requirements. Finally, the staff and funding available to the CON program office have been significantly reduced.[85]

There is nonetheless evidence that states may extend the reach of CON programs into new areas.[86] As legislators have become aware of the need to manage competition, gather outcomes, and provide consumers with data, the CON structure is evolving in some states into an omnibus regulatory body. In Oregon, for example, the legislature has recently linked new capital projects to the institution's patient outcomes. In Vermont and Rhode Island, there have been efforts to use the allocation decisions to drive global budgets. This rediscovery of CON underlines the way programs wax and wane depending on the ardor for competition.[87]

But here we move ahead of our historical narrative. In the early 1970s, physician autonomy and the generally weak authority of hospitals and insurers insulated medical practice from market influences. CON represented a somewhat elliptical effort to rein in costs.

The larger point is that clearly, regulation affects and modifies the market in health care. In fact, CON was intended to reduce the unnecessary technology that the peculiar market in medical care could engender. The regulation was designed to correct the market to socially optimal, rational levels of activity. Any new rules concerning health care quality may have to accomplish similar goals.

Rate Regulation

The history of rate regulation, the other major financing oversight initiative, displays similar themes: the market in medical care can lead to socially suboptimal activity levels, but regulation can fail to bring about the intended corrections. Rate regulation is best defined as state oversight of the per diem rate charged by hospitals. But it has evolved in a variety of directions over the twenty-odd years of its life. By contrast with the CON effort, the federal government never seriously encouraged states to enact rate regulation; nor did the federal government incorporate it into Medicare or Medicaid. Although there were some small but notable exceptions, the federal government generally stayed clear of rate regulation, merely granting the necessary waivers to states that wished to pursue it.[88]

Consequently, experiments with rate regulation were heterogeneous. The most telling examples were those of Massachusetts, New York, Connecticut, Maryland, New Jersey, and Washington. Each state had a different regulatory history, but certain common themes emerge. Consider New Jersey. In the late 1960s, the New Jersey health care economy confronted staggering inflation, inadequate care for the poor, and pressure on the state Medicaid budget. Two powerful interests—insurers uneasy over rising hospital charges and hospitals vying for competitive advantage—began to lobby the legislature for assistance. Blue Cross premiums were subject to the insurance commissioner's approval, and every increase aroused media attention and public resistance.[89] State officials tried to keep

Blue Cross premiums down, but rising hospital prices forced its payments up. Blue Cross in turn sought legislative relief on the grounds
that regulated premiums should be matched by regulated hospital
rates.[90] The hospitals, on the other hand, vigorously opposed government interference with their billing. Predictably, the New Jersey Hospital Association's attempt to appease Blue Cross with
voluntary, nonbinding review of hospital budgets had failed to
reduce the inflation in hospital costs. When the voluntary agreement broke down, the legislature empowered the commissioner of
health and insurance to set the rates that Blue Cross and Medicaid
paid for hospital services.[91] In practice, however, the hospital association simply continued to operate its own review. Hospital officials dominated both planning and rate setting. The state's
commissioners relied on and routinely accepted the hospital association's findings and recommendations.[92]

In 1974, the public learned the shocking news that the hospital
association was conducting government rate reviews. "The regulated were regulating themselves"—another example of capture.[93]
The New Jersey Department of Health took control of hospital rate
review. State bureaucrats swiftly moved to contain Blue Cross and
Medicaid costs with the regulatory apparatus in place. After considerable haggling with angry hospital administrators, the state officials approved rate increases that averaged only 7 percent,
significantly lower than the increases of more than 10 percent permitted by hospital administrators. In short, the state now exerted
stringent control over Blue Cross and Medicaid.[94]

The consequences of regulating some payers and not others
were soon apparent. Blue Cross and Medicaid benefited at the
expense of commercial payers. Most hospitals maintained their
income by shifting costs to commercial insurers. Within five years,
the commercial insurers were paying hospitals approximately 30
percent more than Blue Cross. Commercial insurers soon began to
rally for change.[95]

Hospitals also found the new system burdensome. Urban hospitals treated a disproportionate number of Blue Cross, Medicaid, and uninsured patients.[96] Patients with private coverage lived in the suburbs. As a result, urban hospitals could not shift their losses and bad debts to commercial payers. Even those hospitals able to maintain their revenues found the long rounds of individual negotiation with the Department of Health inefficient. Meanwhile, medical inflation persisted because of cost-shifting.[97] Unable to get a hold on physician practice or hospital cost shifts, rate regulation foundered in New Jersey.

Maryland's less publicized effort to set rates was more successful. At least partially out of a growing concern over escalating health care costs and diminished access for those most in need of health care services, the General Assembly of Maryland established in 1971 the Health Services Cost Review Commission (HSCRC). In its early years, the commission sought to control hospital costs by rate disclosure.[98] In 1974, it initiated a process of mandatory rate setting for Maryland hospitals. Statutory guidelines for establishing rates included consideration of a reasonable correlation between rates, costs, and services. Hospital rates had to be approved by the commission, and a hospital could not charge rates that did not conform to the commission's review decision.[99]

Section 19–216(c) of the Maryland Health General Code authorized the HSCRC to "promote alternative methods of rate determination and payment that are of an experimental nature" in order to promote efficiency and effective use of health care facility services.[100] With this authority, the HSCRC developed sophisticated and comprehensive cost-containment methodologies for Maryland. For example, the commission's "guaranteed inpatient revenue" (GIR) system established preset rates for diagnostic groups, thus giving hospitals a financial motivation to tailor services and hold expenses below the GIR rates.[101] These regulated rates replaced traditional cost-based reimbursement systems that provided little incentive for efficiency.[102]

In 1977, Maryland's HSCRC developed a "market basket"

methodology for setting rates, which was based on an interhospital cost comparison. This methodology, renamed the Interhospital Cost Comparison Methodology (ICC), compared each hospital's aggregate costs with "the average costs of a peer group of hospitals" within the state.[103] This modality proved quite effective as the shift to competition occurred in the early 1980s.

The federal government briefly showed interest in hospital rate regulation during the Carter administration. In its first hundred days, the administration called for federal legislation to limit the annual increases in hospital revenues. Capital reimbursements were also to be reined in. These proposals stalled in Congress, however, as they competed with Democratic bills that called for national health insurance. In November of 1979, Carter's plan was soundly defeated.[104]

Over the past two decades, health services researchers have attempted to gauge the impact of rate regulation on health care costs. Reports are inconclusive.[105] Whereas some states appear to have had limited successes with their regulation, health care inflation in others approaches that of nonregulated states. The apparent lack of efficacy, combined with the perhaps misplaced belief that rate setting could not be integrated with competitive influences in medical care, led some of the leading rate-setting states—most notably Massachusetts and New Jersey—to abandon their programs in the early 1990s.

In summary, both certificate-of-need and rate-setting initiatives, though oriented primarily toward the control of health care costs, have important lessons for regulation of medical care generally, including quality regulation. First, they reveal that regulators have been generally unwilling to challenge physician control over health care practices. Though the physician is clearly the critical economic player, both CON and rate setting employed tangential approaches aimed primarily at the hospital. Regulators avoided economic oversight that would bear directly on the clinical encounter.

Second, the difficulty of obtaining federal consensus led to regulation that was either wholly state-based, like rate setting, or that operated at the state level through federally mediated funding incentives, like the certificate-of-need programs. As the problems of health care costs were dealt with state by state, health care regulation became something of a crazy quilt. In the 1980s, as we shall see, the federal government would attempt to bring some consistency to the patterns of regulation that had developed, and federal influence on health care law would grow dramatically.

Third, and perhaps most important, the tension between government intervention through command-and-control regulation and market-based or competitive solutions began to be felt in medical care as the 1980s approached. As a true market in medical care has never existed, competition advocates have always argued that their programs should be tried and that further regulation compounds existing market failures. The market/regulation dichotomy would deepen in health care financing throughout the late 1970s and 1980s, as cost inflation continued unabated. Only recently has it penetrated the debate over quality of care.

Fourth, cost regulation is more comprehensible in theoretical terms than is traditional quality regulation. The efforts to control technology and set rates seemed to address the failures of a health care market in which consumers were unable to bargain knowledgeably for more inexpensive products. Providers were influenced by the moral hazard of controlling supply and demand. They maintained a monopoly of information, and new regulations were intended to offset the inflationary implications of that monopoly.

The failure of cost regulation is also readily understood. The activities of regulators were generally uncoordinated and intermittent. Furthermore, regulators were not "responsive," in Braithwaite's sense of the term. Their relationship with the regulated entities, especially hospitals, remained antagonistic and authoritarian. On the other hand, the limited successes that did occur with rate regulation may be understood as examples of responsive regulation. The regulators simply set goals (budget limits) and allowed hospitals to meet them. But regulators never tried to induce those hospitals to share information about their successes with other hospitals or to consider new methods for efficient health care delivery. The regulators never acted as teachers. No effort was made to stimulate creativity. Unfortunately, cost regulation set a pattern for health care regulation generally.

Utilization Review and the Professional Standards Review Organizations

There is one place where quality oversight and cost concerns have traditionally come together: utilization review. If tighter control over physician selection of therapies represents a concerted frontal assault on health care costs, the various forms of utilization review are haphazard forays against inflation. Whether in the form of prospective review (especially hospital precertification), concurrent review (oversight of care while it is being provided in hospitals), or retrospective review of treatment decisions, utilization review attempts to overcome the problem of the professional's insensitivity to costs of care, eliminating unnecessary or overly expensive interventions.

Notions of utilization review are more than forty years old. In the 1950s in western Pennsylvania, the Allegheny Medical Society and the Blue Cross program developed voluntary utilization review programs.[106] In the early 1960s, several so-called foundations for medical care were active in several states, offering appropriateness utilization review.[107] These foundations primarily provided hospital certification, using established guidelines of clinical indications for hospital service. Such reviews antedated and anticipated the demonstration of variations in hospitalization rates made by Wennberg and Associates that are discussed in Chapter Three.

It is unsurprising, then, that the Medicare program was introduced with provisions for utilization review. Any hospital (or long-term care facility) receiving Medicare funds was to provide for reviews of sample hospitalizations that would evaluate medical necessity. Retrospective reviews were to be conducted by hospital committees of physicians or by representatives of the local medical society.[108]

The early federal programs evinced two major assumptions about cost regulation that might affect clinical care. First, the regulation had to enroll physician participation; this linked regulation to the professional requirement of self-scrutiny. Second, the regulation had to remain in community hands, at best at the level of the individual hospital, but at least within the control of local medical societies. Only over the next two decades would these assumptions be eroded.

By 1967, initial inflationary warning signals had led Congress to modify the Medicaid program by adding utilization review provisions. In the Social Security Act Amendments of 1967, state Medicaid programs were required to undertake such oversight; some opted to introduce hospital precertification as well as retrospective review.[109]

These early efforts under both Medicare and Medicaid were greatly hampered by the method of administration. As several commentators have noted, the Department of Health, Education, and Welfare decided to cede authority over the review process to existing provider-controlled third-party administrators like Blue Cross, which had little interest in aggressive oversight of costs (a chronic situation in government-sponsored insurance programs).[110] Many Blue Cross plans chose to emphasize education of and discussion with physicians rather than close scrutiny of bills.

Meanwhile, the staff at the National Center for Health Services Research (NCHSR) began to push for more comprehensive oversight. Choosing a strategy of pilot programs, the NCHSR initiated the Experimental Medical Care Review Organization (EMCRO) program. The EMCROs were intended to demonstrate how local organizations could work with hospitals and their staffs to develop thoroughgoing peer review.[111] The staff at NCHSR was eager to incorporate into the EMCRO process the latest thinking about quality of care and utilization review. Eventually, twelve EMCRO grants were made, and these laid the seed for much more far-reaching reform, as will be discussed in Chapter Four.

As the EMCRO experiment proceeded, Congress had become convinced that the existing mechanisms for controlling costs in Medicare and Medicaid were not working.[112] The EMCRO experience had been positive: committees made up largely of physicians could act independently and somewhat aggressively, unlike the Blue Cross–based third-party administrators, yet not alienate the local medical societies. This suggested that regulation could be accomplished with local administrative and physician involvement, and it echoed the virtues of Braithwaite's responsive regulation.

The result was the Professional Standards Review Organizations (PSROs), created by the Social Security Act Amendments of 1972.[113] To be sure, the major factor leading to the formation of the PSROs was fear of cost inflation.[114] Notably, however, the law stated that the purpose of the PSROs included not just cost review, but also quality oversight: "In order to promote the effective, efficient, and economical delivery of health care services of proper quality for which payment may be made [by Medicare and Medicaid], it is the purpose of this part to assure . . . that the services for which payment may be made . . . will conform to the appropriate professional standard."[115] The new order was also clearly intended to supplant existing Medicare and Medicaid regulations on cost and quality.[116]

The major intent of the PSROs, as pointed out by Jost, was to create a review process that would "be made more sophisticated through the use of professionally developed regional norms of diagnosis and care as guidelines for review activities, as opposed to the present usage of arbitrarily determined checkpoints."[117] Because regional variation in care patterns had to be respected and local participation by physicians was deemed necessary, the PSROs were regionally based, each encompassing an area that included at least three hundred physicians and fifty thousand people. In addition, PSROs generally did not cross state lines, although there were some exceptions to this rule.[118]

At least in theory, state authorities played an important role in producing the guidelines on which the PSROs would rely. State

Professional Standards Review Councils (SPSRCs) were intended
to gather data on care practices, disseminate this information, and
provide PSRO oversight. However, owing mainly to relatively inadequate funding, the potential for SPSRCs was never fulfilled; only
six states ever instituted them.[119]

The structure and composition of a PSRO was carefully dictated
by the enabling legislation.[120] It was to be nonprofit, composed of
physicians from a variety of specialties—but not limited to medical society members—and nondiscriminatory with regard to reviews. Congress clearly acknowledged that physician participation
was a *sine qua non* of a successful utilization review process, but it
also wanted to avoid the domination by medical societies that had
characterized the medical licensure boards in many states. This
critical design feature suggests a commitment to responsiveness
without capture.

Although presumably a number of nonprofit hospitals in any one
area could have applied for a contract with HEW, in practice, organized medicine generally took advantage of several provisions in the
act to ensure that multiple applicants did not appear in any one
area. Because 25 percent of the physicians in a particular region
overseen by the PSRO had to enlist as members, it was very difficult for mavericks to hope to attain PSRO status.[121] The polling for
new members was undertaken by the candidate PSRO and HEW
in concert.

The task of the new PSROs was to develop regional norms for
length of hospital stay and appropriate utilization generally.
Regional norms were defined as "typical patterns of patient care for
each diagnosis and by each age group within a region."[122] The
norms were to be approved by the National Professional Standards
Review Council (NPSRC) so as to maintain some uniformity.
They would then be used by the PSROs in mandatory concurrent
screening in the Medicare and Medicaid programs. The PSROs
also had the opportunity—but not the obligation—to do hospital
precertification.[123] Profiles of every patient and every provider were

also to be maintained by the PSRO, so as to allow evaluation of quality, appropriateness, and necessity.[124]

The PSRO program was arguably different from the forms of regulation that had preceded it. First, it was aimed specifically at the critical element in health care inflation: provider (especially physician) decision making. Second, unlike other major regulatory interventions taking shape in the early 1970s, it did not restrict itself to cost considerations but also anticipated analyses of quality. The entire regulatory structure depended on the review of records by physicians and others to uncover episodes of inappropriate usage of health services and of substandard care. But then as now, distinguishing inappropriate care from poor care was difficult.

In theory at least, there is a difference between the concepts of inappropriateness and substandard care. We have posed as a working definition of quality that it is a "match" between the results of the work one does and the needs one intends to meet for a beneficiary. We can conceptually segregate care that does not meet the standard expected of the reasonable practitioner from inappropriate care, which we use here as implying excessive care, while acknowledging that both are related to quality.[125] "Inappropriate" care, when extensive, is a quality defect because it is not needed. "Substandard" care is a quality defect because it fails to meet the need it intended to satisfy. Inappropriate care is superfluous; substandard care represents a mistake. Concerns about health care costs lead to interventions designed to reduce excessive care, but usually without a concern for error or poor execution. On the other hand, technically poor care has traditionally involved not unnecessary care but rather a mistaken or substandard delivery of care. Credentialing committees, state licensure boards, and the JCAHO mandates were designed to reduce the occurrence of substandard care, typically by uncovering "bad apple" doctors who were providing poor medical care more frequently than others.

Allowing the PSROs to engage in technical care review, rather than confining them to appropriateness review, would have been a

clear break with traditional self-regulation of quality. More important, PSROs had little or no experience with such judgments.
Therefore it would have been surprising if this aspect of the law had
not been blunted by physician and hospital opposition and by conservative federal enforcement efforts. Indeed, curbs on the PSROs
were apparent from the outset. First, the law was interpreted widely
as not allowing the use of medical care evaluation studies, as HEW
at the time referred to technical, standard-of-care–based audits of
medical records by reviewers.[126] Rather, reviews were restricted to
the objective appropriateness norms or criteria developed by the
PSRO or the NPSRC.

Second, though no physician could review his or her own
record, or any record that might present a conflict of interest, Section 1155(e) required PSROs to accept the reviews done by the
hospital committee or other local organization. This delegation
clause could be interpreted as institutionalized regulatory capture.
On the other hand, it could also be interpreted as a reasonable alternative to the perceived hostility of the JCAHO and other "external" reviewers.

Third, the sensitive information collected by the PSRO on the
appropriateness of care was protected by a shroud of confidentiality. Though the law itself suggested that physician, hospital, and
patient should be informed of any PSRO interpretations, this
clause appeared to be inserted primarily for purposes of the provider
defense.[127] Moreover, although an offending physician's name could
be reported to the medical licensure authority, even advocates of
PSRO authority suggested that such "options should be used only
in the most severe cases." HEW officials realized that "overly frequent reliance by a peer review group on the 'big guns' of publicity, licensure, accreditation and censure will tend to make the
medical professionals somewhat edgy."[128] Significantly, the Bureau
of Quality Assurance at HEW spent a great deal of effort developing a policy that would allow at least some aggregate hospital data
to be shared with the public, but it never succeeded in creating a

cohesive reporting system.[129] Moreover, HEW firmly stated that PSRO information would be exempt from subpoena from courts considering malpractice actions, and most observers concluded that state law on peer review immunity would cover PSRO data.[130]

Finally, and perhaps most important as a counterweight to the oversight power granted to PSROs, practitioners were able to raise concerns about the appropriateness monitoring function of PSROs by citing the potential conflict between cost reduction and quality improvement. The issue of the cost/quality trade-off was central in the Senate Finance Committee's widely publicized hearings on the PSRO program.[131] Medical societies and organized medicine argued that the PSRO profiles would lead to cookbook medicine and that other methods of peer review would be diminished.[132] Critics suggested that PSRO review would weaken physician autonomy, harming the quality of care.[133]

In the face of such charges, HEW was certain to retreat. For instance, when confronted with the question of restrictions on physician authority, Secretary Weinberger reiterated that any standard setting would remain "in the hands of the local physicians."[134] Government efforts would have to be carefully integrated into a structure responsive to local physicians, in keeping with their tradition of self-regulation. By the mid-1970s, it should have been apparent to advocates of centralized quality regulation that the medical profession's opposition was too formidable to allow PSRO oversight.

That the PSRO initiative lasted eight years is in some ways surprising, given the opposition it provoked from providers, who questioned its efficacy from the outset. Its persistence can be at least partially explained by the different strategies pursued by major opponents. The American Hospital Association wanted review to be delegated entirely to the hospitals. The American Medical Association, on the other hand, wanted oversight of review to be independent of hospitals, ensuring better medical society surveillance of the program.[135] Both wanted to capture the effort.

In any case, by the late 1970s, Congress had become concerned that the program was stalled and acceded in 1981 to the Reagan administration's wish to review the program in detail and to close some of the nonfunctioning PSROs.[136] The administration's pro-competitive tendencies effectively ended any hopes that the program would produce real quality regulation, and in late 1982, it was abolished, with a key Senate committee noting that "over-regulation and too detailed specifications in laws have restricted innovation in new approaches to review. The private sector must be encouraged to institute approaches designed to assure quality while eliminating unnecessary services."[137] The government's inability to control costs through the PSRO program would lead to the prospective payment revolution of the 1980s.

The story of PSROs is quite reminiscent of that of cost regulation. There are greater elements of capture in the former, but both programs reveal poorly coordinated efforts aimed almost solely at addressing the defects of the health care market, especially the consumer's lack of information. In many ways, PSROs were even more dependent than cost regulation on inspections for, and culling of, defects. The hope for collaborative care improvement cultivated in the EMCROs was not realized in the PSROs.

The PSROs, though offering the prospect of independent oversight of the quality of care, were frustrated by provider opposition and by the unwieldy structure that had been put in place, at least in part, to allay provider concerns about external review. The theme is the same as in other areas of regulation in health care. The key providers, physicians and hospitals, were comfortable with self-regulation and perceived any external effort, no matter how rational, as outside meddling. Responsive regulation was not possible, given the antagonism between regulator and regulated. Yet the market in health care, because of its peculiar inner dynamics, did not necessarily provide optimal levels of activity (best quality, most efficient health care). (Some market advocates could blame this on insufficient competition, not lack of regulation.) Cost and quality issues had begun to segregate themselves, with perhaps even greater professional jealousy over quality issues than over cost issues. The result was that the only other source of oversight, apart from self-regulation, was left in the hands of attorneys.

Tort Law

An overview of the regulation of the quality of care through the early 1970s would be incomplete without mention of the law of medical malpractice. Arguably, medical malpractice was the one influence on the practice of medicine that was free of professional control, although it was not recognized as a form of quality oversight then, and even today is rarely given such credit by health care providers.

Medical malpractice, as a species of tort law, plays three social roles. First, it provides a sense of corrective justice for litigants in that the injuring professional pays the injured person. The explicit linkage between a plaintiff and a defendant, some would argue, is critical.[138] Others are less certain, and recent tort scholarship has tended to de-emphasize the corrective justice role.

Second, tort law compensates the injured person. Most victims of medical malpractice will suffer uninsured losses in the form of medical care costs, wage losses, or noneconomic damages. The award from a successful suit is supposed to cover these losses. Of course, tort law in general and malpractice litigation in particular are very inefficient methods for accomplishing compensation, in that the administrative costs are exceedingly high, reaching 50 to 60 percent in some estimates.[139] If our only motivation for malpractice litigation were compensation, it would be far less expensive to employ an administrative compensation plan.

This leaves the third function of tort law: deterrence. The medical malpractice suit is supposed to contribute to the quality of care by sanctioning the physician for injuring a patient with substandard care. The elements of a successful tort claim (dutiful relationship, injury, negligence, and a causal relationship between negligence and injury) are intended to ensure that only practitioners who fail to reach the standard expected of the reasonable medical practitioner can be successfully sued. Because they then must pay the award, economic incentives adhere to the standard of care. Therefore, according to this logic, tort law should deter the practice of substandard medicine.

This critical element of tort law, and hence the role of tort law in quality regulation, has often been overlooked.[140] This is at least in part due to a tendency in health care to emphasize the inaccuracy of tort claims (many claims are not based on negligent injury), rather than acknowledging that the suit may be a signal of poor care. Tort suits are treated as random events that do not clearly reflect on physician competence or hospital quality. When suits are brought, physicians tend not to accept that they may have erred.[141] Of course, often they are correct: relatively few claims are based on episodes of negligent medical injury.

These perceptions were already firmly established more than thirty years ago, even though rates of malpractice were not nearly at the levels known today. Although reliable statistics are difficult to find, it appears that malpractice suits became ever more prevalent from the 1930s through the late 1950s. In 1957, the American Medical Association estimated that 18,500 physicians, or one in seven, had been sued in their career.[142]

The slow but steady increase in malpractice suits can be largely attributed to changes in tort doctrine that lowered previous barriers to suits by patients and other plaintiffs. The middle part of the century witnessed new interpretations of common law principles by judges who were probably influenced by the great professors of tort law.[143] In medical malpractice, these took the form of changes in presumptions, immunities from suit, and evidentiary rules.

The most significant changes in the doctrine of medical malpractice came with the introduction of *res ipsa loquitur*. Literally translated from the Latin as "the thing speaks for itself," *res ipsa* was a relatively well-known device in contract and tort law but was rarely employed in malpractice litigation until the classic decision of the California Supreme Court in *Ybarra v. Spangard*. In that 1944 case, the court ruled that the plaintiff need not bear the burden of proving negligence when the outcome of an operation—in this case, a brachial plexus injury during an appendectomy—was completely unexpected and not likely to have occurred in the absence of negligence.[144] The *res ipsa* instruction in medical malpractice had the effect of exposing to liability surgeons and anesthesiologists, who had previously been protected by a code of silence surrounding injuries in the operating room. It soon became the "legal menace that frightens doctors most."[145] Twenty years later, the California Supreme Court took the even larger step of allowing expert testimony on the *res ipsa loquitur* issue.[146]

To gain better evidence on the standard of care, courts slowly overturned the so-called locality rule, which had prohibited testimony by a medical expert who was not from the same town or city as the defendant on the grounds that the expert would be unfamiliar with the local standard. By 1956, the Supreme Court of Rhode Island had allowed a physician based in Philadelphia to testify in Providence about the standard of care.[147] Within twenty years, many state courts had moved to a national standard of practice, permitting the use of available experts even in rural areas.[148] This effectively overcame the so-called conspiracy of silence among local medical experts when a colleague was sued.

Changes in tort law also affected the liability of hospitals. During much of the first half of the century, hospitals operating on a not-for-profit basis could take advantage of charitable immunity from suits.[149] However, with the recognition that hospitals received payment from many patients, and acted in many ways like other agents of commerce, courts began to chip away at the protection. In a leading 1957 case, the Supreme Court of New York abandoned the doctrine. By 1962, sixteen states had followed suit.[150]

The loss of charitable immunity was, however, only one of the factors opening the hospitals to liability. Perhaps more important was the emerging trend to hold hospitals liable for physician negligence. Although the beginning of this trend is usually dated to 1965, with the decision of *Darling v. Charleston Community Memorial Hospital*, there was a good deal of judicial activism in the decade before that.[151]

The effect of these and other changes in the common law was to increase rates of litigation nationally, and hence to increase the costs of medical malpractice.[152] In 1966, one author noted that "the total amount of court judgments and settlements in malpractice actions is now an astounding $50,000,000 a year. . . . If those statistics alarm, they should."[153] Yet the alarm seemed to be about the litigation rather than about the substandard care that gave rise to it. Typical was the reaction of Carl Wasmuth, chairman of the board of governors of the Cleveland Clinic, who noted in 1972: "Before 1940, medical malpractice suits occurred infrequently. Lawyers had determined that such suits were difficult to litigate successfully. They had alleged the conspiracy of silence and the conspiracy of science. . . . But this conspiracy (if it did exist) like all conspiracies was overcome. . . . The increase in number of malpractice suits soon reached epidemic proportions in Southern California. Unfortunately the disease spread to the East Coast and soon to all large urban centers. Today this problem is endemic."[154]

The problem, according to Wasmuth, was not the substandard care but the spreading disease of malpractice litigation. The disconnection between malpractice suits and quality regulation (with the possible exception of licensure board efforts discussed earlier) was becoming increasingly evident as costs of insurance continued to increase, and as research demonstrated that only a small fraction of potentially compensable medical injuries were leading to suits.[155] As Law and Polan noted perceptively in 1977, "The malpractice debate had focused little attention on the causes of medical malpractice."[156] It is reasonable to see this disconnection between tort law and quality as the natural reaction of a profession to an "uncapturable" form of regulation.

After the mid-1970s, the doctrinal expansion in medical

malpractice would largely come to a close, with courts generally reiterating the role of medical custom in defining the standard of care and refusing to apply principles of strict liability to the medical industry.[157] Indeed, much of the rest of the history of medical malpractice is the story of tort reform, or of the backlash against increased litigation. But the theme of segregation of medical malpractice from the quality debate will remain.

Conclusion

Quality regulation in the United States through the mid-1970s was primarily accomplished through self-regulation by hospitals and physicians. Hospital accreditation by the JCAHO and oversight of medical providers by hospital committees and state licensure boards were the major influences promoting the quality of care from outside the medical industry. Very little concerted governmental effort to regulate medicine was made, except in the area of cost containment, where certificate-of-need and rate-setting laws had limited impact. The federal government's efforts to judge the quality of care, or at least the appropriateness of care, through the PSROs was largely a failure, probably because the providers were never integrated into the program. Medical malpractice litigation was not seen as a source of useful signals about the quality of care.

Perhaps more worrisome than ineffective regulation was the growing perception that existing regulation, rather than contributing to better care, represented needless interference. A negative attitude toward the JCAHO had already begun to incubate by the early 1970s. The connection between quality improvement and the JCAHO's efforts was never realized. The EMCROs' bright start was lost in the concerns about prerogatives that characterized the maneuvering around the PSROs.

The nonresponsiveness of regulation in medical care was due, at least in part, to its being viewed as external. The natural reaction of regulators was to become outsiders, inspectors. The consequences were as adverse as they could be: hostility between regulators and regulated, and increased efforts to capture or avoid capture. In the meantime, however, the market in medical care had not proven capable of guaranteeing socially optimal outcomes.

Nor had the developing science of quality assurance yet penetrated the institutions of quality regulation. Though there are some notable examples of innovation by regulators, the idea that medicine was a complex system that could be improved by concerted effort generally remained unexplored. In the mid-1970s, medicine still remained a matter of the individual provider struggling against the disease of the individual patient. The physician's ethical commitment to the patient, defined by individual providers, was the one major guarantee of high-quality care. But over the next two decades, the science of quality improvement was to blossom, and the medical care system was to be recognized as just that: a complex industry, responsive to influences of the market and governmental regulation.

Notes

1. See, for example, L. R. Jacobs and R. Y. Shapiro, "Public Opinion's Tilt Against Private Enterprise," *Health Affairs* 13 (1994): 285–298.

2. For instance, the Medical Practice Study demonstrated that there might be as many as 100,000 deaths due to negligent injury in American hospitals each year. See P. C. Weiler, H. H. Hiatt, J. P. Newhouse, W. G. Johnson, T. A. Brennan, and L. L. Leape, *A Measure of Malpractice* (Cambridge, Mass.: Harvard University Press, 1993). Of course, as we discussed in the previous chapter, defining quality of care is notoriously difficult. For an empirical view of this issue, see H. R. Rubin, W. H. Rogers, K. L. Kahn, L. V. Rubenstein, and R. H. Brook, "Watching the Doctor Watchers: How Well Do Peer Review Organization Methods Detect Hospital Quality of Care Problems?" *Journal of the American Medical Association* 267 (1992): 2349–53.

3. We will not go into much detail about the history of quality assurance before 1970. This history is discussed in some detail in a series of articles by T. S. Jost, cited in these notes.

4. See D. Blumenthal, M. Schlesinger, and P. Brown Drumheiler (eds.), *Renewing the Promise: Medicare and Its Reform* (New York: Oxford University Press, 1988). For a review of the recent history of physicians' struggle to retain dominance over medical care, see T. A. Brennan, *Just Doctoring: Medical Ethics in the Liberal State* (Berkeley: University of California Press, 1991).

5. See, for example, T. Parsons, "Social Change and Medical Organization in the United States: A Sociological Perspective," *Annals of the American Academy of Political and Social Science* 356 (1963): 21–42; compare E. Friedson, *Doctoring Together: A Study of Professional Social Control* (New York: Elsevier, 1975). See also P. Starr, *The Social Transformation of American Medicine* (New York: Basic Books, 1982). Starr's book is a fairly complete exploration of sociological and economic issues in the development of the medical profession.

6. See Brennan, *Just Doctoring*, chaps. 2, 3.

7. We discuss the role of the Health Maintenance Organization Act and the development of the managed care industry in Chapter Four.

8. The history of the Joint Commission on Accreditation of Hospitals is carefully recounted in T. S. Jost, "The Joint Commission on Accreditation of Hospitals: Private Regulation of Health Care and Public Interest," *Boston College Law Review* 24 (1983): 835–889.

9. See Joint Commission on Accreditation of Hospitals, *Accreditation Manual for Hospitals* (Chicago: Joint Commission on Accreditation of Hospitals, 1976) (hereafter JCAHO 1976), 7, 9.

10. See Joint Commission for Accreditation of Health Care Organizations, *Accreditation Manual for Hospitals* (Chicago: Joint Commission for Accreditation of Health Care Organizations, 1990) (hereafter JCAHO 1990), 1–3, 17–18. Eventually, the JCAHO moved to three-year accreditation. Moreover, the JCAHO applied several levels of grading. For example, a hospital could receive accreditation with Type I recommendations (concerning deficiencies that must be corrected), conditional accreditation with plans for a follow-up survey, or nonaccreditation. See JCAHO 1990, xxvi–xxvii.

11. See JCAHO 1976, 80–88, 109–112. We leave aside here the question of the ethical responsibilities of physicians to ensure and

improve the quality of care. See generally, Brennan, *Just Doctoring,*
chap. 5. For a recent discussion of the physician's duty to report an
incompetent colleague, see E. H. Morreim, "Am I My Brother's
Warden? Responding to the Unethical or Incompetent Colleague,"
Hastings Center Report 23, no. 3 (1993): 19–27.

12. See *St. John's Hospital Medical Staff* v. *St. John Regional Medical Center,* 245 N.W. 2d 472 (S.D. 1976).

13. See JCAHO 1976, 82. See *Barrows* v. *Northwestern Memorial Hospital,* 525 N.E. 2d 50 (Ill. 1988), summarizing the experience of other state courts in review of admitting privileges decisions and noting that only a few states have followed the lead of New Jersey in granting such review.

14. J. D. Blum, "Economic Credentialing: A New Twist in Hospital Appraisal Processes," *Journal of Legal Medicine* 12 (1991): 427–476. For a discussion by courts, see, for example, *Rao* v. *St. Elizabeth's Hospital,* 488 N.E. 2d 685 (Ill. 1986).

15. See JCAHO 1976, 80–82. The later, more detailed standards emphasize education of the staff about bylaws and reporting by committees; see JCAHO 1990, 96–98.

16. JCAHO 1990, 111.

17. C. M. Jacobs, T. H. Christoffel, and N. Dixon, *Measuring the Quality of Patient Care: The Rationale for Outcome Audit,* foreword by J. D. Porterfield, (New York: Ballinger, 1976), ix.

18. As we will see, another effort was to try to measure outcomes, first within the Performance Evaluation Procedure for Auditing and Improving Patient Care, begun in 1972 after being spurred by the Professional Standards Review Organizations.

19. JCAHO 1976, 110, 112, standard IV. Later, all committee activities would be grouped under the reassuring sobriquet *quality assurance.* They included at least monthly reviews by surgical case review committees, particular tissue committees that investigated any cases of normal or surprising pathological specimens, and morbidity and mortality cases in which care provided in particular cases was reviewed (JCAHO 1990, MS.6.1.2.1–3); drug use evaluation, including ongoing evaluation of particular drugs (MS.6.1.3);

medical record review committees that met to assure the integrity of the record (MS.6.1.4); blood usage committees that evaluated use of blood products and serious transfusion reactions (MS.6.1.5); pharmacy and therapeutics committees to ensure that appropriate mechanisms were in place for administration of medicine (MS.6.1.6); and risk management committees to address potential malpractice suits (MS.6.1.7). In addition, the medical staff was to play the leading role in such areas as infection control, administration, and safety in the operating room and elsewhere (SA.1 *et seq.*, 261–267; IC.1 *et seq.*, 65–69).

20. For an especially insightful sociological analysis of the training of surgeons, see C. L. Bosk, *Forgive and Remember* (Chicago: University of Chicago Press, 1974).

21. Ann B. Flood, William R. Scott, W. Ewy, and W. H. Forrest, Jr., "Effectiveness in Professional Organizations: The Impact of Surgeons and Surgical Staff Organizations on the Quality of Care in Hospitals." *Health Serv. Res.* 17 (1984): 341–366.

22. To be sure, on the hotel function side of the survey, some outcome criteria were built into the standards, although hospitals often perceived these as unnecessarily stringent. For example, if chipped glassware was to be discarded, counts of chipped ware provided an outcome measure (JCAHO 1990, DT.4.3). To some extent, this mindset extended to the clinical laboratories where, for example, logs recording daily surveillance were required, (JCAHO 1990, Pa. 5.3.4).

23. See JCAHO 1990, 131, detailing the records necessary for clinical laboratories. Charting in medical records was another area of particular interest to most survey teams. This emphasis no doubt contributed to the near universal acceptance of certain documentation techniques, making medical records quite similar from institution to institution. This in turn makes it possible for physicians to move readily from one hospital to the next. The standardization process that resulted from JCAHO surveys no doubt has made it possible for physicians to admit patients to a variety of hospitals, maintaining economic pressure on hospital administrations.

24. H. R. Burstin, S. R. Lipsitz, and T. A. Brennan, "Socioeconomic Status and Risks for Substandard Medical Care," *Journal of the American Medical Association* 268 (1992): 2383–87.

25. J. S. Roberts, J. G. Coale, and R. R. Redman, "A History of the Joint Commission for Accreditation of Hospitals," *Journal of the American Medical Association* 258 (1987): 936–940.

26. See T. S. Jost, "Medicare and the Joint Commission on Accreditation of Health Care Organizations: A Healthy Relationship?" *Law and Contemporary Problems* 57 (1994): 15–45.

27. 42 U.S.C.A. §§1395x(e) and 1395bb (1992).

28. The exceptions are small, often rural, hospitals (conversation with James Roberts, November 15, 1993).

29. See *Georgia Hospital Association* v. *Ledbetter*, 396 S.E. 2d 488, 489 (Ga. 1990).

30. Mich. Comp. Laws §333.21513(d) (1992).

31. New York CLS, Public Health Law §2803 (1987).

32. Hospital Association of New York, *Recommended Changes in Health Care Regulatory Reform* (New York: Hospital Association of New York, 1993).

33. The universities and medical schools, which had played a role in licensure in the late nineteenth century, largely backed out at this point. The reasons for their actions are discussed in R. H. Shyrock, *Medical Licensing in America, 1650–1965* (Baltimore: Johns Hopkins University Press, 1967).

34. R. C. Derbyshire, *Medical Licensure and Discipline in the United States* (Baltimore: Johns Hopkins University Press 1969), 33, 37.

35. Mich. Comp. Laws §333.17021(1) (1992). Vermont's Board of Medical Practice is composed of twelve governor-appointed members—nine physicians and three persons not associated with the medical field. See Vt. Stat. Ann., Tit. 26, §1351(a) (1989).

36. See *Falcone* v. *Middlesex County Medical Society*, 170 A. 2d 791 (N.J. 1961), 800.

37. *Rogers v. Medical Association of Georgia et al.*, 244 Ga. 151, 259 S.E. 2d 85 (1979).

38. See *Toussaint v. State Board of Medical Examiners*, 329 S.E. 2d 433 (S.C. 1985), but compare *Seidenberg v. New Mexico Board of Medical Examiners*, 452 P. 2d 469 (N.M. 1969), where the court found that it is not an unconstitutional usurpation of the governor's power of appointment to restrict the choice of nominees through a state medical society.

39. See, for example, *In re Wilkins*, 242 S.E. 2d 829 (N.C.1978).

40. See, for example, *Mannan v. District of Columbia Board of Medicine*, 558 A. 2d 329 (D.C. App. 1989), in which a hearing committee composed of two lay members and one physician was appropriately charged with making a determination regarding licensure revocation.

41. See Derbyshire, 77.

42. Colo. Rev. Stat. Ann. §12–36–118(5)(g)(III) (West 1992).

43. Indiana Ann. Code 25–1–9–4(a)(4)(D) (1989).

44. *Raymond v. Board of Registration in Medicine*, 443 N.E. 2d 391 (Mass. 1982).

45. See, for example, *Medical Licensing Board of Indiana v. Robertson*, 563 N.E. 2d 168 (Ind. App. 4th Dist. 1991), where the trial court was found in error for substituting its judgment for that of the medical licensing board.

46. See Derbyshire, 93.

47. See, for example, Vt. Stat. Ann., Tit. 26, §1355 (1989).

48. Office of the Inspector General, Department of Health and Human Services, State Licensure Boards (Washington, D.C. June 1986) (75 percent of all disciplinary actions related to drug and alcohol abuse).

49. Colo. Rev. Stat. Ann. §25–3–107 (1990).

50. *Beth Israel Hospital Association v. Board of Registration in Medicine*, 515 N.E. 2d 574 (Mass. 1987).

51. 243 Code Mass. Regs. §3.07(3)(a) (1987).

52. See "Boston Hospitals Battle State's Move to Take over the Policing of Doctors," *New York Times*, May 17, 1987, 47; D. Kong, "Doctors Get an OK on Bill Restricting the Board of Medicine," *Boston Globe*, May 1, 1993 (funding bill would give the board only 50 percent of the revenues it generates from doctors' fees, as opposed to the 100 percent recommended by a state task force in 1992); I. Van-Tuinen, P. McCarthy, S. Wolfe, and A. Bame, *Comparing State Medical Boards* (Washington, D.C.: Public Citizen, 1993).

53. *Report and Recommendations of the State of New Jersey Commission of Investigations of Impaired and Incompetent Physicians* (Trenton: State of New Jersey, 1987).

54. VanTuinen, McCarthy, Wolfe, and Bame, 18.

55. See T. Kirn, "California Medical Board Slated for Meaningful Reform," *American Medical News*, April 26, 1993, 20.

56. W. P. Burrows, "Incident Reporting: A Hospital's Conflicting Obligations Resolved," *New York State Bar Journal* 58 (October 1986): 10; New York CLS, Public Health Law §2805(1987). See generally, 10 N.Y.C.R.R. pt. 405, §405.8.

57. Hospital Association of New York, *Recommended Changes of Health Care Regulatory Reform* (New York: Hospital Association of New York, 1993).

58. Conversation with Aileen Shinaman, associate counsel, Strong Memorial Hospital, October 8, 1993.

59. See T. S. Jost, L. Mulcahy, S. Strasser, and L. A. Sachs, "Consumers Complaints and Professional Discipline: A Look at Medical Licensure Boards," *Health Matrix: Journal of Law and Medicine* 3 (1993): 333. This is an excellent review of the workings of one board.

60. VanTuinen, McCarthy, Wolfe, and Bame.

61. Mich. Comp. Laws §333.17033 (1992).

62. Hospital Survey and Construction Act, 42 U.S.C.A. §291–291o–1 (1944).

63. A more detailed discussion of this history can be found in J. B. Simpson, "Full Circle: The Return of Certificate of Need

Regulation of Health Facilities to State Control," *Indiana Law Journal* 19 (1986): 1025–88.

64. 42 U.S.C.A. §246 (1991).

65. M. I. Roemer, "Bed Supply and Hospital Utilization: A Natural Experiment," *Hospital* 35 (November 1, 1961): 37–40.

66. This research is discussed in more detail in Chapter Three.

67. Social Security Act Amendments, PL 92–603, 42 U.S.C.A. §1320a–1 (1972).

68. See Simpson, 1037.

69. 42 U.S.C.A. §§300k–300n–5 (1991), repealed by PL 99–660, title VII, §701(a), 100 Stat. 3799 (1986).

70. The structure of the various authorities was quite complex. HSAs were to operate at the local level, so each state would have several of them. A State Health Planning and Development Agency reviewed state plans and coordinated the HSAs. The structure was similar to what the Clinton administration endorsed in the regulatory aspects of its Health Security Act.

    Regarding the components of the CON oversight, review would occur for any construction of hospitals, any capital expenditures of more than $150,000, any increase of beds greater than 10 percent over a two-year period, or any new clinically related service. For more details, see Simpson, 1044.

71. F. Miller, "Antitrust and Certificate of Need: Health Systems Agencies, the Planning Act, and Regulatory Capture," *Georgetown Law Journal* 68 (1986): 873, 874.

72. See Simpson, 1046.

73. On CON effectiveness, see F. A. Sloan, "Regulation and the Rising Costs of Hospital Care," *Review of Economics and Statistics* 63 (1981): 479–487; F. A. Sloan and B. Steinwald, "Effects of Regulation on Hospital Costs and Input Use," *Journal of Law Economics* 23 (1980): 81–109. On courts' reactions to the state agencies, see *North Miami General Hospital, Inc. v. Office of Community Medical Facilities*, 355 So. 2d 1272 (Fla. Dist. Ct. App. 1978).

74. See M. Jee and C. Kent, "Perspectives: States Rediscover Certificate-of-Need Laws," *Medicine and Health*, February 22, 1993. The states that dropped the CON programs included Arizona, California, Colorado, Idaho, Kansas, Minnesota, New Mexico, South Dakota, Texas, Utah, and Wyoming. Many of these states are still rather hostile to regulation.

75. See, for example, J. F. Blumstein and F. A. Sloan, "Redefining Government's Role in Health Care: Is a Dose of Competition What the Doctor Should Order?" *Vanderbilt Law Review* 34 (1981): 849–870; compare R. R. Bovbjerg, "Competition Versus Regulation: An Overdrawn Dichotomy?" *Vanderbilt Law Review* 34 (1981): 965–1002.

76. See Brennan, *Just Doctoring*, 63–65. See also A. S. Relman, "Investor-Owned Hospitals and Health Care Costs," *New England Journal of Medicine* 309 (1983): 370–372. For a discussion of the same issues in environmental policy, see T. A. Brennan, "Environmental Torts," *Vanderbilt Law Review* 46 (1993): 1–73.

77. See Jee and Kent, 2. See generally, R. Pear, "States Are Moving to Re-Regulation on Health Care Costs," *New York Times*, May 11, 1992, A-1.

78. Virginia and Wisconsin both reinstated their CON programs in 1992. See Jee and Kent, 3. Some states have sought to bring doctors' offices within the purview of CON. Other states have followed suit. See T. Johnson, "Certificate of Need Review Targets Doctors," *American Medical News* 36 (1993): 3.

79. See 10 N.Y.C.R.R., pt. 709. The certificate-of-need program has been subject to a certain amount of litigation. See, for example, *Finger Lakes Health Systems Agency v. St. Joseph's Hospital*, 412 N.Y.S. 2d 219 (A.D., 3rd Dept. 1981) (the court warned that injunctions would be granted quickly to ensure that health facilities did not attempt to circumvent CON laws); *Arnot-Ogden Memorial Hospital v. Guthrie Hospital, Inc.*, 505 N.Y.S. 2d 232 (A.D., 3rd Dept. 1986) (hospital lacks standing to sue physicians to require them to obtain a certificate of need for their diagnostic and treatment center).

80. Ind. Code §16–10–4–9.1(9) (West 1992).

81. Ga. Off. Code Ann. §31–6–40 (1991).

82. See *Fulton Community Hospital v. State Health Planning and Development Agency*, 310 S.E. 2d 764 (Ga. App. 1983), and Ga. Off. Code Ann. §31–6–40.1 (1991).

83. Mass. General Law, chap. 111, §25c 1/2 (1987).

84. See J. Clemens, "Oversight of Hospitals Still Needed, Says Panel," *Boston Business Journal,* April 9, 1993, 8 (discussing a six-month analysis by the Hospital Payment System Advisory Commission recommending that the determination-of-need program be altered to reflect the competitive health care environment).

85. J. C. Spring, "A Study of Massachusetts Determination of Need Law as a Tool of Consumer Advocacy" (Cambridge, Mass.: John F. Kennedy School of Government, 1994), 35.

86. In fact, some would argue that CON programs have always had a number of mandates. For instance, a case has recently been made that the Florida CON law has long been used to encourage care for the indigent population, a goal not explicitly stated in the legislation. See E. S. Campbell and G. M. Fournier, "Certificate-of-Need Deregulation and Indigent Hospital Care," *Journal of Health Politics, Policy and Law* 18 (1993): 905–925.

87. See R. B. Hackey, "New Wine in Old Bottles: Certificate of Need Enters the 1990's," *Journal of Health Politics, Policy and Law* 18 (1993): 927–935; Jee and Kent.

88. See L. D. Brown, "Political Evolution of Federal Health Care Regulation," *Health Affairs* 11 (winter 1993): 18–37 (discussing the hospital payment limits built into §223 of the Social Security Act Amendments of 1972).

89. N.J. Stat. Ann. 17:48–49 (West 1963).

90. See J. A. Morone and A. B. Dunham, "Slouching Towards National Health Insurance: The New Health Care Politics," *Yale Journal on Regulation* 2 (1985): 263, 265.

91. 1971 N.J. Laws 300, 310–311 (*codified as amended* at N.J. Stat. Ann. 26:2H–18 [West 1987]).

92. See Morone and Dunham, 266.

93. See Morone and Dunham, 266.

94. See Morone and Dunham, 267.

95. See Morone and Dunham, 267–268.

96. See Morone and Dunham, 268.

97. See Morone and Dunham, 268.

98. See Md. Health Gen. Code Ann. §19–102(a)(1) (Michie 1990)
    (provision of health care to all a priority of the state); §§19–201–222
    (Michie 1990) (authorizes and sets forth the procedures by which
    the commission is to review hospital costs and establish reasonable
    rates) (Act of May 24, 1971, chap. 627, 1971 Md. Laws 1311). See
    C. H. Fleming, M. D. McCauley, and J. D. Wilson, "Survey of Devel-
    opments in Maryland Law, 1983–84," *Maryland Law Review* 4
    (1986): 794; K. D. Savage, "Survey of Developments in Maryland
    Law, 1983–84," *Maryland Law Review* 44 (1985): 571 n. 1.

99. Md. Health Gen. Code Ann. §19–216(b) (Michie 1993) provides:

    (b) Rate Approval Power.
       (1) To carry out its powers under subsection (a) of this section, the
            Commission may review and approve or disapprove the reason-
            ableness of any rate that a facility sets or requests.
       (2) A facility shall charge for services only at a rate set in accordance
            with this subtitle.
       (3) In determining the reasonableness of rates, the Commission may
            take into account objective standards of efficiency and effectiveness.

    The Commission's rate-setting authority has been upheld in *Blue
    Cross of Maryland, Inc.* v. *Franklin Square Hospital*, 352 A. 2d 798
    (Md. 1976). See also *Health Services Cost Review Commission* v.
    Franklin Square Hospital, 372 A. 2d 1051 (Md. 1977).

100. Md. Health Gen. Code Ann. §19–216(c) (Michie 1990). This
     authority was upheld in *Harford Memorial Hospital* v. *Health Services
     Cost Review Commission*, 410 A. 2d 22 (Md. 1980).

101. See *Health Services Cost Review Commission* v. *Lutheran Hospital of
     Maryland, Inc.*, 660 n. 5, 472 A. 2d 55, 59 n. 5 (Md. 1984) (dis-
     cussing GIR).

102. See Savage, 571.

103. See Savage, 571 n. 5.

104. See Brown, 25; Brennan, *Just Doctoring*, 63. Rate setting in Connecticut, Massachusetts, and New York falls between the points on the spectrum represented by New Jersey and Maryland. Connecticut's General Statute §19a–151 provides rate-setting powers for the State of Connecticut. Any hospital wishing to increase its room or aggregate special services rates by more than 6 percent had to file a request with the Commission on Hospitals and Health Care. If the increase was denied, the commission was required to conduct a hearing. Massachusetts's rate-setting authority was created in 1973. See 1973 Mass. App. 1229 §2, creating §32 of Mass. General Law, chap. 6a. It was amended somewhat by the addition of section 37 in 1976, which created the rate approval procedure for nonacute hospitals. See 1976 Mass. App. 409 §4, creating chap. 6a, §32, §37. Subsequent legislation removed most of the rate-setting authority. In New York, rate setting is governed by §2807 and §2807a. See N.Y. Pub. Health Law §2807 and §2807a (McKinney 1993). New York's rate-setting authority is another state law that is threatened by ERISA preemption, as will be discussed in Chapter Five.

105. See, for example, K. E. Thorpe and C. E. Phelps, "Regulatory Intensity and Hospital Cost Growth," *Journal of Health Economics* 9 (1990): 143–166; C. J. Schramm, S. C. Renn, and B. Biles, "Controlling Hospital Cost Inflation: New Perspectives on State Rate Setting," *Health Affairs* 5 (fall 1986): 22–33; M. D. Rasko, "A Comparison of Hospital Performance Under the Medicare Partial Payer Medicare PPS and State All-Payer Rate Setting Systems," *Inquiry* 26 (spring 1989): 48–61; P. B. Ginsburg and K. E. Thorpe, "Can All Payer Rate Setting and the Competitive Strategy Co-Exist?" *Health Affairs* 11 (summer 1992): 73–86. Some would argue that all-payer rate setting has been successful in Germany (Ginsburg and Thorpe, 75).

106. This is recounted in J. D. Blum, P. M. Gertman, and J. Rabinow, *PSROs and the Law* (Germantown, Md.: Aspen Systems Corp., 1977), 2.

107. See Blum, Gertman, and Rabinow, 5.

108. See Blum, Gertman, and Rabinow, 3.

109. See Blum, Gertman, and Rabinow, 14.

110. See Blum, Gertman, and Rabinow, 14. See also Sylvia A. Law, *Blue Cross: What Went Wrong?* (New Haven: Yale University Press, 1974), 120–123.

111. See P. Sanazaro, R. L. Goldstein, J. S. Roberts, D. B. Maglott, and J. W. McAllister, "Research and Development in Quality Assurance: The Experimental Medical Care Review Organization Program," *New England Journal of Medicine* 287 (1972): 1125–28.

112. See, for example, Senate Committee on Finance, 2nd Cong., 2d sess., 1972, S. Rept. 1230, 254–269; Senate Committee on Finance, *Medicare and Medicaid: Problems, Issues, and Alternatives*, 91st Cong., 2d sess., 1970, 105–109. See also T. S. Jost, "Administrative Law Issues Involving the Medicare Utilization and Quality Control Peer Review Organization (PRO) Program: Analysis and Recommendations," *Ohio State Law Journal* 50 (1989): 1, 3–10.

113. See Social Security Act Amendments, 42U.S.C. 1301, PL 92–603, §249F, 86 Stat. 1329, 1429–45 (1972).

114. See Blum, Gertman, and Rabinow, 18 (quoting the Senate Finance Committee's concerns about cost inflation in the Medicare system).

115. 42 U.S.C. 1320c §1151.

116. See Blum, Gertman, and Rabinow, 47, discussing the legislative intent that PSRO decisions were to be binding on Medicare and Medicaid programs.

117. See Jost, "Administrative Law Issues Involving the Medicare Utilization and Quality Control Peer Review Organization (PRO) Program," 20.

118. Some state medical societies balked over the regional nature of PSROs. Indeed, the Texas Medical Association brought suit against the Department of Health, Education, and Welfare for failure to designate the entire state of Texas as a PSRO. See *Texas Medical Society v. Mathews*, 408 F. Supp. 303 (W. D. Tex. 1976).

119. See P. Mellette, "The Changing Focus of Peer Review Under Medicare," *University of Richmond Law Review* 20 (1986): 315–356; see also A. Gosfield, *PSRO's: The Law and the Health Consumer* (New York: Ballinger, 1975), 6–10.

120. See Blum, Gertman, and Rabinow, 23–24

121. See Blum, Gertman, and Rabinow, 26.

122. PL 92–603 §249F(b) (1972).

123. Arguably, such hospital precertification was prohibited for all but voluntary purposes by the AMA's successful suit. See *American Medical Association* v. *Weinberger*, 522 F. 2d 921 (7th Cir. 1975).

124. 42 U.S.C. 1320c §1155(a)(4).

125. On the "reasonable practitioner," see T. A. Brennan, "Practice Guidelines and Malpractice Litigation: Collision or Cohesion?" *Journal of Health Politics, Policy and Law* 16 (1991): 67–85.

126. See Blum, Gertman, and Rabinow, 30–31.

127. 42 U.S.C. 1320c and §1159 set forth notice and also process should a provider wish to dispute the finding.

128. See Blum, Gertman, and Rabinow, 42.

129. Many advocates sought release of hospital data. One of the more interesting efforts was undertaken by the Harvard Center for Community Health, which tried to use state consumer law (General Law, chap. 93A) to lever the PSRO to provide information. See Harvard Center for Community Health, *PSRO Information and Consumer Choice: The Case for Public Disclosure of Health Services Data* (Boston: Harvard Center for Community Health, 1975).

130. C. M. Jacobs and N. D. Jacobs, *The PEP Primer* (Chicago: Joint Commission for Accreditation of Health Care Organizations, 1974).

131. Implementation of PSRO Legislation: Hearings on PL 92–603 before the Subcommittee on Health of the Senate Committee on Finance, 93d Cong., 2d Sess., pt. 1 (1974).

132. Senate Committee on Finance, Subcommittee on Health, *Hearings on Implementation of PSRO Legislation (PL 92–603)*, statement of Dr. R. B. Roth, 71.

133. C. Welch, "PSRO's—Pro's and Con's," *New England Journal of Medicine* 290 (1974): 1319–21.

134. See Senate Committee on Finance, Subcommittee on Health, *Hearings on Implementation of PSRO Legislation (PL 92–603)*, 17.

135. Senate Committee on Finance, Subcommittee on Health, *Hearings on PSRO Proposals*, 97th Cong. 2d sess., 1982, §1250, §2142, 213 (submission of the American Hospital Association). See Gosfield, 180. See also C. C. Havighurst and J. F. Blumstein, "Coping with the Quality/Cost Trade-Offs in Medical Care: The Role of PSRO's," *Northwestern University Law Review* 70 (1975): 6, 46.

136. PL 97–35, 95 Stat. 794.

137. *U.S. Code of Congressional and Administrative News* (1982), 817.

138. See, for example, E. J. Weinrib, "Understanding Tort Law," *Valparaiso University Law Review* 23 (1989): 485–526.

139. G. L. Priest, "The Current Insurance Crisis in Modern Tort Law," *Yale Law Journal* 96 (1987): 1521–1601; P. M. Danzon, "Tort Reform and the Role of Government and Private Insurance Markets," *Journal of Legal Studies* 13 (1984): 517–540.

140. One could argue quite reasonably that the deterrent effect of tort litigation is frustrated by the flat nature of most professional liability insurance, which insulates the practitioner from the economic signal of the claim. See A. G. Lawthers, A. R. Localio, N. M. Laird, S. R. Lipsitz, L. Hebert, and T. A. Brennan, "Physicians' Perceptions of the Risk of Being Sued," *Journal of Health Politics, Policy and Law* 17 (1992): 463–482.

141. See Lawthers and others, 470. See also N. Hupert, T. A. Brennan, L. Peterson, and A. Lawthers, "Physicians' Perceptions of Medical Malpractice," *Social Science in Medicine* (1995).

142. See C. J. Stetler and A. R. Moritz, *Doctor and Patient and the Law*, 4th ed. (St. Louis, Mo.: Mosby, 1962), 304.

143. See Priest, 1530–35.

144. *Ybarra v. Spangard*, 154 P. 2d 687 (Cal. 1944). The court hewed to the three conditions necessary to the *res ipsa loquitur* instruction:

(1) the accident must be of a kind that ordinarily does not occur in the absence of someone's negligence; (2) it must be caused by an agency or instrumentality within the exclusive control of the defendant; (3) it must not have been due to any voluntary action or contribution on the part of the plaintiff (*Ybarra v. Spangard*, 154 p. 2d 689).

145. See H. Hassard, ed., *Medical Malpractice: Risks, Protection, Prevention* (Oradell, N.J.: Medical Economics Book Division, 1966).

146. See *Quintal v. Laurel Grove Hospital*, 41 Cal. Rptr. 577, 397 P. 2d 161 (Cal. 1964).

147. See *Cavallaro v. Sharp*, 121 A. 2d 669 (R.I. Sup. Ct. 1956). See generally, I. M. Gottlieb, "Recent Changes in the So-Called Locality Rule Involving Expert Testimony in Medical Malpractice Cases," in C. H. Wecht, ed., *Exploring the Medical Malpractice Dilemma*, (Mount Kisco, N.Y.: Futura Publishing, 1972).

148. See *Shilkret v. Annapolis Emergency Hospital Association*, 349 A. 2d 245 (Md. 1975).

149. This doctrine was first enunciated in *McDonald v. Massachusetts General Hospital*, 120 Mass. 432 (1876).

150. See, for example, *Bing v. Thunig*, 163 N.Y.S. 2d 3, 143 N.E. 2d 3 (N.Y. 1957); also Stetler and Moritz, 368.

151. *Darling v. Charleston Community Memorial Hospital*, 211 N.E. 2d 253 (Ill. 1965); *cert. denied* 383 U.S. 946 (1965). See generally, Stetler and Moritz, 368, on use of the ostensible agency theory and house officer liability.

152. For a longer discussion of the evolution of medical malpractice law, see P. C. Weiler, *Medical Malpractice on Trial* (Cambridge, Mass.: Harvard University Press, 1991).

153. See Hassard, 3.

154. See C. E. Wasmuth, "Definition and Scope of Malpractice Problem—A National Overview: Its Impact on Inter-Professional Relationships Between Physicians and Attorneys: Physician's View," in Wecht, 1.

155. See P. C. Weiler, H. H. Hiatt, J. P. Newhouse, W. G. Johnson, T. A. Brennan, and L. L. Leape, *A Measure of Malpractice* (Cambridge, Mass.: Harvard University Press, 1993), detailing that liability premiums cost a doctor in New York $360 (1990 dollars) in 1949, $1,000 in 1965, and $7,300 by 1975.

    A study by the California Medical Association revealed that 4.65 percent of hospitalizations in California in 1974 gave rise to medical injuries and that .79 percent would be compensable under the tort system. See California Medical Association, *Medical Insurance Feasibility Study*, ed. D. Harper Mills (San Francisco: California Medical Association. Available from Sutter Publications, 1977).

156. See S. Law and S. Polan, *Pain and Profit: The Politics of Malpractice* (New York: HarperCollins, 1978), 208.

157. See, for example, *Karibjian* v. *Thomas Jefferson University Hospital*, 717 F. Supp. 1081 (E.D. Penn. 1989). The Helling decision is the exception that proves the rule. The Washington Supreme Court was the only panel to approach what would have been the most dramatic change in malpractice law—that is, the replacement of medical custom with a patient-based standard. See *Helling* v. *Carey*, 83 Wash. 2d 514, 519 P. 2d 981 (1974).

. . . .

3

The History of Research
on Health Care Quality

T o design new rules that regulate for improvement of the quality of care, the regulator must understand how quality is defined and measured. This is surprisingly difficult because quality has not always been carefully defined in medicine. In fact, as is the case in many professions, quality has been treated as a matter to be judged by the practitioner, and specifically not by the beneficiary of care.

Yet even at the turn of the last century, ideas concerning the systematic measurement and improvement of quality were incubating. They have matured slowly but steadily, eventually giving rise to the modern conception of good medical care, which places the technical definition of quality more firmly in the experience and outcomes of those who depend on care and increasingly views the enterprise of medicine as accountable to the public that it is meant to serve.

Understanding how modern conceptions of health care quality have evolved during this period of maturation is essential if regulators are to contribute effectively to the continuous improvement of medical care in the modern era.

Unfortunately, only a limited portion of the modern scientific understanding of quality has been embraced by regulation. Our discussion of the history of health care regulation in the first three-quarters of the century made little explicit reference to science, largely because research has had so little impact on that history until recently. This disconnection between quality science and quality regulation is a recurrent theme throughout this book, and a problem that we believe needs remedy. If, as we have suggested, regulation based on antagonism is to be replaced by a responsive variety, regulators must understand the science of quality improvement as it has evolved in the twentieth century; and, they must incorporate these understandings into their own efforts.

In this chapter, we review the evolution of modern scientific knowledge about quality in health care, especially in America, and especially during the first three-quarters of the present century. During this fertile period, the seeds were planted for the truly scientific study of quality of care. In the last quarter of the century, we have seen the flowering of that field. Meanwhile, as the sciences of health care quality were developing, a separate and almost totally independent science was developing in other industries, leading to practical approaches to the management of quality in complex production systems. That other history—the history of industrial quality management techniques—is also described in this chapter, as it has become increasingly significant and promising for the improvement of health care in the years ahead.

The intellectual history of the study of health care quality by American researchers is rich, but it is not orderly. In trying to summarize it, we will be describing more a tangle of vines than a family tree. Nonetheless, the twentieth century included many important advances in approaches to the definition and assessment of the quality of care, and although no single author came close to articulating a comprehensive theory of quality management by today's standards, many writers anticipated the key elements of such a theory.[1]

Several excellent historical reviews are available that trace the evolution of research on quality in health care. John Williamson has analyzed the development of quality assurance methodologies as a series of intertwining efforts among various players on the American health care scene: professional societies, hospitals, payers, government, and others. At each phase in the development of methodologies for quality assurance, Williamson claims, one or another of these voices predominated in the leadership of relevant research and development. (We are greatly indebted to Williamson for sharing with us a superb but so far, unfortunately, unpublished 1975 paper, "Quality Assurance: A Historical Perspective," which we have relied on liberally for the summary provided here. Williamson's review is, overall, the best we have encountered.)

The dean of American researchers in the field of health care quality, Avedis Donabedian, has offered an alternative framework describing five different but interconnected "schools" of investigators whose work composes the majority of research on quality in the mid- and late twentieth century. Some of these schools were centered, according to Donabedian, at Johns Hopkins University (John Williamson, Kerr White, and Paul Lembcke, among others), at the University of Michigan (Beverly Payne, Thomas Lyons, and Donald Reidel), in the New York City area (Mildred Morehead, Sam Shapiro, and others), at Yale University (a group including I. S. Falk), and more recently, at the Rand Corporation in Santa Monica, California (Robert Brook, Mark Chassin, and John Ware, Jr., among others). In this chapter, we will use a somewhat more simplistic chronological analysis, reviewing key contributions decade by decade. Our aim is not to supplant the other fine reviews, but rather to describe a series of highlights of particular relevance to the proper regulation of quality in the future.

For the greater part of the century, the names of individual investigators rather than recognizable, substantive lines of inquiry draw our attention. From the turn of the century until the mid-1970s, quality assurance in health care was an immature science. It was shaped and controlled by the acts and ideas of individual investigators, often iconoclasts, who were seeking to define a new field that lacked the stable vocabulary, organizational structures, academic titles, and even professional journals that characterize a fully formed scientific discipline. Only in the mid- and late 1970s, largely because of a crucial concentration of senior researchers at the Rand

Corporation, did these efforts begin to acquire the real hallmarks of a modern science. Until then, our narrative describes not the history of a field but a history of people struggling to create a field.

Unlike other authors, we provide this history to illuminate the failure of regulation of quality and to suggest a pathway to new responsive rules. The incubation of methods of quality improvement occurs largely apart from the antagonism between the regulated and the regulator, which we have already reviewed. Its incorporation into medical care and regulatory efforts in the recent past suggests the solution to obstructive regulation.

1900–1920: Discovering the "Product" of Health Care

All histories of concern for quality in health care in the modern era seem to begin with Ernest Codman. A surgeon at Massachusetts General Hospital in Boston, Codman emerged as a controversial figure in the first two decades of the century by suggesting, in sometimes strident tones, that hospitals in general, and surgeons in particular, should measure and report the effects of their own work.[2] Codman urged the keeping of simple epidemiologic records of the immediate and longer-term outcomes of surgical procedures, so that surgeons and organizations could be compared on the basis of their "end results." Codman appears to have had two objectives in mind. First, he suggested that those who use health care have a right to information on the results of practice, so that they can make choices among providers. Second, he believed that the study of end results would be a necessary condition for a productive exchange of information among providers of care, on the basis of which each could improve the care they gave.

From the viewpoint of quality management, Codman's arguments are astounding in their modernity. In his key 1914 paper "The Product of the Hospital,"[3] he specifically recounts his own conversations with industrial engineers, which helped him to formulate his views of the hospital as a production system. He is careful to show the important interdependencies among the hospital's several missions of service, teaching, and research, and with the sensibility of the modern systems thinker, he emphasizes that teaching people how to carry out processes of work without underlying knowledge of the effects of that work on its intended beneficiaries is actually a form of waste. Teaching surgery, he argued, was futile without the means for ongoing study of the effects of surgery on patients. His understanding of the deep relationship between ignorance and waste, and therefore of the positive relationship between quality and efficiency, is absolutely modern. But it appears to have been forgotten, or at least underestimated, by many of the researchers who followed Codman for decades afterward. The dominant paradigm of individual doctors committed to individual patients did not leave much intellectual room for Codman's grander perspectives on systematic data analysis and professional learning as a response to the need for better health care.

But Codman was not alone in these concerns. In fact, he is only the best known among a large number of American and European surgeons in the early twentieth century who were creating arguments for the construction of results-oriented data bases, epidemiologic study of the effects of care, comparative analyses of performance of organizations and individual physicians, and in some cases, public release of information on results of care. Other voices, disconnected from each other but consistent in their views, included those of Haidenthaller[4] in Germany, Bassini[5] in Italy, and Bowman, Cabot, Cushing, Morris, and Martin in the United States.[6]

Although Codman does not appear to have become especially popular for his views among his professional colleagues, he was not ignored. Indeed, through the second and third decade of the century, it was primarily Codman's colleagues, American surgeons like John G. Bowman, who took up the challenge to study and act on information on the results of health care. In 1913, the American College of Surgeons (ACS) launched a major effort to understand

and improve supports for effective surgery in American and Canadian hospitals, and in 1914, the Committee on the Standardization of Hospitals reported at the Fifth Clinical Congress of Surgeons on an "End Results Record System" that was designed to support assessment of the outcomes of surgery in American hospitals.[7] By 1920, on-site visits by trained surveyors under the Hospital Standardization Program of the American College of Surgeons had yielded data on 697 hospitals with more than 100 beds.[8] Specifically, the Hospital Standardization Program addressed five dimensions of hospital performance:

1. Medical staff organization
2. Qualifications for medical staff membership
3. Rules and policies governing professional work in the hospital
4. Medical records
5. Diagnostic and therapeutic facilities

The reports uncovered an astounding degree of nonconformity among American hospitals in their approaches to medical care. Apparently, hospitals were exerting little effort to bring individual doctors into compliance with standards of best practice, a finding consistent with the ascendance of physicians and the passivity of hospitals characteristic of those times.

In the 1917 proceedings of the American College of Surgeons Conference on Hospital Standardization, Dr. John Hornsby noted:

> In perhaps 75 percent of the hospitals in this country . . . the [medical] record as it is kept today is practically valueless. . . . In 75 percent of the hospitals there is no examination whatever on the admission of the patient. . . . In 75 percent of the hospitals the records do not show a diagnosis even after examination, and up to the moment that the patient goes to the operating room

for surgical procedure; and in many hospitals this lack is premeditated and is actually intended to cover up and hide carelessness or incapacity on the part of the surgeon to diagnose the disease for which he is about to subject his patient to a serious major surgical operation. . . . In Bellevue Hospital, New York, . . . in 58 percent of the cases that went to autopsy the diagnosis was wrong.[9]

It is important to realize that these remarks, and many others like them, were published in the *Bulletin of the American College of Surgeons* in 1917, and were part of a firm and public commitment by leading surgeons to the discovery and correction of defects in care, exactly as counseled by Codman (who spoke at the same 1917 conference). In a follow-up conference at New York's Waldorf Astoria Hotel on October 24, 1919, J. G. Bowman, director of the college, reported that of 692 surveyed hospitals with more than 100 beds, only 89 had met the new ACS standards.[10]

This era of ACS review through the Hospital Standardization Program offers an unusually impressive example of a medical discipline actually taking responsibility for the assessment of its own work. Unfortunately, it also has given us a vivid tale showing how difficult the path of self-regulation can be. Several authorities tell, with apparent foundation, of a bizarre episode at that 1917 conference, in which the ACS leaders, concerned that the identities of the noncomplying hospitals (some of which were among the leading institutions of the time) might become public, met together at midnight at the furnace of the Waldorf Astoria and incinerated the original reports.[11]

Though it may have burned the data, the American College of Surgeons did not, in truth, back away from the disturbing information. Instead, it intensified its efforts to review and certify surgical programs in American hospitals (albeit in less public ways), and it established a series of standards for the proper management of hospitals and of surgical units within them. Understandably, these

standards focused more on the recruitment, certification, and interaction of surgeons themselves than on the hospital as a system for
the support of surgery.

Although the work of the Hospital Standardization Program of
the ACS has been criticized by some as failing to address variation
in performance either publicly enough or aggressively enough, it
represents the most important effort in the first half of the century
to link intellectually grounded forms of standard setting and audit
with the actual conduct of day-to-day care. This effort was the direct forerunner of the more comprehensive and rigorous methods
of accreditation and certification that were to develop under the
Joint Commission for Accreditation of Hospitals (later the Joint
Commission for Accreditation of Health Care Organizations, or
JCAHO) beginning in the early 1950s.[12] Unequivocally, however,
the ACS's efforts represented self-regulation and not the progression of external scrutiny or public accountability to those outside
the profession of medicine. In the early part of the century, there is
little evidence of public authorities becoming involved in oversight
of the quality of care being given by doctors or hospitals. As Starr
has suggested, therapeutic medicine had already faced down the
challenge of public health.[13] The lack of external oversight was to
persist more or less intact until the 1960s, when the JCAHO began
to find its own, slightly antagonistic voice.

1920–1940: From Standardization
to Resource Planning

Codman's pleas for the measurement of end results and the Hospital Standardization Program of the ACS were facets of a larger trend
that dominated the evolution of American health care in the first
quarter of the twentieth century: the increasing formalization of
medicine as a profession and of health care as a system. The same
formalization was occurring in American medical education, as it
moved from a model of apprenticeship to institutionally based train-

ing in university settings. Supported by a grant from the Carnegie
Foundation, Abraham Flexner and his colleagues visited every medical school in the nation, obtaining data on curricula, budgets, staff,
and facilities, and in their 1910 report,[14] provided (as John Williamson recounts in his unpublished historical account of quality assurance in health care) the first "detailed exposure of medical schools
by name."[15] Between 1900 and 1915, 92 of approximately 165 medical schools in the United States closed their doors, leaving behind
as training settings only those medical schools that could match the
more stringent image of medical training in a scientific environment—an image first developed at Johns Hopkins University and
then made an American standard through the Flexner report. The
American Medical Association formed a Council on Medical Education in 1904, which ranked (and publicized the performance of)
medical schools in four classes according to failure rates on state
board examinations. In 1913, the AMA extended its attempted
oversight to postgraduate medical training by establishing a committee on graduate education within its Council on Medical Education, eventually leading to standards and accreditation procedures
for specialty training. Specialty boards began to form, beginning
with the American Board for Ophthalmic Examinations in 1917,
and to assume responsibility for the certification of their own professional members.

On the whole, however, these advances in quality regulation
and oversight were structural, not scientific or intellectual. Codman's suggestions for a data base that could be used for judgment of
outcomes were elegant, but by modern standards extremely simple,
and few if any breakthroughs in approaches to the measurement
of quality were proposed during the three or four decades following
his work. The survey procedures of the ACS and the accreditation
procedures of the AMA and specialty boards became increasingly
formal and professionalized but were not themselves the object of
research and careful development. A blossoming of quantitative,
scientifically tested methods for the study of health status and

outcomes would have to wait until the mid-1940s—and then it would occur not in the United States but in England, and not for the study and improvement of the quality of health care as a profession or system, but rather for the study of the causes of disease and for the assessment of the efficacy of cures.

The educational reforms of the first two decades of the century also tended to place control more exclusively in the hands of the medical profession. Physicians dominated the medical schools and ran the specialty boards. Like the leaders of the ACS, the reformers of medical education were advancing the power of self-regulation, not the voice of external accountability. This was progression, but progression within the boundaries of professional control.

In an important and unusual exception to the overwhelming dominance of the medical profession in the study of quality of care, the 1930s did witness the planning and completion of a professionally organized study, now nearly legendary, of the resource needs for the health care system of the United States as a whole, the so-called Lee-Jones Report of the Committee on the Costs of Medical Care.[16] Funded by private philanthropies, the Committee on the Costs of Medical Care was (as its charge reads) "organized to study the economic aspects of the prevention and care of sickness, including the adequacy, availability, and compensation of the persons and agencies concerned." It produced a comprehensive, bottom-up analysis of the total demand for health care services in the American population, including physician services, public health services, hospital facilities, and nursing services. The committee itself, though numerically still dominated by doctors (who occupied twenty-five of the forty-nine seats on the committee), comprised a rich array of other interested groups, including ten Ph.D.'s (most of whom were public health professionals), two nurses, two dentists, and eight nonprofessional members from "the public."

The study team, headed by I. S. Falk, used a methodology that would today be characterized as consensus-driven or expert-based to develop a model of the patterns of morbidity and needed treatments for the American population as a whole. Their model inevitably engaged the issue of standards of care, because the investigators sought to base their recommendations not on existing patterns of care but rather on images of care that the experts regarded as ideal based on the scientific knowledge available at that time. For example, in contrast to the prevailing investment in acute and curative services (as much a characteristic of yesterday's medicine as of today's), the Lee-Jones Report recommended a far greater emphasis on preventive medicine and public health practice in an idealized American health care system.

Almost as a by-product of the work of the Committee on the Costs of Medical Care, the Lee-Jones Report listed the following characteristics according to which the quality of a health care system or provider ought to be assessed:

1. Good medical care is limited to the practice of rational medicine based on the medical sciences.

2. Good medical care emphasizes prevention.

3. Good medical care requires intelligent cooperation between the lay public and the practitioners of scientific medicine.

4. Good medical care treats the individual as a whole.

5. Good medical care maintains a close and continuing personal relationship between physician and patient.

6. Good medical care is coordinated with social welfare work.

7. Good medical care coordinates all types of medical services.

8. Good medical care implies the application of all the necessary services of modern, scientific medicine to the needs of all the people.

This list, impressive in its understanding of the systemic nature of health care, was well known and highly regarded among students of quality assurance in health care for decades following the report.

Even today, the Lee-Jones criteria read as a vibrant, defining vision of the ideal properties of a system of care as a whole. But in the 1930s, they struck many physicians as revolutionary and drew their ire. Much of American medicine was not ready for such broad thinking about the quality of the system as a whole.

The work of the Committee on the Costs of Medical Care is more properly classified as policy development than as research, although the committee did break some new ground in the use of expert estimation in the development of a policy model. In the early 1930s, however, it stood nearly alone as an example of significant intellectual work dealing with the quality of health care. Furthermore, the Lee-Jones Report was the last major study involving quality of health care before a stunning silence descended on the field in the latter part of the 1930s. That silence was to persist throughout the 1940s. The Progressive era was ending, and with it was passing a progressive phase in professional medical self-regulation.

The reasons for the dormancy of academic interest in quality of care in this period are not altogether clear. The war years intervened. Professional societies consolidated their hegemony over the right to judge the quality of the work of medicine—a right exercised mostly in secret. And biomedical science began its rapid ascendancy, drawing the attention of the major intellectual forces in medical care away from the less crystalline challenges of health care policy, systems, and day-to-day work. Whatever the cause, a wide and durable chasm began to open between the real workings of health care—its management, financing, and provision—and the concerns of those few and scattered academicians who continued to make the quality of health care an object of their investigations.

In the time of Codman and the era immediately following him, the center of intellectual activity regarding the quality of care had been very much within the traditional leadership structures of American medicine, or at least surgery. It was the American College of Surgeons that took on the task of developing and leading the study of hospital standardization; few others could have. By con-

trast, the groundwork laid for the JCAHO, state and local certification boards, and specialty boards in the 1940s appears to have
been little guided by any specific traditions of formal research. The
methodologies of inspection and certification of specialists and facilities that were employed, such as those in the Hospital Standardization Program, were based far more on opinions, beliefs, assumptions, and traditions of review than on any recognizable
technologies for assessing and assuring the quality of care through
science. Slowly, licensure boards and survey authorities began to
take shape, but they were hardly informed by a clear, factually
grounded understanding of the nature of the medical care system
and of the sources and patterns of its flaws. The disconnection of
quality regulation from clinical activity had occurred.

1940–1960: A Field Takes Form

Most histories regard Ernest Codman as the first significant American proponent of the scientific study of the quality of health care.
Our candidate for the second position is Paul Lembcke. As a surgeon at Johns Hopkins University Medical School, Lembcke, much
like Codman fifty years before, became concerned about evidence
of extreme degrees of variation in the utilization rates and patterns
of care among surgeons in the United States. And like Codman,
Lembcke believed that the study of the results of care was an essential component of any intellectually sound effort to assess and improve the care. Lembcke, however, went far beyond Codman in
suggesting specific methodologies through which relevant information could be collected, analyzed, and built on, so that lessons could
be learned from variation in clinical practice.

Lembcke proposed criteria through which the data themselves
could be improved and verified, and he suggested a design for what
he called *medical audit*—a specific, tested method through which
individual institutions and physicians could be compared with each
other. He further attempted to establish standards of performance

through the use of comparative data from audits, identifying benchmark organizations whose levels of performance on specific criteria could set a realistic although stringent standard for others to match.

Lembcke's papers of the 1950s and 1960s document his careful development of methods for the review and judgment of records of care.[17] His 1956 article "Medical Auditing by Scientific Methods Illustrated by Major Female Pelvic Surgery" was a watershed in the history of medical quality assurance. In this paper, Lembcke reported on the application of his model of medical audit to the specific case of female pelvic surgery. His findings were impressive in their solidity and disturbing in their implications. Through the application of specific criteria for the appropriateness of female pelvic surgical procedures (a form of study that would later come to be known as "explicit review"), Lembcke found that in the initial phase of audit, only 30 percent of the operations reviewed were, in his word, "justified." Even more surprising, Lembcke reported that even though the identities of individual physicians were strictly protected, the mere existence of medical audit procedures in the facilities under review resulted over a period of months in dramatic improvement in the rates of "justified" female pelvic surgery—from 30 percent at the beginning of audit to more than 80 percent in subsequent audit periods. Through sophisticated use of his data base, Lembcke was able to show that the reductions in rates of surgery in these facilities were achieved almost exclusively through a decrease in inappropriate cases, the number of appropriate surgical procedures remaining relatively constant over the period of the study.

In this single breakthrough paper, Lembcke anticipated not only methods of explicit review of care that were to become conventional within a decade, but also approaches both to data base development and to the assessment of appropriateness of care that were not to see further vigorous work until nearly twenty years after his untimely death. The dramatic improvements in appropriateness of surgical procedures apparently achieved through his simple system of audit and feedback would later become the object of consistent investigation by a generation of health services researchers led by Jack Wennberg.

One by one, there followed in Lembcke's steps a series of individual academicians who were to constitute by the late 1960s a recognizable and active community of scholars specializing in quality of health care. They were an unusual, untraditional group of investigators—eager, mostly young, quite isolated from each other, and even more isolated from the mainstream intellectual affairs of the universities in which they did their early work. In their relative disconnectedness and intensity, they were nearly monastic. If they were the monks, their abbot was Donabedian.

Donabedian, a Lebanese physician who came to the United States in the early 1950s, intended to study health services administration at the Harvard School of Public Health. There he came under the influence of academicians—especially Franz Goldman and Leonard Rosenfeld—interested in quality of care as a research topic. They introduced Donabedian to the works of Lembcke and Falk, and to the Lee-Jones Report. In 1966, Donabedian, by then at the University of Michigan, published his generative article "Evaluating the Quality of Medical Care," in the *Milbank Memorial Fund Quarterly*,[20] a classic now regarded as the manifesto of the discipline of quality assurance in its modern academic form. In that key paper, Donabedian offered the first competent summary of academic work on quality of care in the decades preceding him and set out for future investigators the now standard typology of *structure*, *process*, and *outcome* of care as the three main objects of study and assessment in the pursuit of quality.

Donabedian acknowledged his debt to colleagues working in relative isolation from each other on similar matters. In particular, he cited the work of Mildred Morehead in New York City,[21] Osler Peterson in North Carolina,[22] and Mindel Sheps.[23] These and other researchers,[24] working in the tradition of Lembcke, were busily engaged in developing specific methods of explicit review of the processes of care and in applying those methods to real-world health care systems, including the Health and Hospitals Department in New York City and the rural general practices of North Carolina. But these applications by regulators were as isolated as the researchers themselves. Only slowly did quality regulators become aware of the academic progress.

By the time of Donabedian's manifesto for the field of quality assurance in medicine, significant research groups had begun to form at several academic centers in the United States, including the University of Michigan, Yale, Harvard, and Johns Hopkins. At Michigan, for example, Beverly Payne[25] had taken the work of Lembcke to an altogether new scale, applying the methodologies of medical audit to nonsurgical conditions and publishing a series of reports on applications of these methods—for example, to discharge records from twenty-two hospitals in the state of Hawaii in 1968. Payne and his colleagues were able to demonstrate not only that methods of explicit assessment could be widely deployed, but also that they could be made more and more reliable through repeated efforts at refinement of criteria, definitions, and record abstracting.

At Yale University, building on the work of the Lee-Jones Report, Falk and his colleagues were revisiting the issue of standard setting in health care through the use of implicit methods and expert judgments from faculty and associates at the Yale University School of Medicine.[26] By 1975, Falk and his colleagues had published criteria for the appropriate care of more than 260 medical conditions. According to today's standards, the methods of the Yale group in eliciting expert opinions on appropriate medical practice were primitive, but they remain impressive in their scope. Like the authors of the Lee-Jones Report (Falk himself included), the Yale investigators were primarily interested in using expert judgment to develop idealized criteria for appropriate care, with the ultimate purpose of planning resource allocation.[27] They were thus setting in place methodologies that would later be incorporated into the largely unsuccessful efforts at regional health planning of the late 1960s and early 1970s.

Of all the centers of intellectual activity on quality assurance, none equaled Johns Hopkins University in its range and importance through the late 1960s. At Johns Hopkins, an outstanding group of investigators had assembled, foremost among them John Williamson and Kerr White. As chairman of medicine at Johns Hopkins, White had become enamored of the scientific approaches to epidemiology and clinical investigation that were taking shape in England through the middle part of the century.[28] Influenced especially by the work of J. N. Morris,[29] White began to realize that the formal methods of epidemiology that Morris and others had been using to study risk factors for illness could be applied with equal power to modern problems of health systems assessment and public health management.[30] Whether or not he actually coined the phrase, White provided leadership in the early 1960s for the formation of a field soon to be called *health services research*. He suggested to Williamson and others that these modern quantitative methods could be applied with profit to the study of quality of care, and Williamson took on the task with a vengeance. White thus provided a stimulus for the melding of two fields—the study of quality and the study of epidemiology—that together would become the central methodologies for academics concerned about the quality of care.

In his own right, Williamson represented another melding of interests.[31] Strongly influenced by George Miller and other scholars of adult learning, Williamson's initial interest in health care research had been in the study of continuing medical education and adult learning among physicians. As White contributed the perspectives of epidemiology to the field, so Williamson contributed the perspectives of modern social and cognitive psychology. He wanted to know the processes and social systems through which knowledge grows in individual human beings. "Tools not rules" was among the aphorisms Williamson coined in an effort to emphasize that the key issues in the assessment and improvement of quality of care had to do with the ways physicians think rather than with the ways they are controlled or judged. This viewpoint on quality is entirely consistent with the theories and approaches of Walter

Shewhart, W. Edwards Deming, Joseph Juran, and others associated
with the modern quality management movement, and perhaps no
other investigator in the entire academic terrain of quality assurance in health care anticipated more thoroughly than Williamson
the understandings of quality improvement sciences as they were
developing in other industries.

As interested as he was in approaches to human learning,
Williamson spared no efforts in his equal devotion to mastering the
methods of measurement. Codman, Lembcke, and others had noted
an important gap between what was scientifically achievable in
health care systems and what was being achieved in fact. Williamson formalized an understanding of this gap in his definition of
achievable benefits not achieved, which he proposed should become a
standard metric to guide priorities and progress in the improvement
of health care.[32]

Perhaps the key element in Williamson's view of the problem of
quality in health care is what he called the "cybernetic" model linking measurement and feedback to the processes of learning—his
own version of what people in other industries were coming to call
the "Shewhart Cycle" of improvement, or the Plan-Do-Check-Act
Cycle.[33] What Lembcke had observed only as a "black box" effect—
the improvement of appropriateness of pelvic surgery as a result of
the feedback of measures of appropriateness from medical audit—
Williamson illuminated by linking the feedback model with a model
of adult learning. Williamson placed audit in a deeper and more
powerful context of individual adult growth and development.

In the mid-1960s, Williamson took on the task of supervising
the work of a young Johns Hopkins medical resident named Robert
Brook, who was soon to emerge as the leader of his own generation
of quality researchers in health care. Like his mentor, Brook was as
undaunted by warnings that the field of quality assurance would
become an intellectual backwater as he was fascinated by evidence
of extraordinary variation both in approaches to care and in the
quality of outcomes.

Among Williamson's first assignments to Brook was to analyze systematically more than fifteen thousand medical records in order to classify and study patterns of problems in the quality of care. Brook was captivated, and in the quantitatively sophisticated environment of research at Johns Hopkins, he was able to bring to bear the full force of modern epidemiologic methods on his analysis of the assessment of health care outcomes. Donabedian's 1966 paper had codified theory and language in the study of quality. Brook's 1973 dissertation "Quality of Care Assessment: A Comparison of Five Methods of Peer Review" did the same for the empirical study of approaches to the assessment of quality.[34] To this day, Brook claims (and he may well be right) that the methodologies he compared in his dissertation compose the full range of approaches feasible in the assessment of quality of care. In this single piece of work, Brook leaped to the forefront among methodologists equipped to study the quality of health care.

Thus from Johns Hopkins in the 1960s came the two leading streams of health services research on the quality of health care in America. One, epitomized by Williamson, we may call the "learning tradition." It sought to link tightly the methods of assessment of care to models of learning, feedback, and personal change by exploring systems of education, leadership, and management. The second, which we may term the "assessment tradition," focused primarily on the collection and use of information on results and processes of care, permitting appropriate selections to be made on the basis of quality and enabling market forces to operate. Although Brook straddled these camps, his subsequent work at the Rand Corporation became more and more clearly centered in the assessment tradition.[36] Along with Joseph Newhouse (the principal investigator of the Rand Health Insurance Experiment), John Ware, Jr., and others, Brook continued there his pathfinding explorations of methods through which standards for processes of care could be set and compliance assessed.

A third arm of influence from the Johns Hopkins camp also

emerged in the early 1960s, although it was soon to become increasingly disconnected from its own intellectual roots and more closely associated with the "other history" summarized in Chapter Two: the history of regulation. Again, it was White whose vision and influence catalyzed events, eventually establishing a home for health services research in the federal government. White played a key role in forming the National Center for Health Services Research (NCHSR), and one of his colleagues and protégés, Paul Sanazaro, became its first director.

Sanazaro's familiarity with Williamson's work and with other leading investigations of quality assessment in health care were quickly demonstrated in the focus of the new agency.[36] Through NCHSR, Sanazaro sponsored the Experimental Medical Care Review Organizations[37] (EMCROs) to develop and improve approaches to the assessment of quality in settings where health care was actually being delivered. The need to identify assessment methods had become increasingly important since 1964, when the federal government began paying for a significant proportion of health care for the American elderly in the Medicare program. With a sudden new stake in the financing of American health care, the U.S. government became acutely interested in assuring the quality of what it was buying.

At this crucial stage, however, it appears that an opportunity was missed. On the one hand, health services research on the quality of care had entered a new phase of maturity in the theoretical work of Donabedian and in the practical applications of Williamson, Payne, and soon thereafter, Brook. The field was ready to be used. On the other hand, the need for sophisticated assessment and improvement methodologies was becoming concentrated in the federal Medicare system. Both a new science and an excellent customer for that science were being born at exactly the same time. But the promise of that conjunction was largely unfulfilled; the match was never really made.

In our interviews with them, each of the key figures in the field of quality assessment at that pregnant time—Williamson, Donabedian, Brook, Sanazaro, and others—offered a somewhat different view of the chain of events that followed in the mid- and late 1960s. All, however, agreed on what ultimately happened: a disconnection between public policy and science. The chasm that had existed between academic quality assurance and health care delivery in the second quarter of the twentieth century was recreated between public policy on regulation of health care and the best available approaches to its assessment and improvement developed in academic environments. By the early 1970s, the distance was enormous between what was known to academic investigators about the epidemiology, assessment, and improvement of health care quality and the specific activities endorsed and supported through mechanisms of regulation and financing, largely in the Medicare system. A field had indeed been born, but it was an orphan. More important, an opportunity was lost to build a system of responsive regulation of health care quality.

The 1970s and 1980s: The Reign of Methods

The infant sciences of quality in health care, albeit disconnected from the real world of delivery and regulation, began to grow quickly in the 1970s, largely owing to three interrelated factors. First, federal grant dollars began flowing through the National Center for Health Services Research into the hands of health service investigators, some of whom were interested in the assessment and improvement of quality. Second, both private foundations and government sponsors of research were becoming more and more concerned about slowing the rate of increase in medical care costs. Their initiatives to increase the energy of research on cost-effective medical practices inevitably steered researchers toward judgments about quality of care. Third, focused training programs, such as the Robert Wood Johnson Clinical Scholars Program (which produced Robert Brook), began spawning generalist clinical investigators who combined the skills of quantitative assessment with strong backgrounds in clinical care. This new generation of scholars was thus well equipped to address issues of clinical quality.

In the rapidly burgeoning collection of research activities during this period, it is difficult to discover a few strong threads of inquiry as cogent as, for example, the cybernetic models proposed by Williamson in the early 1960s. One exception was an effort of particular excellence developed at the University of North Carolina under the leadership of a sociologist, Barbara Hulka. Hulka's 1979 monograph "Peer Review in Ambulatory Care: Use of Explicit Criteria and Implicit Judgments," which compared the reliability and validity of two methods for the review of care, is a landmark of health services research.[38] Hulka added new levels of rigor to both explicit and implicit methods for the assessment of care, and showed how both approaches, appropriately designed and administered, could support accurate judgments of quality of care by both researchers and policy makers. By the late 1970s, however, the chasm between the real world of care giving and the academic investigation of the quality of care had widened so greatly that the major forces using both explicit and implicit review to judge quality (such as the JCAHO and state accreditation offices) remained largely unaffected by Hulka's findings.

What helped more than anything else to bind the academic field together in the 1970s and 1980s was the emergence of a new leading center for the investigation of quality in American health care, at the Rand Corporation in Santa Monica, California. Rand's preeminence in this field developed in the context of the Health Insurance Experiment (HIE), one of the largest social experiments ever undertaken in the United States. Headed by Newhouse, who was an economist, the HIE intended to offer policy makers and others information on the relationship between various approaches to financing health care insurance—especially variations in the levels of copayments and deductibles in insurance policies—and the health status and utilization profiles of the covered populations.[39]

The remarkable research team assembled by Newhouse for the experiment (it included Ware, Brook, Mark Chassin, Allyson Ross Davies, and Sheldon Greenfield) poured out through the 1970s and early 1980s evidence and instruments supporting plausible methods of assessing the quality of both outcomes and processes of care. The Rand team proved that dimensions of quality as subtle as patient satisfaction, functional health status, emotional health, and appropriateness of care could be measured in ways that were, by the most stringent standards, reliable, apparently valid, and eminently practical, at least in a research environment.

Within five years of its inception, the HIE had become the standard against which to judge all other academic efforts to measure, define, and assess quality in health care systems. It produced a rich array of measurement instruments, albeit initially cumbersome ones; and even more important, it defined stable and significant dimensions of quality and translated them into operational terms. The HIE investigators made each subdimension of health, such as physical functioning, emotional well-being, general well-being, and social and role functioning, measurable characteristics of individuals and populations through the development of specific assessment instruments. They showed how patients themselves could be sources of valid and reliable information on their own functional status, and they explored relationships between these patient-centered measurements and more classical medically oriented measurements of physiological status and function. In addition, in their definition of quality, they included measurements of patient satisfaction and ease of accessibility of health care services.[40] In their sophisticated economic analyses, they developed cogent metrics of system cost and efficiency, centering particularly on the concept of episode of illness rather than on a resource-by-resource assessment of costs and effectiveness. These methods for assessment of quality of care and outcomes became even more practical in a successor study to the HIE, the Medical Outcomes Study,[41] supported through Rand by the Kaiser Family Foundation and other private and public philanthropies.

In the decade following the end of the HIE, both the original researchers and others throughout the world refined the instruments developed by the HIE team into shorter and simpler questionnaires of equal or greater precision and reliability. One of the derivative instruments, the SF-36, has become one of the most widely used general questionnaires for assessment of the experiences and functional status of patients, both in the United States and abroad.[42]

Rand's SF-36 is a tool for measurement of general health status that is applicable across a wide variety of health care conditions and types of encounter. Meanwhile, other researchers have developed more disease-specific assessment instruments targeted at symptoms, outcomes, and experiences associated with particular diagnoses. Important advances in disease-specific measurement have occurred, with applicability to such conditions as arthritis, coronary heart disease, depression, and neurological impairment. Altogether, today's health services research has transformed the simple and elegant measurements of survival proposed by Codman in the early twentieth century into a robust and elegant "tool kit" for the measurement of quality in its many and subtle dimensions.[43] In comparison with Codman's "end results" index cards, the modern armamentarium for assessment of functional status and outcomes of health care is impressive.

While the Rand Health Insurance Experiment was reshaping the measurement of the results of health care, equally important research, with Dartmouth professor Jack Wennberg at the forefront, was reshaping our knowledge about the activities of health care professionals—the content of care itself. Wennberg was not the first to suspect that enormous variations existed in the rates and patterns of use of health care practices and procedures (such as hospital bed days, tests, surgical procedures, and diagnostic images) among regions, organizations, and practitioners of care. At various levels of detail, Codman, the American College of Surgeons, Lembcke, Payne, Archibald Cochrane, and many others had long ago documented surprising degrees of variability in medical practice—variations without apparent scientific foundation.[44] What Wennberg added, in association with his colleague Klim MacPherson and others, was a level of precision and a sophistication of statistical adjustment in the study of these variations that left no doubt about the extraordinary pervasiveness and the lack of epidemiologic explanation for these "small area variations" in the use of medical resources.[45]

Wennberg showed that the use of health care resources varied greatly, and that this variation could not be accounted for by differences in medical needs among populations. Although it was not possible to conclude from Wennberg's research designs exactly where the quality of care was high and where it was low, his accumulating corpus of evidence made it untenable to believe that the quality of care could be *consistently* high across the entire range of variation that he observed. Hospitals and obstetricians within sixty miles of each other in Maine varied in their rates of hysterectomy on a population basis by 250 percent. It was impossible to claim that both the highest rates and the lowest ones equally represented the best available quality of care. Numerous researchers followed on Wennberg's heels, documenting variation as large or greater and raising equally profound questions about the implications for overall quality.[46]

The research on variation in utilization of health care conducted by Wennberg and colleagues built on Roemer's original observations showing that hospital bed availability strongly determined local rates of medical and surgical procedures.[47] Certificate-of-need legislation was erected on the same foundation, but Wennberg's research was rarely if ever incorporated into regulatory models. The deep, decades-long disconnection persisted between research and regulation.

Whereas Wennberg's work was focusing on variation in rates of *utilization* in health care, other scholars at the Rand Corporation and elsewhere were becoming interested in variation in the *appropriateness* of care, building on their experience from the Health Insurance Experiment.[48] Brook, Chassin, and others developed group process techniques through which they could assess the probability that particular health care procedures would help particular patients. They defined an appropriate procedure as one of likely or possible benefit to patients, whereas an inappropriate procedure was one that, on scientific grounds, stood little or no chance of helping the patient. This group of investigators discovered variations in rates of appropriateness that were every bit as large as Wennberg was documenting for utilization. For some procedures, such as carotid endarterectomy, rates of inappropriateness in some geographical areas exceeded 50 percent.

It was logical to suspect that these two key findings from health services research of the 1980s—that rates of procedures varied widely and that inappropriateness levels were high for many procedures—were closely related. It makes obvious sense that high levels of inappropriateness would correlate with high utilization rates. But in fact, this turned out not to be the case. By the early 1990s, it had become evident that these two important characteristics of health care systems, rate and appropriateness, varied nearly independently of each other. The apparent dissociation between utilization and appropriateness still begs explanation and has raised important questions about the validity and meaning of both measurements.[49]

Unlike most previous findings from quality-oriented research, however, these cumulative findings about the high levels of variation and the high levels of inappropriate care eventually prompted action in regulatory and marketplace initiatives in health care. Three responses in particular acquired momentum during the decade following publication of these important results.

First, health care payers seized upon the issues of variation and inappropriateness to refine and reinvigorate their approaches to utilization review. Insurers and government agencies responsible for providing care had begun to institute wide-ranging utilization review practices in the 1960s. But now new programs were designed to put pressure on high utilizers of care, even without direct evidence that such rates of utilization were unfavorable for outcomes. In our opinion, a direct relationship exists between the vigorous activity in health services research documenting variation in practice and the even more vigorous activities in utilization review that now affect the lives of virtually every health care provider and organization that deals with the medical insurance industry and managed care.

Second, a host of health care consultancies began selling their services to review utilization rates, measure levels of appropriateness of care, and create and provide software packages and other data systems for the analysis of variations in resource use among providers. A virtual subindustry has developed since the 1980s involving inspection of rates of use of procedures to support both internal management activity in health care organizations and selection of "preferred providers" from among them. Such inspections are now among the cornerstones of managed care and utilization review, which are discussed in the next few chapters.

Partly to quell claims of unfairness in selection among providers of care and partly to support studies comparing outcomes among providers for the purpose of identifying "best practices," another branch of quality measurement developed in the 1980s and 1990s under the general rubric *case-mix adjustment* or *severity adjustment*.[50] Researchers in this field have tried to segment sources of variation in resource use or outcomes into two general categories: causes of variation attributable to the health status or needs of the patients being served (and therefore not directly due to activities of the care providers), and causes of variation that are at least plausibly attributable to the nature and quality of the care given to those patients. For example, fair comparisons of the survival rates of patients in different intensive care units require models that accurately stratify patients according to their condition at the time of admission to the hospital and that thus allow estimation of their probability of survival *assuming equivalent quality of care*. In the language of sports that so often (and so revealingly) marks discussions of ratings and comparisons among health care providers, the severity adjustment model "levels the playing field" on which comparisons of performance are to be made. Severity adjustment models have reached a high level of refinement in recent years, especially as purchasers of care have pursued "report cards" that they can use as a basis for choosing providers.

The third response to the research on appropriateness was greater interest, in both public and private quarters, in the development of standardized guidelines, algorithms, and protocols for care that might help to reduce and control variation. Specifically, the Agency for Health Care Policy and Research was given a mandate in the late 1980s to develop and promulgate scientifically based guidelines for the care of conditions of high cost or widespread impact. In addition, private insurers and even some larger corporations have supported the development of guidelines for care. As will be shown, guidelines emanating from sources both internal and external to the organization have now become part of the daily life of administrative and clinical leaders in many sectors of the health care system, although little research has yet documented the effect of guidelines on either cost or quality at a systemic level.

Thus in this era of relative maturation of statistical and epidemiological research on the quality of health care, at least seven well-developed themes can be identified, each now pursued at a level of scientific rigor not seen earlier in the century:

1. Research on the measurement of health status overall and in its component dimensions, including satisfaction among users of care (drawing largely on the Rand Corporation's HIE and Medical Outcomes Study)

2. Research on classification systems for severity of illness and on diagnostic categories with common features, primarily to support fair comparisons among providers and among treatments

3. Research on variations in procedure rates and resource utilization, permitting comparisons among regions, small geographical areas, and providers of care (largely motivated by Wennberg's pathfinding epidemiologic studies)

4. Research on methods to develop and refine guidelines for care, so as to permit standardization of approaches to diagnosis, treatment, and prevention (pursued largely under the recent agenda of the Agency for Health Care Policy and Research)

5. Research aimed at facilitating judgments about the appropriateness of care (drawing on earlier studies by Gertman and colleagues,[51] and on later research at Rand)

6. Econometric research, studying possible trade-offs between incentives and resource-allocation decisions on the one hand and health status and costs of care on the other (the most significant such study being the HIE.)

7. Ongoing development of methods of medical decision making, building on the quantitative methods first championed in the United States by White and by Alvin Feinstein[52] and leading today to research in such varied areas as clinical decision sciences, clinical epidemiology, and computer-based expert decision systems.

These streams of research are competently pursued, scientifically intriguing, and on their face, pertinent to the needs of regulators. However, as technically powerful as this research has become, especially with respect to methods of assessment of quality, the chasm remains wide between the sciences of quality on the one hand and the practice of regulation and (to a large extent) medicine on the other. Throughout the 1980s and into the 1990s, with the important exceptions of Wennberg's studies of variation and recent techniques for severity adjustment, the findings of research on quality of care have remained almost exclusively in the hands of researchers.

A sociologist examining the methods of assessment being employed by the mainstream regulatory and review organizations in American health care throughout this period (professional standards review organizations, peer review organizations, utilization review organizations, managed care executives, and other private

certifiers of care) might well be astounded by the lack of connection between the methods for regulation and judgment in actual
use and the elegant investigations of the best of our modern scholars of quality: Newhouse, Ware, Brook, Palmer—and still active
and at the forefront, Williamson. To cite but one example, in the
Rand Health Insurance Experiment and Medical Outcomes Study,
Ware and his colleagues developed a set of strong, practical, and
well-validated measures of patient satisfaction (an outcome dimension of increasing importance in the competitive health care market of the 1980s), yet it remains a virtual certainty that among one
hundred randomly selected hospitals in America, one hundred different measurement instruments for patient satisfaction will be in
use, only a few of which will draw explicitly on the work of Ware
and the HIE team.

It would be easy to dismiss this disconnection as merely the consequence of a lack of curiosity on the part of practitioners and regulators or of ambition among the researchers. Indeed, we can see
examples of bridges built when curiosity and ambition have both
been great enough. For example, in the mid-1990s, a consortium of
major corporations has supported the development of an Employee
Health Care Value Survey, in which companies have asked their
own employees to rate care that they have received from major
managed care systems. This system has been designed in collaboration with a first-rate team of academicians skilled in modern psy-
chometric methods for obtaining quality ratings from patients. The
National Committee on Quality Assurance (NCQA) has led the
collaborative development and testing of the Health Plan and
Employer Data and Information Set (HEDIS), an array of specific
performance measures for process and outcome formulated by payers and producers in managed care plans. The HEDIS team has
sought involvement from a wide range of health services researchers
to define and refine their measures.

On the whole, however, knowledge of quality and regulation of
quality still are worlds apart. We believe that this gap reflects a

problem more fundamental than the differences in sociology between the worlds of regulation and research. What is missing, we think, is a sustainable, credible *theory of improvement*, in light of which the quality scientists and the action-oriented regulators would discover a need for each other. At its best, the prevailing theory of improvement is a theory of selection—a market theory resting on the belief that *measurement alone will be sufficient to assure the improvement of the health care system* because it will foster informed market behavior and support definitive regulatory actions. Under this theory, the link between quality sciences and quality regulation is relatively simple: the link is measurement. Research supplies sound measurement, and regulation uses it. If this alone were enough to bond research and regulation, however, we would see a much tighter relationship than we do, for as we have shown, health services research has already produced quality measurement tools that are precise, valid, reliable, and convenient. Yet in the practice of regulation, those tools—the key supply from research under the prevailing theory of regulation—are almost nowhere in active use.

The tools are not enough. Even with the best measurements available, regulation for improvement cannot achieve its intended aims unless it works from a far more powerful and comprehensive theory of improvement than it currently has. To understand the basic flaw in reliance on measurement as the key to regulatory action, we must first elaborate on a better theory of improvement. That theory, it so happens, comes from outside health care. Its history, though grounded in science, is strikingly different from the stories of both quality research and quality regulation that we have told so far. To hear it and learn from it, those of us in health care must drop our guard a bit, and become curious about events in this century that occurred very far from medicine and that have so far had much more to do with improvements in our cars, our telephones, our computers, and our material world than with improvements in the health care on which we so deeply depend.

The History of a Better Theory: Modern Quality Management

While professional quality review and audit were evolving slowly in American health care through the first half of this century, a different, parallel, and almost totally separate evolution was taking place in some quarters of American manufacturing. Whereas the health care efforts were primarily focusing on methods for the review of outcomes and processes of care and for inspection of underlying structures such as medical staff organization, efforts in other industries—which came to be labeled "Total Quality Management," "Continuous Quality Improvement," and so on—addressed deeper questions about the nature and causes of variation in the production processes themselves. To oversimplify, whereas health care was primarily developing methods through which the results of care could be *assessed*, manufacturing was developing methods through which the *causes* of results could be more deeply understood and modified.

This shift in the management of manufacturing processes from a focus on assessment of results to a focus on understanding and managing fundamental causal systems did not occur quickly. Indeed, refocusing the attention of American management on the continuous improvement of processes of production has taken the greater part of the middle of the twentieth century, and even today, the shift is far from complete. Systems of reliance on inspection and strict adherence to standards to assure quality are deeply rooted in American manufacturing, especially in the assembly-line process designs pioneered by Henry Ford and Frederick Taylor at the turn of the nineteenth century.

What Ford discovered and Taylor housed in a theoretic framework was the immense power of standardization when the central aim is mass production of reliable products. Before Ford and Taylor, the production of any but the simplest manufactured product was essentially an act of craftsmanship. Each single item—bed, dresser, coach, gown, or car—was the product of a single craftsperson or team of craftspersons, and each was in sequence, one at a time. Ford and Taylor recognized the undesirable economic consequences of this form of production: slow pace and relatively high unit cost.[53]

Their remedy was standardization of parts and of processes for assembly. In mass production, speed was the goal and variation was the enemy. Individual craftspersons making individual cars had to assure, for example, that each individual axle correctly fitted each individual wheel. Whereas the integrity of each individual assembly mattered a great deal, the similarity of axles to each other mattered little. Even today, variation is a hallmark, an essential ingredient, of the product of real craftsmanship. Each handmade vase or woven rug is noticeably different from every other one; it had better be, or we would not regard it as craftsmanlike. The minor blemishes that are the signature of a handmade piece make the piece more valuable, not less.

But variation of this type, the variation of the craftsman, is not compatible with effective mass production. On an effective assembly line, we cannot have individual axles created for individual wheels. Instead, we must have bins of axles and bins of wheels from which individual units can be randomly selected and reliably fitted together. We must have specifications, strictly adhered to, for size, shape, weight, and so forth. The alternative is waste and delay.

A management theory follows from this. If speed depends on standardization, and if variation produces waste, then mass production implies a management system capable of producing sound designs, and once such designs exist, capable of assuring strict adherence to them. In an era of craft, each worker must solve problems at the point of production, trimming the axle or reshaping the wheel until each separate unit fits exactly. In an era of mass production, each individual worker had better *not* solve problems at the point of production, as this would lead to variation and waste. In Taylor's view, workers' behaviors, like the parts of machines, are objects for standardization.

Mass production achieved what craft could not: it made the automobile a consumer good. Furthermore, the theoretical and practical approach was generalizable, placing an enormous range of goods and services economically within the reach of the vast majority of the American population, who could never have afforded these same goods and services if produced by craft. Taylor's theories, put into action, yielded unprecedented benefits in quality of life for the average consumer of products and services. Taylor himself believed that his new understanding of work as a system and his formulation of "Principles of Scientific Management" would allow both workers and their managers to realize such a vast improvement in productivity and profit that the troublesome antagonisms between workers and managers could be dissolved by the sharing of this rich "surplus." He had evidence. "Scientific management" at the Simonds Rolling Machine Company allowed 35 women to do work that formerly required 120. Wages doubled, and the length of the workday was reduced by two hours. In the resulting work environment, Taylor wrote, "each girl [sic] was made to feel that she was the object of especial care and interest on the part of the management, and that if anything went wrong with her she could always have a helper and teacher in the management to lean upon."[54]

But in the hands of others, the costs of mass production in human terms were higher than Taylor intended. His management system opened the door for many to treat individual workers no longer as people invited to be craftspersons, but rather as "hands" to carry out faithfully the instructions of others, draining energy and spirit from the workplace. The assembly line, even while improving the connection of parts of products to each other, was disconnecting workers from the meaning of their own work. This disconnection was, of course, not new. The sweatshops and toil that Charles Dickens described did not benefit from or need the theories of "scientific management" to guide their managers. What was new in the approach of Ford and Taylor was not toil itself but rather the strong, and essential, emphasis on standardization as the underlying managerial objective and on the need to control exactly how, not just how much, workers did their jobs. Taylor's own writings bear witness to his respect for the well-being of workers, but "Taylorism" more broadly applied did not.

It was, in the end, the economic toll of mass production, not its human cost, that eventually led to a rethinking of the management systems designed by Ford and Taylor. The gains of mass production, and the fortunes made thereby, were so impressive that at first the superiority of this method of production seemed incontrovertible. Walter Shewhart, a statistician and physicist at Western Electric Laboratories and often regarded as the father of scientific methods of quality management in industry, was among the first to raise powerful technical questions about the costs and benefits of Taylorism as a system of production.

In the mid-1920s, Shewhart became a self-taught student of the economic costs of obtaining quality in manufacturing processes. He began by studying variation in the characteristics of manufactured products from the Western Electric system—mostly telephone switching equipment. In his early work, he achieved three important insights. First, he observed that the levels of quality, such as the defect rates, of the switching equipment emerging from the assembly-line processes were relatively constant. That is, rates of failure (product by product, or interval by interval) followed a relatively orderly mathematical distribution, which Shewhart, as a statistician, could easily model. Furthermore, he showed that these rates of defect as a whole remained stable over time. In other words, he documented that the statistical distribution of defect rates over time was often a highly predictable characteristic of the process of production itself.

Second, as a student of management as well as statistics, Shewhart observed highly inefficient behaviors among the supervisors and managers within the production system. Even though they were observing in defect rates the results of an essentially randomly distributed variable, managers tended to overreact to this random variation with senseless and costly overadjustments. Through such overreaction, managers were actually adding to the level of variation already occurring in the process of production itself. Even more important, by reacting to individual instances of random fluctuation from average performance, managers were diverting their own energies and the energies of others away from the more central question of how to improve the basic characteristics of the process of production. They were treating every defect as if it had a special cause, without understanding that the overall rate and distribution of defects over time were themselves properties of the process of production. Reacting to defects case by case was usually a form of pure waste.

Third, Shewhart documented that the production system, unable to improve the defect rates characteristic of its own work, had no ultimate recourse for protection of the consumer other than endpoint inspection followed by repair or discarding of the final product prior to delivery to the customer. Inspection, in fact, was the main process by which Western Electric Laboratories maintained the quality of its own product. In the middle of the 1920s, 25 percent of all the employees of Western Electric Laboratories were inspectors.

Shewhart thus recognized three important sources of cost added to the production system as a result of naive approaches to standardization: 1) costs associated with the stable defect rates that were embedded in the processes of production; 2) costs associated with overreaction and overadjustment by managers to random fluctuations in those stable defect rates; 3) high costs of inspection and rework of finished goods, both of which were needed to protect the ultimate customer.

Shewhart proposed a better way, with profound implications for the activities of managers and workers. He suggested, first, that it was extremely important for managers in production systems to be able to classify accurately the variations that they observed. When those variations were truly of special cause, that is, due to events that were not part of the usual system of production, managers could support workers and others to correct those special circumstances. On the other hand, when the variation in rates of defect or other measures of quality were purely random, Shewhart suggested that it would be more prudent for managers not to react to individual events but rather to analyze and, if necessary, improve the production process as a whole. Activities to improve production processes were management's responsibility, according to Shewhart, and workers could not be held responsible for improvements of sources of variation and defect that they could not control.

Shewhart further pointed out that inspection alone could not improve the basic characteristics of production processes. He encouraged managers to make improvement rather than standardization their primary aim. This would necessarily involve changing designs and production processes on the basis of deeper understanding of the causes of defect within those processes. Shewhart's statistical and economic insights implied that improvement and redesign—*changes*, not just standardization and control—were essential activities for managers and leaders in complex systems of production. In the words of Shewhart's student, W. Edwards Deming, "reliance on inspection alone to improve quality" could not possibly succeed. If defect rates were characteristics of processes, then only changes in processes could produce sustained reductions in defect rates.

Shewhart's seminal work was completed by the end of the 1930s,[55] but it appears to have had little impact on American management in the thirty years that followed. Instead, and almost by accident, Shewhart's work found itself exported to Japan in the early 1950s as part of the American activities in postwar reconstruction of the Japanese economy. Teachers sent to Japan by the American government during that period, notably W. Edwards Deming[56] and Joseph M. Juran,[57] had been schooled by Shewhart and his immediate successors in the statistical and economic principles that had been developed for the management and improvement of quality.

For reasons that remain unclear even today, the small group of key leaders of Japanese industry during the period of postwar recovery seized upon the teachings of Shewhart as conveyed by Deming, Juran, and others, and appear to have used these principles as foundational guides for the redesign of Japanese industry.

Many others have documented the steady progress of Japanese industry from the rubble of the late 1940s to its position of emerging worldwide dominance by the early 1970s.[58] Numerous factors account for this success, only some of which relate to the disciplined use of methods of statistical process control (as the approaches championed by Shewhart came to be known) and modern quality management. The Japanese themselves evinced a remarkable degree of pragmatism as they developed their own management approaches through the 1950s, 1960s, and 1970s. Indeed, a great deal of the "Japanese theory of management" so widely studied by worried American businesses in the last quarter of this century are theories only in retrospect. Japanese corporations appear to have built their management methods as they went along, learning from each new effort to guide, control, and improve production and design. Theoreticians did emerge, most notably Taiichi Ohno, the genius who designed the "just-in-time" production system that became the hallmark of Toyota as it emerged to dominate its industry.[59] Kaoru Ishikawa, another leading Japanese quality theorist, helped to translate the statistical and engineering principles of quality improvement into a series of tools and approaches that everyone in an organization, at all levels, could use in their daily work.[60] Ishikawa especially encouraged ongoing studies and experiments on causes of variation within production processes and urged that such studies be defined as part of everyone's work, not just as the concern of the research and development department.

In the United States, pockets of statistical research and engineering science and occasional teachers of management (Deming and Juran primary among them) continued to build on the pathfinding work of Shewhart. On the whole, however, the American manufacturing and service sectors remained unimpressive in their strategies for managerial reform during the third quarter of the century, while the Japanese moved to a position of global market dominance. The wake-up call came during the 1970s, as many American corporations found themselves well behind their new Japanese competitors in the cost and quality of their products. For many, survival was at stake, which stimulated widespread curiosity among American industrial leaders about the methods of management and production that were allowing the Japanese to achieve results beyond any ever seen in American industry.

By the late 1970s, a number of prominent American corporations were proclaiming a need for fundamental transformation of the approaches to management and production that had dominated their operations throughout the century. Declarations in favor of new managerial methods that would focus on improvement of quality and efficiency came from the chief executives of Xerox, Ford, Motorola, McDonnell-Douglas, and others. The "new theory" that each leader embraced varied in its details, but all shared in common at least the following attributes:

1. A revivified focus on the needs of external customers
2. A goal of continuous improvement of performance (not just adherence to standards)
3. The appropriate use of statistics and data on variation (building especially on Shewhart's insights)
4. The involvement of the workforce throughout the organization in the effort to improve
5. A new emphasis on training and education of the workforce as a primary organizational investment
6. An ongoing organizational focus on innovation and experimentation (including experiments in daily work)
7. Long-term improvement strategies

8. Continuous reduction in the costs of production while maintaining or improving quality

9. The most important element: a new definition of leadership
   as a form of organizational coaching, going well beyond the
   more classical emphasis on control as a primary process of
   leadership

Interestingly, these corporations were largely responding to market pressures, especially competition from Japan. Regulatory incentives or pressures had very little to do with the adoption of quality
improvement techniques. Unlike Japanese companies, American
firms had little or no governmental assistance in innovating or in
improving management methods.

Today, as the century nears its close, these basic principles form
the core for the modern management of quality and quality improvement in most industries in the global marketplace, even if the
exact framing of the principles—and the ways they are implemented—tend to vary from one consultant to another or from
teacher to teacher. Significant codifications of principles of quality
management exist, for example, in the work of Deming (in his
"Fourteen Points for Top Leadership of Improvement"),[61] Armand
Feigenbaum (in his seminal book on companywide Total Quality
Management),[62] Juran (in his concept of managerial breakthrough
and in his many technical books on leadership for quality),[63] Philip
Crosby (beginning with his landmark call to arms, *Quality is Free*),[64]
and in the continuing technical work of scholars such as George
Box at the University of Wisconsin, Harry Roberts at the Univer-
sity of Chicago, and in Japan, Genichi Taguchi and Noriaki Kano.

A particularly powerful and eclectic image of a modern, "world-
class" system for the management of quality appeared in the United
States in the mid-1980s, in the form of the examination criteria for
the Malcolm Baldrige National Quality Award. The Baldrige Award
system established an evolving set of criteria through which its
board of examiners and judges could assess and score the maturity

of quality management systems in large manufacturing companies, the service industry, and small businesses. The Baldrige Award criteria have become a *lingua franca* for conversations in much of American industry today about the development of organizational capacity to achieve rapid improvement and enhanced efficiency.

Although Continuous Quality Improvement (CQI) took root in a number of industries, we have very little information on its being adopted by regulators. The model of CQI, as we have portrayed it, is that market competition forces industries to adopt this set of innovations. Regulation does not play a role. Yet it could. Regulator adoption of principles such as focus on customers, use of statistics, and emphasis on coaching could lead to responsive regulation in many industries, including health care.

Quality Management and Health Care: An Early Courtship

Between Shewhart's work beginning in the 1920s and the development of the Baldrige Award system in the United States in the mid-1980s, only a few thin, nearly invisible fibers connected the "industrial quality management movement" and American health care. Shewhart's key book *Economic Control of Quality of Manufactured Product*[65] uses many medical metaphors and images to describe underlying causal systems that, in his view, exist in production processes and need to be "diagnosed" and "treated" in order to support the improvement of products and services. Indeed, his particular statistical approach to understanding variation is similar to methods of epidemiology that were beginning to take shape among his medical contemporaries. Both Shewhart's own work on production as a system and later contributions by general systems theorists such as Russell Ackoff[66] at the University of Pennsylvania had strong parallels in the medical world. Examples include the systems thinking visible in the Lee-Jones Report of the 1930s,[67] Williamson's views of improvement as a "cybernetic" learning process,[68] and

George Engel's important work at the University of Rochester on understanding medicine as a biopsychosocial system.[69] Larry L. Weed's visionary explorations of the nature of medical reasoning also resonate strongly with the insights of Shewhart and Deming.[70] Shewhart's specific research on statistical approaches to variation in production systems appears to have escaped the notice of health care leaders for several decades. However, it is intellectually related to the improvements in the use of quantitative reasoning in medicine led by White,[71] Feinstein,[72] and others who have contributed to the development of the modern fields of clinical epidemiology, decision theory, and improved research designs in health care. Vergil Slee,[73] who did pioneering work in developing data bases and systems to assess performance of hospitals on a national scale, has had a long-standing friendship with Juran; and White was briefly acquainted with Deming in the 1960s. Juran's major technical text on quality, *The Quality Control Handbook*,[74] makes specific references to medication errors and other medical examples in explaining statistical interpretation and process failures, and one section of Deming's key 1984 book *Out of the Crisis*[75] was written by Paul B. Batalden, who several years earlier had met Deming and become intrigued with his theories and their potential application in health care.

So far as we know, however, no specific applications of modern industrial quality management methods, explicitly identified as such, occurred in the health care sector—at least in the United States—until approximately 1984 or 1985. In those years, executives at two American hospitals—Meritor Hospital in Madison, Wisconsin, and Norton-Kosair Children's Hospital in Louisville, Kentucky—independently encountered the work of Deming and saw its possible application to their own organizations. At about the same time, executives from several American corporations already engaged in quality management transformations were serving on boards of trustees of various health care organizations around the United States and were using those positions to encourage local executives to explore quality improvement methods for their potential application to health care. Examples include executives from the IBM Corporation, Johnson & Johnson, and Eastman Chemical Company, who involved themselves in leadership functions in hospitals, respectively, in Kingston, New York; Toms River, New Jersey; and Kingsport, Tennessee.

In 1987, Donald Berwick, one of the authors of this book, while serving as vice president of the Harvard Community Health Plan in eastern Massachusetts, met A. Blanton Godfrey, who was then head of the quality systems and theory division at AT&T Bell Laboratories. The two of them approached The John A. Hartford Foundation, a medical philanthropy, with a proposal for a trial of applications of modern quality improvement methods in health care settings. With the foundation's support, Berwick and Godfrey organized what came to be known as the National Demonstration Project on Quality Improvement in Health Care (NDP). Godfrey identified twenty experts from industrial quality management circles (industrial and academic settings), and Berwick enlisted twenty-one health care organizations interested in this experimental venture. An eight-month project, in which quality professionals worked on a volunteer basis with health care organizations on chronic performance problems, culminated in a national meeting in June 1988 at which initial reports were made on progress in this attempted transplantation of industrially developed methods into health care settings. The results were promising enough to warrant a book, *Curing Health Care*[76] (which has since sold more than twenty thousand copies) and to interest the John A. Hartford Foundation in a further three-year demonstration project whose aim was to expand teaching, research, and demonstration efforts on the application of quality management methods to health care.

Meanwhile, the application methodologies themselves had progressed quickly under the leadership of Paul Batalden, who in 1986 become vice president for medical care at the Hospital Corporation of America. There he developed the Quality Resource Group, which rapidly became the leading source of writing and experience in the application of quality management methods in health care settings.

By the 1990s, quality improvement in health care had become virtually a national movement, with its rhetoric and activities appearing in the work of almost every major health care organization and association in America. Hundreds, if not thousands, of American hospitals and health maintenance organizations were setting up quality management functions internally, and industrial consultants skilled in teaching various components of quality management saw rapid growth in the number of health care clients seeking their services.

However, fundamental differences persist between health care and other industries in the depth and strategic centering of their quality improvement methods. Whereas the mastery and application of such methods was a mandatory strategic thrust in globally active manufacturing companies by the mid-1980s, the health care industry, even in the mid-1990s, has kept its work on quality improvement, as opposed to the inspection of quality, at a relatively low, nonstrategic, and programmatic level.

More important, the use of CQI techniques by regulators has lagged behind even the slow-moving health care industry. Since the early 1980s, the major quality-oriented initiatives in American health care (the Health Care Financing Administration's peer review organizations, the accreditation processes of the JCAHO, the guidelines efforts of the Agency for Health Care Policy and Research, and the emerging managed care accreditation procedures of the National Committee for Quality Assurance) remain firmly entrenched in the battlefields of inspection. Though the rhetoric of health care leaders in the 1990s moved toward the jargon of quality improvement and quality management, the behaviors evident throughout the industry at a strategic and policy level remained far more closely connected to the views and ambitions of Ford and Taylor than to the insights and reforms of Shewhart and his intellectual descendants. Many leaders in both management and regulation of American health care talk of improvement, but most of them still walk in inspection.

In the search for better performance, leaders in other industries have changed the ways they manage; health care leaders, both inside and outside the system of care, have primarily changed the ways they measure. Why have health care systems lagged so far behind other systems of production in their openness to improved ways of managing their work? The most common reply is that the work of health care must be different in fundamental ways from the work of other industries. Skeptics abound who believe that the processes through which patients receive diagnostic and therapeutic care differ so much from the processes of production of other goods and services that experience with the latter provides few lessons that can help improve the former.

However, practitioners who have explored improvement in both terrains have almost universally come to doubt that the differences are so deep. Important principles of modern quality management map immediately and well into the health care context:

The imperative to focus on meeting external needs

The importance of managing interdependencies well

The essential role of sound statistical analysis in guiding improvement

The need to focus on continuous improvement as an aim

The potential value of involving all participants in the improvement of the processes in which they work

The crucial role of leaders in supporting systemic improvement

One of the core structural forms in industrial quality management, the quality improvement project team—described especially well in the work of Juran—has found almost immediate success in

many health care settings. Quality improvement teams in health care
have been able to achieve breakthroughs in performance of processes
on which they work, using methods that would be immediately recognizable to Juran, Ishikawa, and other teachers not formally involved
in health care. These breakthroughs occur in cost, in service characteristics such as waiting times, and in clinical outcome areas such as
morbidity, mortality, and pain control. The admittedly minor successes reported in the first phase of the NDP have now been followed
up by much more impressive results in many settings. On a project-
by-project basis, the skeptics lose; quality improvement teams achieve
results in health care every bit as remarkable as those in other industries through the use of similar methods.

Summary

The science of quality measurement, the science of quality improvement, and the regulation and oversight of medical care have developed independently of each other. This is both extraordinary and
unfortunate. Only recently have health care leaders begun to appre-
ciate the importance of drawing on all of these traditions at once
to shape a sound, scientifically informed approach to improvement.
Regulators face the same challenge: to ground their own activities
in the best available knowledge about the measurement, management, and improvement of quality of care. Because regulators are
behind in their understanding of quality improvement, they take
initiatives that obstruct rather than promote quality.

We believe that regulation truly responsive to the needs of the
day would integrate knowledge from the modern scientific fields of
quality measurement and quality management, as well as the best
of pertinent knowledge from health services research about the
quality of care. Such regulation would be an active force for encouraging improvement. Before describing how this can occur,
however, we must explore in some more detail the structure and
key issues of today's health care system, and we must examine more

precisely the influences currently exerted on it by regulation. The landscape of medical care is reordering itself at a breathtaking pace, and responsive regulation must take full account of the new order if it is to succeed.

Notes

1. See E. A. Codman, *A Study in Hospital Efficiency: As Demonstrated by the Care Report of the First Five Years of a Private Hospital* (Boston: Thomas Todd, 1916).

2. Codman, *A Study in Hospital Efficiency.*

3. E. A. Codman, "The Product of a Hospital," *Surgery, Gynecology, Obstetrics* 18 (1914): 491–496.

4. J. Haidenthaller, "Die Radicaloperationen der Hernien in der Klinik des Hofraths Prof. Dr. Bilroth 1877–1889," *Archiv für Chirurgie* 40 (1890): 493–555.

5. E. Bassini, "Neue Operations-Methode zur Radicalbehandlung der Schenkelhernie," *Archiv für klinische Chirurgie* 47 (1894): 1–25.

6. See H. B. Devlin, "Professional Audit; Quality Control; Keeping up to Date," *Bailliere's Clinical Anaesthesiology* 2 (1988): 299–324; L. Davis, *Fellowship of Surgeons: A History of the American College of Surgeons* (Chicago: American College of Surgeons, 1973).

7. American College of Surgeons, "Conference on Hospital Standardization," *Bulletin of the American College of Surgeons* 2 (1917): 1–54.

8. See J. G. Bowman, "Hospital Standardization Series: General Hospitals of 100 Beds or More: Report for 1919," *Bulletin of the American College of Surgeons* 4 (1920): 3–36; J. G. Bowman, "Hospital Standardization Series: General Hospitals of 100 Beds or More: Report for 1920," *Bulletin of the American College of Surgeons* 5 (1921): 3–16. See also American College of Surgeons, "Hospital Standardization Series: Conference on Hospital Standardization: New York, October 24, 1919," *Bulletin of the American College of Surgeons* 4 (1919): 3–9; American College of Surgeons, "Hospital Standardization Series: Report of Hospital Conference held at Chicago, October 22–23, 1923," *Bulletin of the American College of Surgeons* 8 (1924): 1.

9. American College of Surgeons, "Conference on Hospital Standardization" (1917), 1–54.

10. American College of Surgeons, "Hospital Standardization Series: Conference on Hospital Standardization: New York, October 24, 1919," 3–9.

11. See Devlin, 299–324; Davis, J. S. Roberts, J. G. Coale, and R. R. Redman, "A History of the Joint Commission on Accreditation for Hospitals," *Journal of the American Medical Association* 258 (1987): 936–940.

12. See Roberts, Coale, and Redman, 937.

13. P. Starr, *The Social Transformation of American Medicine* (New York: Basic Books, 1982), 180–197.

14. A. Flexner, *Medical Education in the United States and Canada: A Report to the Carnegie Foundation for the Advancement of Teaching* (Boston: Merrymount Press, 1910).

15. J. W. Williamson, "Future Policy Directions for Quality Assurance: Lessons from the Health Accounting Experience," *Inquiry* 25 (1988): 67–77.

16. R. I. Lee and L. W. Jones, *The Fundamentals of Good Medical Care* (Chicago: University of Chicago Press, 1933).

17. See P. A. Lembcke, "Measuring the Quality of Medical Care Through Vital Statistics Based on Hospital Service Areas: 1. Comparative Study of Appendectomy Rates," *American Journal of Public Health* 42 (1952): 276–286; P. A. Lembcke, "Medical Auditing by Scientific Methods Illustrated by Major Female Pelvic Surgery," *Journal of the American Medical Association* 162 (1956): 646–655; P. A. Lembcke and O. G. Johnson, *A Medical Audit Report* (Los Angeles: University of California, Los Angeles School of Public Health, 1963).

20. A. Donabedian, "Evaluating the Quality of Medical Care," *Milbank Memorial Fund Quarterly* 44 (3) part 2 (1966): 166–203.

21. See E. F. Daily and M. A. Morehead, "A Method of Evaluating and Improving the Quality of Medical Care," *American Journal of Public Health* 46 (1956): 848–854; M. A. Morehead, *Quality of Medical*

Care Provided by Family Physicians as Related to Their Education, Training, and Methods of Practice, (New York: Health Insurance Plan of Greater New York, 1958); J. Ehrlich, M. A. Morehead, and R. E. Trussell, *The Quantity, Quality and Costs of Medical and Hospital Care Secured by a Sample of Teamster Families in the New York Area* (New York: Columbia University, School of Public Health and Administrative Medicine, 1960); M. A. Morehead, *A Study of the Hospital Care Secured by a Sample of Teamster Family Members in New York City* (New York: Columbia University, School of Public Health and Administrative Medicine, 1964); M. A. Morehead, "The Medical Audit as an Operational Tool," *American Journal of Public Health* 57 (1967): 1643–56; M. A. Morehead, "Evaluating Quality of Medical Care in the Neighborhood Health Center Program of the Office of Economic Opportunity," *Medical Care* 8 (1970): 118–168; M. A. Morehead, R. S. Donaldson, and M. R. Seravalli, "Comparisons Between OEO Neighborhood Health Centers and Other Health Center Providers of Ratings of the Quality of Health Care," *American Journal of Public Health* 61 (1971): 1294–1306; M. A. Morehead and R. Donaldson, "Quality of Clinical Management of Disease in Comprehensive Neighborhood Health Centers" *Medical Care* 12 (1974): 301–315.

22. See O. L. Peterson, L. P. Andrews, R. S. Spain, and B. G. Greenberg, "An Analytical Study of North Carolina General Practice, 1953–54," *Journal of Medical Education* 31 (1956): 1–165; O. L. Peterson and E. M. Barsamian, *Diagnostic Performance: The Diagnostic Process* (Ann Arbor: The University of Michigan Press, 1964), 347–362.

23. See M. C. Sheps, "Approaches to the Quality of Hospital Care," *Public Health Reports* 70 (1955): 877–886.

24. See H. B. Makover, "The Quality of Medical Care: Methodology of Survey of the Medical Groups Associated with the Health Insurance Plan of New York," *American Journal of Public Health* 41 (1951): 824–832; S. Shapiro, L. Weiner, and P. M. Densen, "Comparison of Prematurity and Perinatal Mortality in a General Population and in the Population of a Prepaid Group Practice, Medical

Care Plan," *American Journal of Public Health* 48 (1958): 170–187; S. Shapiro, H. Jacobziner, P. M. Densen, and L. Weiner, "Further Observations of Prematurity and Perinatal Mortality in a General Population and in the Population of a Prepaid Group Practice Medical Care Plan," *American Journal of Public Health* 50 (1960): 1304–17; A. Ciocco, G. H. Hunt, and I. Altman, "Statistics on Clinical Services to New Patients in Medical Groups," *Public Health Reports* 65 (1950): 99–115; I. S. Falk, H. K. Schonfeld, B. R. Harris, S. J. Landau, and S. S. Milles, "The Development of Standards for the Audit and Planning of Medical Care. I. Concepts, Research, Design and the Content of Primary Physician's Care," *American Journal of Public Health* 57 (1967): 1118–36.

25. B. C. Payne, F. T. Lyons, L. Dwarshius, M. Kolton, and W. Morris, *The Quality of Medical Care: Evaluation and Improvement* (Chicago: Hospital Research and Education Trust, 1976).

26. See Falk and others.

27. See H. K. Schonfeld, J. F. Heston, and I. S. Falk, *Standards for Good Medical Care*, vols. 1–4 (Washington, D.C.: U.S. Dept. of Health, Education, and Welfare, Office of Research and Statistics, 1975).

28. See R. W. Revans, *Standards for Morale: Cause and Effect in Hospitals* (Oxford, England: Oxford University Press, 1964).

29. See J. N. Morris, *Uses of Epidemiology* (Edinburgh: E & S Livingstone, 1957); L. Lipworth, J.A.H. Lee, and J. N. Morris, "Case-Fatality in Teaching and Non-Teaching Hospitals, 1956–59," *Medical Care* 1 (1963): 71–76.

30. K. L. White, T. F. Williams, and B. G. Greenberg, "The Ecology of Medical Care," *New England Journal of Medicine* 265 (1961): 885–892.

31. See J. W. Williamson, M. Alexander, and G. E. Miller, "Continuing Education and Patient Care Research: Physician Response to Screening Test Results," *Journal of the American Medical Association* 201 (1967): 938–942; J. W. Williamson, "Evaluating Quality of Patient Care: A Strategy Relating Outcome and Process Assessment," *Journal of the American Medical Association* 218 (1971):

564–569; J. W. Williamson, *Assessing and Improving Health Care Outcomes: The Health Accounting Approach to Quality Assurance* (Cambridge, Mass.: Ballinger, 1978); J. W. Williamson, "Formulating Priorities for Quality Assurance Activity: Description of a Method and Its Application," *Journal of the American Medical Association* 239 (1978): 631–637; J. W. Williamson, H. R. Brasswell, and S. D. Horn, "Validity of Medical Staff Judgments in Establishing Quality Assurance Priorities," *Medical Care* 17 (1979): 331–346. J. W. Williamson, H. D. Braswell, S. D. Horn, and S. Lohmeyer, "Priority Setting in Quality Assurance: Reliability of Staff Judgments in Medical Institutions," *Medical Care* 16 (1978): 931–940; J. W. Williamson, "Future Policy Directions for Quality Assurance: Lessons from the Health Accounting Experience," *Inquiry* 25 (1988): 67–77.

32. See Williamson, "Future Policy Directions for Quality Assurance."

33. See Williamson, Alexander, and Miller; Williamson, "Future Policy Directions for Quality Assurance."

34. R. H. Brook, "Quality of Care Assessment: A Comparison of Five Methods of Peer Review" (Rockville, Md.: Department of Health, Education and Welfare, Bureau of Health Research, 1973).

35. See R. H. Brook, A. Davies-Avery, S. Greenfield, L. J. Harris, T. Lelah, N. E. Solomon, and J. E. Ware, "Assessing the Quality of Medical Care Using Outcome Measures: An Overview of the Method," *Medical Care* 15 (Suppl.) (1977): 1–165; R. H. Brook, J. E. Ware, A. Davies-Avery, A. L. Stewart, C. A. Donald, W. H. Rogers, K. N. Williams, and S. A. Johnston, "Overview of Adult Health Status Measures Fielded in Rand's Health Insurance Study," *Medical Care* 17 (7) (Suppl.) (1979): 1–131; K. N. Lohr and R. H. Brook, "Quality Assurance in Medicine," *American Behavioural Scientist* 27 (1984): 583–607.

36. P. J. Sanazaro and J. W. Williamson, "End Results of Patient Care: A Provisional Classification Based on Reports by Internists," *Medical Care* 6 (1968): 123–130; P. J. Sanazaro and J. W. Williamson, "Physician Performance and Its Effects on Patients: A Classification Based on Reports by Internists, Surgeons, Pediatricians and Obstetricians," *Medical Care* 8 (1970): 299–308.

37. P. J. Sanazaro, R. L. Goldstein, and J. S. Roberts, "Research and Development in Quality Assurance: The Experimental Medical Care Review Organization Program," *New England Journal of Medicine* 287 (1972): 1125–31.

38. B. S. Hulka, F. J. Romm, G. R. Parkerson, I. T. Russell, N. E. Clapp, and F. S. Johnson, "Peer Review in Ambulatory Care: Use of Explicit Criteria and Implicit Judgments," *Medical Care* 17 (3) (Suppl.) (1979): 1–73.

39. See W. G. Manning, A. Leibowitz, G. A. Goldberg, W. H. Rogers, and J. P. Newhouse, "A Controlled Trial of the Effect of a Prepaid Group Practice on Use of Services, *New England Journal of Medicine* 310 (1984): 1505–10; J. P. Newhouse, W. G. Manning, C. N. Morris, L. L. Orr, N. Duan, E. B. Keeler, A. Leibowitz, K. H. Marquis, M. S. Marquis, C. E. Phelps, and R. H. Brook, "Some Interim Results from a Controlled Trial of Cost Sharing in Health Insurance," *New England Journal of Medicine* 305 (1981): 1501–07; J. P. Newhouse, R. W. Archibald, and H. L. Bailit, *Free for All? Lessons from the Rand Health Insurance Experiment* (Cambridge, Mass.: Harvard University Press, 1993); E. B. Keeler and J. E. Rolph, "How Cost Sharing Reduced Medical Spending of Participants in the Health Insurance Experiment," *Journal of the American Medical Association* 249 (1983): 2220–22.

40. See J. E. Ware and M. K. Snyder, "Dimensions of Patient Attitudes Regarding Doctors and Medical Care Services," *Medical Care* 13 (1975): 669–682.

41. See A. R. Tarlov, J. E. Ware, S. Greenfield, E. C. Nelson, E. Perrin, and M. Zubkoff, "The Medical Outcomes Study: An Application of Modern Methods for Monitoring the Results of Medical Care," *Journal of the American Medical Association* 262 (1989): 925–930.

42. See A. L. Stewart, R. D. Hays, and J. E. Ware, "The MOS Short-Form General Health Survey: Reliability and Validity in a Patient Population," *Medical Care* 26 (1988): 724–732.

43. See E. C. Nelson and D. M. Berwick, "The Measurement of Health Status in Clinical Practice," *Medical Care* 27 (Suppl.) (1989): s77–s90.

44. See Codman, *A Study in Hospital Efficiency;* American College of
    Surgeons, "Hospital Standardization Series: Report of Hospital
    Conference held at Chicago, October 22–23, 1923"; Payne and oth-
    ers; J. A. Glover, "The Incidence of Tonsillectomy in School Chil-
    dren," *Proceedings of the Royal Society of Medicine* 31 (1938):
    1219–36; R. S. Hooker, *Maternal Mortality in New York City: A
    Study of All Puerperal Death 1930–1932* (New York: Oxford Univer-
    sity Press, 1933); C. E. Lewis, "Variations in the Incidence of
    Surgery," *New England Journal of Medicine* 281 (1969): 880–884.

45. See J. E. Wennberg and A. Gittelsohn, "Small Area Variations in
    Health Care Delivery: A Population-Based Health Information Sys-
    tem Can Guide Planning and Regulatory Decision Making," *Science*
    182 (1973): 1102–08; J. E. Wennberg, J. L. Freeman, and W. J.
    Culp, "Are Hospital Services Rationed in New Haven or Over-
    Utilized in Boston?" *Lancet* 1 (1987): 1185–1189.

46. See R. H. Palmer, R. Strain, J.V.W. Maurer, J. K. Rothrock, and
    M. S. Thompson, "Quality Assurance in Eight Adult Medicine
    Group Practices," *Medical Care* 22 (1984): 632–643; E. Vayda, "A
    Comparison of Surgical Rates in Canada and in England and
    Wales," *New England Journal of Medicine* 289 (1973): 1224–29.

47. M. I. Roemer, "Hospital Utilization and the Health Care System,"
    American Journal of Public Health 66(10): 953–955 (1976).

48. See J. Kosecoff, M. R. Chassin, and A. Fink, "Obtaining Clinical
    Data on the Appropriateness of Medical Care in Community Prac-
    tice," *Journal of the American Medical Association* 258 (1987):
    2538–42; R. H. Brook, R. E. Park, M. R. Chassin, D. H. Solomon,
    J. Keesey, and J. Kosecoff, "Predicting the Appropriate Use of
    Carotid Endarterectomy, Upper Gastrointestinal Endoscopy, and
    Coronary Angiography," *New England Journal of Medicine* 323 (1990):
    1173–77.

49. L. L. Leape, R. E. Park, D. H. Solomon, M. R. Chassin, J. Kosecoff,
    and R. H. Brook, "'Does Inappropriate Use Explain Small-Area
    Variations in the Use of Health Care Services?' A Critique" *Journal of
    the American Medical Association* 263 (1990): 669–672; G. Davidson,

"Does Inappropriate Use Explain Small-Area Variations in the Use of Health Care Services?" *Health Services Research* 28 (1993): 389–400.

50. See L. I. Iezzoni, "Measuring the Severity of Illness and Case Mix," in *Providing Quality Care: The Challenge to Clinicians*, N. Goldfield and D. B. Nash, eds. (Philadelphia: American College of Physicians, 1989), 70–105.

51. See P. M. Gertman and J. Restuccia, "The Appropriateness Evaluation Protocol: A Technique for Assessing Unnecessary Days of Hospital Care," *Medical Care* 19 (1981): 855–871.

52. See A. R. Feinstein, *Clinical Biostatistics* (St. Louis, Mo.: Mosby, 1977).

53. See F. W. Taylor, *The Principles of Scientific Management* (New York: Harper and Brothers, 1911).

54. C. D. Wrege and R. G. Greenwood, *Frederick W. Taylor: The Father of Scientific Management: Myth & Reality* (Homewood, Ill: Business One Irwin, 1991), 194–195.

55. See W. A. Shewhart, *Economic Control of Quality of Manufactured Product* (New York: Van Nostrand, 1931).

56. See W. E. Deming, *Out of the Crisis* (Cambridge, Mass.: Massachusetts Institute of Technology-Center of Advanced Engineering Study, 1986).

57. See J. M. Juran, *Managerial Breakthrough: A New Concept of the Manager's Job* (New York: McGraw-Hill, 1964); J. M. Juran, *The Quality Control Handbook* (New York: McGraw-Hill, 1988).

58. H. M. Wadsworth, Jr., K. S. Stephens, and A. B. Godfrey, *Modern Methods for Quality Control and Improvement* (New York: Wiley, 1986); D. A. Garvin, *Managing Quality: The Strategic and Competitive Edge* (New York: Free Press, 1988); I. M. Kaisen, *The Key to Japan's Competitive Success* (New York: Random House, 1986); J. P. Womack, D. T. Jones, and D. Roos, *The Machine That Changed the World: How Japan's Secret Weapon in the Global Auto Wars Will Revolutionize Western Industry* (New York: Harper Perennial, 1991).

59. See T. Ohno, *Toyota Production System: Beyond Large-Scale Production* (Cambridge, Mass.: Productivity Press, 1988).

60. K. Ishikawa, *What is Total Quality Control?* (Englewood Cliffs, N.J.: Prentice-Hall, 1985).

61. See Deming, 80–85.

62. A. V. Feigenbaum, *Total Quality Control* (New York: McGraw-Hill, 1983).

63. See Juran, *Managerial Breakthrough;* Juran, *The Quality Control Handbook;* J. M. Juran, *Juran on Leadership for Quality: An Executive Handbook* (New York: Free Press, 1989).

64. P. B. Crosby, *Quality is Free: The Art of Making Quality Certain* (New York: McGraw-Hill, 1979).

65. See Shewhart.

66. R. L. Ackoff, *Redesigning the Future: A Systems Approach to Societal Problems* (New York: Wiley, 1974).

67. See Lee and Jones.

68. See Williamson, "Future Policy Directions for Quality Assurance."

69. See G. L. Engel, *Psychological Development in Health and Disease* (Philadelphia: Saunders, 1962).

70. L. L. Weed, "Medical Records That Guide and Teach," *New England Journal of Medicine* 278 (1968): 593–600, 652–657.

71. See White and others.

72. See Feinstein.

73. C. W. Eisele, V. N. Slee, and R. G. Hoffmann, "Can the Practice of Internal Medicine Be Evaluated? *Annals of Internal Medicine* 44 (1956): 144–161.

74. See Juran, *The Quality Control Handbook.*

75. See Deming.

76. D. M. Berwick, A. B. Godfrey, and J. Roessner, *Curing Health Care: New Strategies for Quality Improvement* (San Francisco: Jossey-Bass, 1990).

4

The Evolution of Health Care
and Its Regulation

As has been shown, the practice of medicine was relatively isolated from the intrusions of a regulatory state for the first three quarters of the twentieth century. The major oversight of physicians was provided by state licensure boards that rarely undertook proceedings against doctors for failure to provide high-quality care. The inspection and regulation of hospital care was largely turned over to the private, physician-dominated Joint Commission on Accreditation of Health Care Organizations (JCAHO). In theory, both physicians and hospitals were attuned to the deterrence signal sent by the tort system, but in reality, there was little evidence that the threat of malpractice suits produced higher-quality care or prompted serious efforts to prevent medical injury. Federal authorities provided some scrutiny of care for patients in the Medicare and Medicaid programs, especially through peer review, but this oversight was fairly limited. Society relied primarily on the ethical commitment of the provider to the patient for high-quality care. This in turn meant that developing notions of quality improvement through analysis of trends and rates, similar to that undertaken by other industries, had little or no niche in the health care industry. Innovations in quality measurement and improvement could not easily find organizational or structural platforms for application and remained largely a matter of academic interest. The blame largely lies with the professional dominance of medical care, not with regulators. Nonetheless, regulation had not prompted change.

As both regulatory theory and a review of the history of health care regulation suggests, providers actively engaged in capture of regulators. Those regulators who could not be co-opted were treated as meddlers who contributed little to the everyday work of health care. In turn, regulators were forced into a hostile inspection mode. This constellation of perceptions precluded any responsive regulatory efforts. Regulators and regulated could not work together toward socially optimal goals. Nor was there sufficient market competition, independent of professional influence, that could lead to competition on quality or to a movement toward modern quality improvement techniques.

Now the regulatory landscape has changed. Three of the four pillars of regulation of quality—federal government oversight through the Professional Standards Review Organizations (PSROs), medical malpractice, and JCAHO accreditation—have or are undergoing profound transformation, while medical licensure has fallen further into desuetude over the past decade. Meanwhile, a host of other mechanisms has begun to emerge, from self-regulation and public data initiatives to new federal antitrust efforts and crackdowns on fraud and abuse. The result is a much more complicated regulatory environment that intertwines with medical practice. The isolation of the doctor-patient relationship that persisted in the first three quarters of the century has ended.

There are many explanations for this upheaval. One important factor has been the increasing acceptance of industrial methods of quality improvement discussed in Chapter Three, prompting great changes in the way regulators and regulated entities operate. Another is the influence of three Republican administrations that have advocated market mechanisms in health care. In the tug-of-war that we have described between regulation and competition, market proponents have gained the upper hand.

The third major factor contributing to the change in quality-of-care regulation has been the significant reconstruction of medical care. Twenty years ago, the managed care industry still had meager influence. Strengthened by the Health Maintenance Organization Act of 1973, the managed care industry has thrived and today is rapidly growing, largely because of its success in controlling cost. Indeed, cost control is the major motivation in the health care sphere.

In this chapter, we explore the rise of managed care and the evolution of the structures of quality regulation that were discussed in Chapter Two.[1] In Chapter Five, we will review the federal law that has infiltrated medical care and laid the groundwork for movement toward a market-based system of delivery. We will then report on providers' perceptions of the regulatory state—especially those providers who have been actively involved in modern approaches to quality improvement.

Each step of the way, we will be aware of our original thesis and prescriptions: that health care and health care regulators must labor to remove the perception that regulation obstructs true quality; that to do so, regulation must become responsive, adopting the methods of modern quality improvement; and that the challenges facing new attempts to regulate for improvement will lie in the market's sometimes inappropriate emphasis on cost control.

A Changing Medical Industry: The Rise of Managed Care

Perhaps the most striking development in the structure of American health care since the mid-1970s has been the emergence of managed care organizations. The history of health maintenance organizations (HMOs) since the 1930s has been widely discussed.[2] Though their penetration of the health care market remained relatively shallow through the beginning of the 1970s, since that time, their growth has been explosive, especially in the early 1990s.[3] Much of this growth can be ascribed to federal incentives introduced in the HMO

Act of 1973. Passed by the Nixon administration as an alternative
to more thoroughgoing reform in the health care industry, the act
has had a subversive, revolutionary effect on American health care.

Under this act, still in effect today although modified periodi-
cally over the past twenty years, HMOs had to provide basic health
services for a periodic payment assessed without regard to the date,
frequency, extent, or kind of services required.[4] So defined, the
HMO contrasted sharply with indemnity insurance and fee-for-
service medicine that were still the rule in 1975. The basic services
that HMOs had to provide in order to qualify under federal law
included physician care, hospital inpatient and outpatient care, crisis intervention, treatment or referral for alcohol or addiction services, home health services, and preventive services. Supplemental
health services such as podiatric care were also mandated when the
act was first passed, although in 1976 these became optional.

HMOs were not required to be federally qualified, but most
sought this status because of a competitive advantage that was the
result of two critical provisions. First, the act prohibited all state
laws or practices that served as barriers to the formation of HMOs,
regardless of whether there was a direct conflict with federal regulation or not. This prohibition included any state regulations requiring the approval of a medical society before an HMO could be
licensed, provisions that physicians make up a certain percentage
of an HMO's governing body, and insurance regulations concerning capitalization or financial reserves to prevent insolvency.[5] States
were also prohibited from regulating advertising by HMOs.

In addition, federal law required a mandatory dual choice policy. Any employer with more than twenty-five employees and
required by law to pay the minimum wage had to offer an HMO
option as part of its health benefits and could not charge less than
was charged for indemnity insurance. This requirement meant that
employers could not discriminate via payroll deductions or contributions against those who chose to receive coverage through an
HMO rather than through a fee-for-service plan.[6] The indemnity

plan would provide a floor for HMO premiums.[7] Employers were originally forced to offer the HMO option if there was a federally qualified HMO in their area, but in 1976 the act was modified so that an HMO had to request that it become part of an employer's health plan.

Before 1973, many state laws had enforced a ban on the corporate practice of medicine (employment of physicians by corporate entities). This stymied HMO development in many jurisdictions. Moreover, benefits managers simply were not used to offering the managed care organization as an option. The 1973 legislation therefore opened the door for HMO development and ensured that there would be a niche for them in the marketplace.

Perhaps more significantly, the HMO Act was an example of regulation that modified the peculiar medical care market so as to allow a more socially optimal delivery system to emerge. Existing market forces themselves might not have been sufficient.

The HMO Act included several other provisions. The federal government insisted that there be adequate protection against risk of insolvency and that certain administrative and managerial arrangements had to be satisfactory to the secretary of the Department of Health and Human Services.[8] It required financial disclosure, including a report to the secretary, on a yearly basis. The new legislation took one further step to aid managed care. It provided seed money for new HMOs through grants and loans. Loans could be provided to private concerns to assist them in meeting operating costs for the first sixty months or during times of significant expansion in a membership or service area.[9] In distributing these loans, special consideration was given to those HMOs that treated medically underserved populations.

The legislation slowly evolved. As already mentioned, amendments in 1976 made availability of supplemental services optional. To encourage existing health care plans to move to an HMO status, a forty-eight-month phase-in period for community rating (rating premiums based on the health of communities, not individuals) was offered for plans already offering prepaid health services. It is notable that the federal legislation has consistently maintained that HMOs must "community rate" patient premiums, with only certain modifications available.[10]

In 1978, in order to maintain the integrity of HMOs by encouraging an exclusive and responsive staff, contracts with physicians were limited by law to those physicians already in an independent practice association (IPA) or medical group. To accommodate the growing variation in HMOs and promote the development of point-of-service plans (managed care plans in which enrolled patients may opt to receive care from an out-of-plan physician, usually at an additional cost), Congress allowed HMOs to impose a reasonable deductible when members obtained a basic service from a physician who was not a member of a staff IPA or a group HMO plan. However, 90 percent of services still had to be provided by an affiliated physician.

In the past decade, Congress (and Republican administrations) have acknowledged that HMOs are ready to compete in the marketplace and have removed some of the advantageous protections given to them under the 1973 legislation. In 1983, Congress decided that it was no longer necessary to provide loans to HMOs. More important, amendments required that the attractive dual choice provisions be eliminated by 1995 and relaxed the equal contribution requirement that obliged an employer to make the same financial contribution to an HMO as would be made to a traditional health plan.

Federal preemption of state laws provided a rich culture for the growth of HMOs. The preemptive effect of the federal HMO Act of 1973 has been challenged several times, but courts have largely deferred to the federal government's grant of authority. The only exceptions are those cases in which state courts have sought to coordinate benefits with other state programs, thereby limiting the applicability of the HMO Act.[11]

Under the protections provided by the HMO Act, managed care

organizations have grown and evolved. The original HMOs were largely *staff model*, employing their own physicians who often practiced in the same clinical center. Very few HMOs were *open panel*— that is, consisted of physicians in solo practice who had banded together into an independent practice association.[12] Over the course of the 1980s, a variety of new organizational forms took shape, giving rise to a confusing set of acronyms.[13] The critical remodeling of the traditional staff-model HMO consisted of some loosening of ties of physicians to the managed care organization and the introduction of financial risk-sharing arrangements with physicians, individually and in groups. To give consumers a greater choice among medical providers—often including the opportunity to retain their own ongoing physician relationship while moving into managed care coverage—more and more managed care organizations found a competitive advantage in allowing some independent physicians to affiliate loosely with the HMO. These so-called *open HMOs* essentially had relations with a number of preferred providers. The preferred providers were not full members of the HMO staff, but they did follow certain guidelines in caring for patients referred by the HMO. Patients paid premiums that to some extent reflected the point of service of the medical care. As indemnity insurers evolved in the direction of preferred provider organizations, and staff-model HMOs evolved in the direction of independent practice associations, both headed toward a mixed system offering a variety of different options for the participating patient and a variety of different contractual relationship with physicians.

By 1990, HMOs controlled 18 percent of the United States marketplace; preferred provider organizations, 17 percent; and managed indemnity plans, 40 percent.[14] Since that time, growth of the hybrid managed care organizations has been dramatic. It was estimated in 1995 that more than fifty million Americans had their care provided through some sort of managed care organization. With increasing capitation (insurer transfer of risk to providers by paying providers for all health care costs on a "per capita" basis) of health care premiums providing significant competitive advantages to managed care, at least in terms of lower premiums, most observers now anticipate continued significant growth over the next decade. Indeed, it seems safe at this point to predict that the managed care organization—or its offspring, the integrated delivery system (IDS), discussed later in this chapter—will be the dominant model of health care delivery in the early years of the twenty-first century. As a result, the quality of medical care may very well depend on how managed care organizations promote quality. Clearly, from our perspective, the regulation of quality in managed care organizations is essential.

Preemptive federal law has not obstructed all state regulation of HMOs. States are able to regulate any aspect of managed care organizations that is not addressed by the federal law (and little of the federal law addresses quality of medical care). Moreover, fewer and fewer HMOs are seeking federal qualification as its benefits wane, and increasingly the state regulations alone are applicable.

There is a good deal of variation between states in their regulatory approach, with some encouraging and others restricting the growth of managed care organizations. Each state tends to define managed care in explicit detail.[15] Most definitions embrace the complete panoply of managed care organizations but still eliminate fee-for-service financing.

Maryland offers an excellent example of how state regulatory structures can encourage HMOs to provide high-quality care. Maryland requires that HMOs

have regular hours

provide for twenty-four-hour access to a physician

assure that each member seen for a medical complaint is evaluated under the direction of a physician

give each member an opportunity to select a primary care physician make available primary care services, including enrollment history and physicals

offer appropriate preventive services as well as periodic health education

Each managed care organization must have a written plan providing for implementation of these standards. The plan is also required to review statistics on the health care needs of its patients and to identify any vulnerable groups such as the poor, the elderly, or the mentally ill. Each organization must have an internal peer review system that in many ways is modeled on peer review in hospitals, but the state also requires the systematic collection of data on performance and patient results.[16] In addition, each HMO must provide information to all subscribers on available services and on potential responsibility for payment of services by subscribers. The secretary or commissioner of insurance must be informed if an HMO undertakes any important change or rearrangement of these systems of quality assurance.[17]

Fiscal oversight also looms large for managed care organizations. Most state's HMO statutes were updated in the late 1980s, following the bankruptcies of large managed care organizations in several jurisdictions. For instance, Maryland requires that any HMO formed after July 1, 1989, must have an initial surplus that exceeds liabilities by at least $1.5 million. In addition, each HMO must maintain a surplus greater than $750,000 or 5 percent of the subscription charges. These financial requirements complement those set forth by the federal government and have proven to be acceptable to the managed care industry. In a significant break with the federal government, some states allow their (non–federally qualified) HMOs to operate under experience rating (as opposed to community rating).[18] However, most jurisdictions have generally mandated that HMOs not set rates that are excessive, inadequate, or discriminatory.[19]

Many states maintain separate regulatory structures for preferred provider organizations. In Massachusetts, any such organization seeking approval to operate must submit certain information about providers to the commissioner of insurance; this includes a description of the health services offered, the location of the services, and copies of any contracts with providers.[20] The arrangement must also provide standards for maintaining quality of health care and for controlling health care costs. As a compromise with organized medicine, the preferred providers must not be paid more than 120 percent of fees paid to nonpreferred providers.

Some states, especially in the southeast, are quite antagonistic toward managed care organizations. Their regulations generally reflect this antagonism, which is often fueled by the local medical societies' interests. For example, in Texas, the protections against insolvency are much more thoroughgoing (some would say oppressive) than in other states. In addition, HMOs must not refer to themselves as insurance or mutual organizations. Perhaps most important, the enabling legislation for HMOs specifically states that "this Act should not be construed to authorize any person other than a duly licensed physician or practitioner of the healing arts, acting within the scope of his or her license, to engage, directly or indirectly, in the practice of medicine or any healing art."[21] The hostility of some Texas doctors to managed care is reflected in ongoing lawsuits in which physicians are suing the managed care divisions of Aetna Life Insurance and Prudential Insurance Companies for deselecting physicians from their approved panels.[22] Yet even a harsh regulatory environment probably will not outweigh the comparative economic advantages of managed care.

California, with perhaps the most advanced managed care industry, also has the most advanced regulation. The state's Department of Corporations sets high standards for financial accounting and disclosure to patients under the Knox-Keene Health Care Services Plan of 1975. In addition, the state health authorities may undertake on-site surveys of plans to evaluate peer review mechanisms, internal procedures for oversight of quality of care, and overall performance of a plan.[23] Several other states reserve such authority.[24]

In 1994, California authorities fined a managed care organization $500,000 for failing to follow its own procedures in a patient referral matter.[25]

For our purposes, it is sufficient to note that HMOs and other managed care operations are subject to regulation—some of which applies to quality—both at the federal and the state level. In many ways, this regulation may seem as far-reaching as that which applies to hospitals and doctors. However, most of the quality regulation is relatively bland, except with respect to the information passed along to potential beneficiaries. This should not be surprising, because the federal regulation of HMOs was largely designed to promote the concept of managed care, rather than to provide oversight of quality. Somewhat more surprising is the fact that in 1995, thirty-one states reported to the Physician Payment Review Commission that they used CQI techniques to regulate managed care plans.[26] We found little evidence of such techniques in the nine states we studied (see Chapter Six), even though all but one indicated in the survey that they used CQI.

Managed care organizations are now accepting a self-regulation framework similar to the JCAHO. In 1979, the Group Health Association of America and the American Managed Care Review Association, the major trade associations in the industry, founded the National Committee for Quality Assurance (NCQA). Through much of the 1980s, the NCQA lay dormant, but slowly HMOs began to recognize the need for an accreditation process parallel to that provided by the JCAHO. In 1990, the NCQA was spun off as an independent not-for-profit organization, helped by a grant from the Robert Wood Johnson Foundation.[27] This action constituted a presumptive strike against the JCAHO, which had declared its intention to develop accreditation standards for HMOs. The NCQA board presently consists of industry representatives but also includes quality experts and employers. It operates an accreditation program that reviews all types of HMOs, including those with point-of-service plans. (Preferred provider organizations are excluded.)

The NCQA has formulated a series of accreditation standards that focus on six areas:

1. Preventive health services
2. Medical records
3. Utilization management
4. Members' rights and responsibilities
5. Credentialing
6. Quality improvement

According to NCQA president Margaret E. O'Kane, the accreditation process is imbued with the ideas of Continuous Quality Improvement.[28] Members pay between twenty and thirty thousand dollars for an accreditation visit. An organization that seeks accreditation sends the NCQA complete information on quality improvement plans, utilization review techniques, physician panels, and credentialing information. About six weeks later, an NCQA team made up of three individuals, two of whom are HMO medical directors, arrives on-site for a two-to-four-day visit. Approximately six weeks after a visit, the NCQA team sends a report back to the HMO. A draft of this report is usually evaluated by the NCQA Review Oversight Committee before being transmitted back to the organization seeking accreditation. There are four levels of accreditation decision: full accreditation for three years, accreditation with recommendations, provisional accreditation for one year, and denial or revocation of accreditation.

Much of the accreditation process is now focused on the so-called HEDIS criteria. The Health Plan and Employer Data and Information Set is a list of performance measures that were intended to respond to the simple employer question, "How do I understand the value of what my health care dollars are purchasing, and how do I hold a health plan accountable for its performance?"[29] HEDIS provides a core set of measures and also systematizes the measurement process. The NCQA would like the HEDIS criteria to become the single standard by which all quality in managed care organizations is judged. The HEDIS measures were selected on the basis of three criteria: value and relevance to employers; the ability of health plans to provide the requested data; and the potential for improvement of quality of care.

The specific components of HEDIS are quality; access and patient satisfaction; membership and utilization; and finance. Each of these components contains detailed subcriteria. Most managed care organizations have well-developed programs assuring patient rights and addressing grievances.[30] HEDIS concentrates on preventive medicine, prenatal care, acute and chronic disease, and mental health and substance abuse. Under preventive medicine, for example, health plans must report rates of childhood immunization, cholesterol screening for particular populations, mammography screening for women over the age of forty, and pap smears for women aged fifteen to seventy. Regarding prenatal care, the criteria measure rates of low birth weight and the amount of prenatal care in the first trimester. Under acute and chronic disease, the specific issues are asthma admissions and readmissions to both emergency rooms and hospitals, the use of retinal examination in the diabetic population, and therapy after myocardial infarction. In each case, the health plan must calculate rates using the specific denominators prescribed by HEDIS. Most health plans gather this data through chart reviews of sample patients, but increasingly, better-organized plans are finding ways to analyze the information from computer data sets. Managed care organizations that participate in HEDIS are able to receive comparative information from competing plans. The criteria are intended to indicate areas of deficiency, and it is to be hoped that they will promote quality improvement teams and projects. At the least, HEDIS criteria promise to provide some of the epidemiological information that can guide quality improvement.

The NCQA/HEDIS accreditation process may constitute

self-regulation. Like the JCAHO, the accrediting organization has arisen from the industry itself. There is little external validation of the accrediting process, and regulator and regulated sit cheek by jowl at least as much in the NCQA as in the JCAHO. Little of the information of the accreditation visit is made public. Nevertheless, the NCQA does appear to be committed to sharing at least some information. For example, in the fall of 1993, the organization launched a Report Card Pilot Project involving twenty-one health plans. The NCQA's intention is to produce a report card for each participant, based on selected HEDIS measures. Providing consumers with information from regulatory oversight represents an exciting new step, one that suggests basic changes in assumptions about regulating for improvement. Some plans, in particular U.S. HealthCare and Kaiser Permanente, have already begun to share their scores on report cards.[31] However, there are questions about this information, arising from charges that some plans may have reported the best performance by one participating group, not overall performance.

Generally, our conversations with leaders in the managed care industry reveal much the same sort of attitudes toward regulation as is found among traditional hospitals and providers: outside regulation is obstructive, self-regulation is better. But no matter how they are regulated to provide high-quality care, it is clear that managed care organizations are transforming the health care industry. Indeed, partially owing to pressure from managed care organizations, most hospitals and physicians are considering new and different organizational models to obtain the same kinds of advantages. A much more cohesive approach than that found in the traditional independent hospital and among medical staff is necessary to contract with large groups of patients or to accept capitated payments from insurers. Physicians, hospitals, and their lawyers are responding with a variety of new institutions. These new organizations are variously called *management service foundations, physician-hospital organizations*, and *integrated health delivery systems*.[32] Their *raisons d'etre* are to develop patient referral bases and to manage care. They are the newborn cousins of traditional managed organizations.

In large degree, the primary movers of physician-hospital organizations (PHOs) are hospitals fearful of being eliminated by larger health systems. They recruit physicians, often by acquiring group practices, and develop a tightly integrated working structure. Many of the physicians in these arrangements are salaried by the hospitals, allowing the hospitals to take on capitated risk for patient care.[33] In this way, physician-hospital organizations emulate the managed care organizations' ability to control costs and perhaps use guidelines to provide higher-quality care.[34]

Large numbers of hospitals and doctors are considering forming PHOs, which are legal entities created by a joint venture between one or more hospitals and the members of the hospital medical staff.[35] The physician-hospital organization itself does not provide medical services but instead contracts with its members for medical service. Typically, a PHO consists of two classes of members, the physicians and the hospital, with each member electing a certain percentage of the directors. PHOs lay the groundwork for integration in such areas as coordinated billing and accounting, quality assurance and utilization review, and cost-effective approaches to managed care programs, including those that capitate.

Hospitals that do not want to create a PHO can test the integration waters with a hospital-based clinic allowing the hospital to gain experience with physician reimbursement. (In many cases, academic institutions already operate such hospital-owned clinics.) They can also simply acquire the practices of physician groups. In this situation, the hospital is the only legal entity, and it employs physicians to provide care.

There is also the option of a *medical foundation*—usually a nonprofit tax-exempt organization set up by a hospital, its parent, or a physician group. Medical foundations can own and operate facilities and employ nonphysician personnel. In some cases, the medical foundation is used as a vehicle for acquiring the assets of physician practices. It is usually the first step beyond a PHO toward the creation of a true vertically integrated system of health care delivery. The foundation receives all revenues from managed care plans and third-party payers and then contracts with physicians and others. In this fashion, it can readily accept capitation payment.

The other forms of integration are driven by the identity of the primary movers. In the *physician equity model*, an independent group practice purchases a hospital and its related facilities. The physicians then create a parent corporation—often a *management services organization*—that owns the hospital.[36] The physician group usually maintains its status as a separate medical group and has the potential to merge with other group practices, while the management services organization provides administrative services to the medical group and the hospital. The management services organization also negotiates managed care contracts including capitation payments, on behalf of the physician organizations and the hospital. The physician owners bear most of the financial risk of the operation of the hospital.

The reverse situation is a *hospital-affiliated independent practice association*. In this case, the hospital develops, finances, and manages an independent practice association.[37] The IPA is usually open-panel, the members being physicians who have staff privileges at the hospital. Managed care organizations can contract simply with the hospital or the IPA, but the joint venture usually offers a capitation option. The IPA and the hospital typically set up their own risk pool to share the risk of overutilization for inpatient services.

The most mature integrated model is the single-corporation *integrated delivery system*. This model usually develops from a single umbrella parent organization; in some cases, it is a hospital; in others, a group practice or a management services organization. Physicians are employed on a salary basis by the parent corporation, and the corporation receives all payment, including capitated payment. The IDS can contract directly with employers and assume all risk for health care delivery. It is safe to say that today, some model of integration is being considered by almost all hospitals and many physicians.

Here, we should pause to distinguish the IDS from the traditional managed care organization. The latter had its roots in the traditional staff-model HMO, which underwrote health care risk but usually did not have a hospital component integrated into the organization. The organization was at financial risk for excess care.

IDSs most often start with a hospital or a group practice as a foundation. Vertical integration characterizes them, as hospital and providers come together to offer more cost-effective care. In some cases, the care is managed through protocols or critical pathways, specifications of standard care with schedules and expectations regarding documentation. The organizations do not typically underwrite risk (they assume the risk that is underwritten in a formal insurance policy between beneficiary and insurer). Thus, they provide managed care, but are not what we have been referring to as managed care organizations. The latter are the traditional HMOs that have usually written formal insurance policies.

The distinctions are historical and increasingly anachronistic. All health care organizations are evolving toward vertical integration and toward assumption of risk. The rush to integration is especially strong where managed care organizations are dominant. This is especially true in California and Minnesota. In Minnesota, the Park Nicollet Group Practice and the Mayo Clinic both have moved quickly to integrate with hospitals to be in a position to assume risk for capitated payment. Meanwhile, the number of independent hospitals has fallen from thirteen to five in eleven years.[38] The Mullikin Group Practices in Southern California have taken similar courses, although the Mullikin IPA is not very different from the traditional managed care organization. These examples reinforce our prediction that both group practices and staff-model HMOs will move toward integrated delivery systems that can accommodate various arrangements between patients and providers (the so-called point-of-service plan).

Oversight of these emerging delivery systems is rather thin. The federal government has shown some interest in defining integrated delivery systems and has provided a good deal of scrutiny regarding their nonprofit tax exemption, as will be discussed in the next chapter. In at least two instances, the IRS has declared that there must be a 20 percent ceiling on physician representation on a foundation's board of directors.[39] In many cases, this will make it more difficult to organize integrated delivery systems, especially insofar as physician-dominated group practices are the primary motivating force. Both the IRS and the Office of the Inspector General are raising questions about the economic incentives provided under integrated delivery systems, an issue addressed in more detail in Chapter Five.[40] In many states, statutory law does not directly address the integrated system or medical foundation.[41] Only Minnesota and Iowa have rewritten insurance laws to address physician-hospital organizations, although more than two dozen other states have some kind of oversight of integrated delivery.[42]

The IDS, and the management of care that it brings, is in philosophical conflict with the traditional physician-focused practice of medicine. The system holds the risk and manages the doctor's practice on the basis of more effective protocols or guidelines. Driven by cost containment pressures, the IDS oversees utilization carefully.

The emergence of such systems adds a new dimension to our study of regulation and our search for new rules for quality. In a sense, the IDS internalizes the cost containment incentives that previously had been the domain of rate regulation and certificate of need. Another way to characterize the change is to say that a better-functioning market in medical care has emerged, cultivating the new systems through price competition. But this metamorphosis also gives rise to concerns that price competition could become too intense, leading to decrements in quality.

New rules to address such concerns could be a double-edged sword. On the one hand, they could dampen the market's overly aggressive price competition by assuring quality. On the other hand, they could be used by providers to shield themselves from appropriate competition.

Any-willing-provider laws are a good example of the double-edged sword. In theory, an any-willing-provider statute would require managed care organizations to admit into their provider networks any individual or institutional provider willing to meet a plan's financial and educational criteria. No state statute is quite this stringent, but many do make it difficult for managed care organizations to maintain a cohesive panel of practitioners. Some states allow managed care organizations to maintain reasonable selection criteria as long as these standards are openly published. Managed care organizations can also exclude geographically remote providers.

But other any-willing-provider statutes require notice to all providers of the opportunity to become network participants, creating large expenses and formidable obstacles for managed care organizations. Any-willing-provider statutes also create appeals structures based on rules of due process. Some statutes insist on patient freedom of choice, so that patients can see out-of-network providers, often with a cap at 20 percent of the costs of service. Also prominent is the any-willing-pharmacy provision, which protects small independent pharmacies from losing their customers to the large chains that dominate the managed care pharmaceutical market. At least twenty-seven states have one or more any-willing-provider provisions as part of their preferred provider/HMO enabling acts. Only two states, Maine and Wisconsin, appear to have authorized unrestrained selective contracting with preferred providers.[43] The any-willing-provider statutes are not new. All but two were enacted before 1988. Recently, more than a few have been materially amended, and many states are now considering emulating the more restrictive models.[44]

Among the more restrictive statutes are those in Texas, Utah, Montana, and Michigan. Texas requires an alternative delivery system to notify each licensed health care provider in a geographical area of his or her opportunity to participate in a plan. Notifications must be continued annually: providers "may apply for and shall be afforded fair, reasonable and equivalent opportunity to become pre-ferred providers."[45] Presumably, the any-willing-provider provision is intended to protect patients' freedom of choice, which is seen as a major quality issue under the Texas legislation.[46] The Michigan statute contains similar provisions regarding the initiation of an alternative delivery system, including specific procedures like writ-ten notification of all physicians in the pertinent geographical area.[47]

Other states have less severe legislation. Indiana, for instance, provides for open admission of providers who agree to the alterna-tive delivery system's terms—and those terms should not discrimi-nate unreasonably against or among providers. However, selection criteria can include price differentials and other economic charac-teristics.[48] New Hampshire law does not even mention the need for open submission or admission procedures.[49] In some states, such as Colorado, physicians and managed care organizations have reached a set of compromises on oversight of the organizations.[50]

The any-willing-provider laws are most probably an effort to turn the clock back on medical care. In the long run, such legisla-tion is not a workable solution to today's health care problems, but the concern that lies behind them must be recognized—namely, that management of care has the potential to produce ethical con-flicts as quality could suffer as cost containment is emphasized. Inte-grated and managed care plans may create incentives to provide low-cost care without sufficient attention to the welfare of the pa-tient. Limiting physician control is central to cost containment through managed care, but with these limits comes dilution of physician responsibility for the patient. Economic gains may loosen the moral bond between doctor and patient.[51]

In the past, as we have discussed, theory had it that the physi-cian's commitment to the patient ensured the provision of appro-priate care—care that meets the standard of the reasonable medical practitioner. Although research has demonstrated significant vari-ations among health plans in appropriateness and quality of care, the advocates of managed care and managed competition set forth the following benign scenario.[52]

Health plans will compete for contracts with employers and voluntary alliances. In this new health care system, the patient will become an informed consumer of medical care. Incentives to contain costs will be largely the result of market pressures. In addition, a great deal of data on the quality of care will be made available to consumers.[53] Consumers or their representatives will be able to review data on satisfaction, outcomes, and the like before selecting a health plan or a provider. The new health care system will therefore ensure that plans are accountable to patients for their costs, their services, and the quality of their care. Consumers will not select those plans that receive failing grades; those providers who fail will presumably undergo remedial education or drop out of the system. Health will be treated like any other commodity: consumers will make decisions informed by price and quality.

According to current wisdom, as a result of changes in the past twenty years, health care is now an industry with a variety of important institutional structures. There is much more opportunity for consistent application of scientific methods of quality improvement. Significant new methods of regulating for improvement will continue to present themselves. Perhaps more important, the notion of consumer information or report cards on plans and providers will take advantage of the advances made in quality measurement that were discussed in Chapter Three. With such information in hand, organized, integrated systems of care can undertake real quality improvement. We are therefore at the dawn of a new era in health care, with minimal regulation necessary.

As suggested earlier, this scenario has a darker side. The new framework shifts the focus from the professional-patient relationship to that between patient and health plan. It may be difficult to maintain the continuity of the caring relationship—a relationship that has been fundamental to the ethical integrity of the medical care system—if health plans are going to manage care aggressively and bring about cost savings. Nor will physicians as employees of health plans be able in every case to do what their clinical judgment dictates.[54] Of course, patients and doctors who want to follow the traditional path can choose a fee-for-service arrangement, but this will be more costly.

Neither any-willing-provider laws that destroy managed care nor physician-dominated networks fit well with the benign scenario. Consider the movement toward capitated care, or payment of an integrated medical group on a per capita basis. The insurer or other intermediary that collects premiums from beneficiaries simply passes the risk along to the integrated system. This changes physicians' incentives: rather than rendering all care necessary, they are motivated to render minimal care. Jacque Sokolov estimates that a fee-for-service system requires 35 to 50 primary care physicians and 175 specialists to provide care for 100,000 covered lives. The budget is $350 million. A capitated system needs only 50 primary care physicians and 50 specialists for the same population. The budget is $150 million.[55]

In the capitated plan, the savings are gained by placing the risk at the level of the provider. Utilization of all tests drops, specialist referrals wither, and aggressive hospital admission wanes. In a competitive market, the utilization slashing becomes ever more radical. The well-integrated plans are able to pass costs directly to the providers.

But where does cost reduction begin to affect quality? The capitated physician group may be liable for all utilization of outpatient tests and referrals. When will the profit motive begin to lead to inadequate diagnostic workups? Who will monitor the potential trade-offs between cost and quality?

In short, the scene may be set for significant quality problems. Consider the following example:

An integrated health plan employs physicians and other health professionals. The plan has average marks on a variety of quality measures, including patient satisfaction and health status. Yet these

measures do not identify failures to diagnose disease in the outpatient setting—failures considered secondary to the satisfaction of
new productivity requirements for primary care practitioners. What
is a health care professional to do? She can tell patients to seek
other plans, although that only helps the particular patients she in-
forms, and furthermore reduces the market share of the organization that employs her. Moreover, she might not consider it ethical
to leave the problem in place for the host of other patients in the
plan. Does the physician then assist the patient in bringing a federal action against the plan, or against the state government for cer-
tifying the plan? Health care quality may suffer unless new
mechanisms for addressing issues arising from the capitated plan
paradigm are identified.

Physician concerns about managed care are compelling. We do
not, however, advocate a return to the past. The weaknesses of the
traditional doctor-patient relationship have been well documented.[56] Patients should have the choice that occurs in a market
setting, and the professional relationship should be reshaped in a
manner that fits modern notions of patient autonomy.[57] But the
potential quality concerns must be addressed.

The American Medical Association has offered a comprehensive,
if quite conservative, answer to these questions, in the form of the
proposed Patient Protection Act of 1994.[58] The Patient Protection
Act would incorporate much of what is found in state any-
willing-provider laws, requiring managed care organizations to contract with any licensed provider who meets reasonable predetermined
standards. The act would rely on federal certification of managed care
plans. Managed care organizations would be required to provide
enrollees with all terms and conditions of the plan in easily understood, truthful, and objective terms. Physician credentialing within
the plans would also be subject to oversight, in particular the credentialing criteria based on economic factors such as the physician's
past expenditure per patient. Case mix, severity of patient illness, and
patient age adjustments would all have to be incorporated into such

credentialing. The same sort of scrutiny would be focused on utilization review programs. Finally, all enrollees in a health benefit plan would have to be offered a selection of plans, including at least one traditional fee-for-service plan. In addition, managed care plans would have to resemble point-of-service plans and there would be severe restrictions on the amount of copayment.

The proposed Patient Protection Act, again revised in 1995 and competing with Senator Paul Wellstone's proposed Health Quality and Fairness Act of 1995, represents an important effort to ensure that trade-offs between cost and quality under managed care programs do not injure patient care; it can also be characterized as a carefully crafted attempt by the medical profession to retain certain economic prerogatives at the expense of managed care organizations. Clearly, these discussions will continue as pressures for cost-effective care lead to new efforts to restrict providers' decision-making power and to remove expensive providers.

The latter is the issue in ongoing battles over "economic credentialing" in hospitals and at managed care organizations. Economic credentialing is simply a matter of retaining physicians who practice in a cost-effective manner and removing, or decredentialing, those who do not. Although the concept is old, legal battles over the ability of hospitals and managed care organizations to decredential have only just begun. Certain cases in the mid-1990s have suggested that the courts will be sympathetic to decredentialed physicians.[59]

Interest in the problem of limits on professional responsibility has also focused attention on the ownership of health plans. Relman has thoughtfully recommended several steps that would facilitate physician ownership and encourage not-for-profit models.[60] Though these suggestions have merit, physician ownership may not be the solution. Many of the problems noted earlier could recur in physician-owned plans, especially if only a few providers control the plan and are profit-driven. It is also unlikely that physicians can easily generate the capital necessary to initiate a plan. Finally, even if physician-owned plans solve some of the problems of a diminished doctor-patient relationship, ethical conflicts will persist in profit-driven plans.

The last portion of our three-part thesis about the need for new rules to regulate for improvement has now come into clearer focus. We have previously asserted that antagonism between regulators and regulated and failure of regulators to adapt to new methods of quality improvement have led to a perception that outdated techniques of regulators obstruct quality improvement. Our solution is to move away from hostility and efforts to capture, toward responsive regulation. The latter might entail the development of a theory of regulation for improvement.

That effort might have been sufficient for the traditional medical care system. But the traditional system is fading fast, replaced by an industry that presents a different set of challenges. New rules must address the potential conflicts between cost and quality that are inherent in managed care.

As patterns of health care delivery evolve, regulation of quality must do so as well. Since the early 1970s, the industry has moved well beyond the simple, traditional system. Individual providers, fee-for-service reimbursement, independent hospitals, and indemnity-based insurance have been replaced by a growing welter of managed care organizations. Insofar as these organizations affect and modify care practices, they also affect the quality of care.

Regulation is accommodating these new organizations slowly. States appear eager to increase patient and consumer information by requiring HMO reporting of care protocols and incentives for cost containment. The NCQA has suggested a course for responsive regulation, but unfortunately without yet addressing the need for punitive action should the regulated fail or dissemble. The notion of creative fulfillment of HEDIS criteria and the possibility of learning substantive improvement techniques are very encouraging. One suspects that the major prospect for improved quality oversight will be in the evolutionary development of institutions that regulate managed care organizations; this will provide the opportunity to avoid the mistakes made in the traditional system. It is necessary now to turn to that traditional system of regulation of quality, to see how it has evolved over the past twenty years.

Evolving Regulatory Institutions

Having reviewed the rise of quality improvement and the movement toward managed care, we return to the original structures of quality regulation introduced in Chapter Two. In particular, the JCAHO, PSROs, and tort law have all evolved under the influence of modern quality improvement and, to some extent, the emerging role of managed care. Most of this has been for the good—a movement in the direction of responsive regulation. But as we shall argue, new rules would require much greater change.

Joint Commission for Accreditation of Health Care Organizations

Many of the traditional review criteria of the JCAHO would be considered part of the "structure" of health care quality, as defined by Donabedian.[61] However, in the early 1970s, the JCAHO moved toward nonstructural measures, setting forth a series of systematic review procedures, and attempted to define thorough criteria for measuring the quality of care. These procedures were known as its *audit methodology*. Through the late 1970s, the JCAHO's medical audit criteria were refined and consolidated.[62] In addition, the JCAHO began to tighten up the relationship between clinical privileges and quality assurance by asking hospitals to delineate relevant quality assurance data in the granting of privileges to medical staff.

The JCAHO itself, however, acknowledged that many of these audit measurements were merely paper exercises undertaken for the sake of meeting basic requirements.[63] In 1979, the commission eliminated numerical audit requirements and instead asked hospitals to undertake integrated quality assessment activities. However, the shift toward a systematic quality assessment process did not apparently change hospital perception of the JCAHO as an external regulator performing inspections in hospitals. (This is perhaps paradoxical in view of the JCAHO's beginnings as a physician- and surgeon-dominated institution.) The commission's emphasis on targeting "bad care" and on using punishment or corrective actions as the major responses to such care, as well as physician presumption that mistakes are not the rule, contributed to a negative image of the JCAHO in the eyes of providers. As one commentator observed, "Not surprisingly external QA/PR (quality assessment/ performance review) systems tend to be loathed and deeply resented by the vast majority of practitioners, who perceive themselves as committed high quality practitioners."[64]

In 1985, Dennis O'Leary became president of the JCAHO. He was committed to changing both the methodology of the commission and provider perceptions. O'Leary's initiative became known as the "Agenda for Change."[65] The Agenda for Change intended to modernize the accreditation process in three ways. First, reasonable standards would be retained and new ones designed. Second, the JCAHO would demand evidence that the effect of these standards was being monitored and evaluated by hospitals. Finally, hospitals had to take steps to convert this information into real improvements in quality.

Of course, these changes were not easily brought about in a system that relied on an experienced staff of surveyors constantly on the road, visiting hospitals. O'Leary and others admitted that they had underestimated the challenges of implementing the Agenda for Change, and that the program's goals would not be attained in the three to four years that had been projected.[66] However, the JCAHO remains fully committed to moving from quality assurance to quality improvement, embracing the Total Quality Management philosophy.

The JCAHO's first recommendation was for hospitals to break down their simplistic organization. Instead of thinking of various "boxes"—one for the medical staff, one for dietary administration, and so on—the hospital was advised to think in terms of organizational tasks (like patron rights or infection control). Once these tasks were identified, key steps for improving care could be determined. In turn, a system of evaluation of the key functions could be designed, making use of an appropriate data base. The proposed regrouping would require strong leadership and a commitment to quality improvement from the top down.

In the 1990s, this agenda has meant rapid change in the accreditation manual for hospitals. Whereas in 1991 there were just a few changes, in 1992 about 25 percent of the standards were deleted and new ones added.[67] The revisions were intended to hasten the functional approach to quality assessment and improvement. In addition, the JCAHO committed to designing performance indicators. A new survey process was promised in the near future.[68] The commission also endorsed the use of practice guidelines as a method for providing more appropriate and better-quality care.

By late 1993, the JCAHO had begun to shift a great deal of its emphasis to outcome measures. In May of that year, its board of commissioners approved policies that would lead to measurement of provider performance and public dissemination of such information.[69] The JCAHO had been working since 1986 on an evaluation system, one component of which was the Indicator Measurement System (IMSystem). The IMSystem consists of a number of sentinel events and aggregate data indicators that are associated with quality of care. For example, the system computes cesarean sections per live births and central-line infections per days of central-lines use. A limited group of health care organizations evaluated the indicators in an alpha testing period in the early 1980s. In 1992 and 1993, several hundred organizations used the indicators in a beta testing phase. This phase was intended to indicate the capability of the JCAHO to analyze data, the ability of health care organizations to gather the data and then to integrate the indicators into their monitoring activities, and the reliability of the data elements.[70]

In 1994, the JCAHO announced that it planned to require

accredited hospitals to participate in the system by 1996. Essentially, hospitals were to transmit information to the JCAHO, which would process the data and provide feedback. The JCAHO maintained that it was important for all accredited hospitals to participate, for the sake of consistency and fairness to individual institutions. The commission was convinced that the benchmarking data would be helpful to hospitals' quality improvement processes. Furthermore, breaking with past confidentiality, the JCAHO decided to publicly release organization-specific data on accreditation visits. Thus the commission has struggled to make its surveys more responsive to providers and to develop measures with greater face validity. It has also reaffirmed the relevance of its survey process as a source of information that consumers may want to draw on.

The parallel to the evolution of peer review organizations, discussed in the next section, is striking. The JCAHO, long wedded to the inspection model of accreditation, has wholly endorsed the outcomes movement and attempted to provide feedback to organizations that can be used to make real improvements in the quality of care. This is the theme of quality assurance and quality improvement efforts in the mid-1990s—one that, as the rest of this chapter will show, is repeated under other regulatory formats. In O'Leary's words, "Report card day is coming."[71]

However, many hospitals were not happy with the JCAHO's agenda. Hospitals balked at the financial requirements of the IMSystem, citing deficiencies in their computer systems that made it difficult to participate. They argued that the process of providing the data has been time-consuming and perhaps counterproductive.[72] Indeed, some reports suggest there was a major revolution under way within the hospital industry against the JCAHO's mandate.[73] In early 1995, the American Hospital Association demanded action by the JCAHO on a series of reform measures, with the implied threat that the hospital industry could seek accreditation elsewhere.

The JCAHO hired several public relations firms to try to change the hospital industry's opinion about the Agenda for Change generally and the IMSystem in particular. But these efforts did not slow the rate of hospital withdrawal from beta site participation.[74] Many hospitals were upset that there did not seem to be a linkage between the IMSystem indicators and quality of care improvement. Moreover, other indicator sets were now available. For example, more than 750 hospitals were voluntarily using the Maryland Hospital Association indicator set in the summer of 1994.

It would seem, then, that the JCAHO's efforts at joining the outcome measurement movement have been frustrated by ongoing perceptions of a narrow inspection focus and punitive authority. One must therefore question whether the JCAHO will survive as the traditional regulator of hospitals in a changing health care market. Though the commission's financial health has remained quite vigorous, mandatory accreditation may become an anachronism.

But perhaps this assessment is overly gloomy. The JCAHO has been tremendously successful in moving away from its punitive inspection model. Ongoing liaison, more flexible standards, and an orientation toward understanding how institutions can best position themselves for improvement all suggest a sea change in the organization's self-concept. An observer gets a sense that at least the leadership of the JCAHO, and increasingly the surveyors themselves, want hospitals to comply creatively.

In the sunshine of public scrutiny of hospital results, consumers may find it easier to make informed choices. In the spring of 1995, the JCAHO was actively seeking competitors in the field of accreditation.[75] The next decade will be critical for the commission as it struggles to become a responsive regulator.

The Peer Review Organizations

In 1982, the Reagan administration had decided to eliminate the professional standards review organizations, but some members of Congress managed to stave off the inevitable temporarily. In October 1983, the advent of the prospective payment system for Medicare payment of hospitals through the diagnosis related groups system finally sounded the death knell for PSROs. The Tax Equity and Fiscal Responsibility Act (TEFRA) abolished the PSROs and replaced them with Peer Review Organizations (PROs), intending more effective and leaner regulation.[76] Under TEFRA, the 195 PSRO regents were reduced to 54 territory or statewide programs.[77] Biennial and triennial contracts were awarded to PROs by competitive bidding. Those found to be ineffective would be terminated by the Department of Health and Human Services.

The PRO program was less controlled by physicians than the PSROs had been. The Department of Health and Human Services was required to offer PRO contracts initially to physician-sponsored organizations but could turn to insurance companies or other fiscal intermediaries if the initial contractors proved to be ineffective. Moreover, the PROs were no longer allowed to delegate review responsibilities to hospitals before a review. New powers were given to the PROs for sanctioning physicians and denying payment authority.[78] The PROs were also exempted from Freedom of Information Act reporting requirements. In many ways then, the PRO program represented a swing of the pendulum away from self-regulation. If anything, the structure of the PRO program seemed to highlight potential antagonisms with physicians.

The health policy backdrop to the PRO program was perhaps even more important than the structural changes. The federal government had decided to reduce health care costs and to rely, in the Medicare program, on a prospective payment system based on diagnostic groups. The prediction was that excessive length of stay would cease to be a problem, and this has generally proved to be the case. The PROs were thus expected to be much less attentive to concurrent review and more interested in appropriateness of hospitalization and quality of care. Indeed, PRO program officers have come to characterize quality of care as their primary concern.[79]

This quality review function was built into the PRO enabling legislation by the Social Security Act Amendments of 1983. The House bill for the Social Security Amendments had included explicit provisions requiring PROs to monitor hospital admissions, in part to "review admissions and discharge practices and quality of care."[80] The conference agreement between the House and the Senate struck this provision, but did include PRO authority to review patterns of admissions and quality of care when this was deemed necessary. Had House provisions taken root, it is possible that the PROs might have moved in the direction of institution-based analyses of the quality of care in the mid-1980s.

Unfortunately, little effort had been made to address the criteria by which PROs would review medical records. Without a systematic basis for gathering and analyzing data from hospitals, a rigorous, modern strategy based on quality improvement proved impossible. Moreover, an initiative that includes sanctioning authority must provide evidence that sanctions have been applied to be considered successful; but as has been shown, overemphasis on sanctions and inspections frustrates real reform. By the mid-1980s, commentators were suggesting a strong possibility that the PROs would be hampered by inaccurate and incomplete discharge data and would also suffer from the emphasis on individual cases that might lead to sanctions.[81]

Somewhat surprisingly, Congress took some halting steps to address these concerns. The Budget Reconciliation Act of 1986 had the important effect of expanding PRO review of early readmissions, considering them signals of possible poor care in the previous inpatient hospitalization.[82] In addition, the act required each PRO to devote a reasonable proportion of its time to systematic reviews of quality of care.[83] Both of these changes had the effect of shifting PRO attention from individual sanctions to systematic analysis. However, the 1986 act also required PROs to review all written complaints by beneficiaries about quality of services. A further provision was that before declaring a physician's care to have been substandard, the PRO had to provide him or her with reasonable notice and opportunity for discussion. The latter points clearly emphasized sanctions; the former a more modern analysis of quality. This bifurcated strategy for the PROs was further extended by the Medicare and Medicaid Patient and Program Protection Act of 1987, which emphasized protection of patients from incompetent practitioners and inadequate care.[84]

The PRO sanctioning authority slowly became more expansive. If a PRO determined that a health care practitioner failed to comply with obligations regarding appropriate and high-quality care, it was required to notify the physician in writing and state the sanction it recommended. The physician then had an opportunity to respond, either in writing or at a meeting with the PRO. If the PRO continued to believe that the doctor had violated Medicare standards, a report and a sanction recommendation were made to the Office of the Inspector General of the Department of Health and Human Services. That office would then determine whether the PRO had properly followed procedure, whether a violation had occurred, and whether the practitioner lacked the ability to substantially comply with obligations. Physicians dissatisfied with the imposition of a sanction could request an evidentiary hearing before an administrative law judge. Further levels of appeal included the departmental appeals council and the federal district court. Sanctions included nonpayment for services, fines, and exclusion from the Medicare program. The PROs' use of their authority produced a great deal of litigation.[85]

The effect of PRO sanctions on the overall quality of health care was and is unknown. We have every reason to believe, however, that it is weak and very wasteful. In conflating the institutional analysis of quality with sanctioning authority over physicians, the PRO meets the same problems that plague medical malpractice litigation—at least with regard to its role as a promoter of quality improvement. Isolated events are simply not as helpful for quality improvement as is systematic analysis. It is widely held by advocates of Continuous Quality Improvement that the inspector role, if overplayed, can impede true improvement efforts. The PRO, insofar as it produces sanctions against individual physicians, falls into this trap. It is impossible for physicians to cooperate with and promote the PRO process when the search for "bad apples" is the mainstay of PRO strategy.

In the mid-1990s, this situation may be changing somewhat. The PROs have taken several steps toward gathering more satisfactory utilization and quality data, which may in the future provide the basis for true industrial-style investigations of care. During successive contract cycles, the screening criteria and the shape of PRO activities have traditionally been restructured in the so-called *scope of work*. The scope of work was essentially the contract between the Department of Health and Human Services and individual PROs. Under the third scope of work, established in 1988, the PROs were to review a 3 percent random sample of all discharges, 50 percent of transfer cases, 25 percent of all readmissions within thirty-one days, and certain percentages of cases within specific problem DRGs (diagnostic related groups). If there were errors in more than 5 percent of cases in any one category, the PRO was to boost its review— to 100 percent of cases if necessary. In addition, the PROs were to launch new community outreach efforts, including establishment of beneficiary hotlines. They were also to review outpatient care rendered between two hospital stays where the second admission was within thirty-one days of the original one. This scope of work reflected PRO priorities and an epidemiological strategy for uncovering poor care.

The PROs have also been active in promoting new patterns of review, in particular those that can be accomplished through a computerized system. For example, the Uniform Clinical Data Set (UCDS) initiative was introduced in the late 1980s. Pilot-tested in seven PROs, the UCDS collected up to 1,600 data elements on each case, including vital signs at admission and discharge, medications, laboratory findings, treatment details, and socioeconomic information. These data elements were then put through a set of computer algorithms in order to identify particular quality problems. The Health Care Financing Administration (HCFA), which oversees the PRO program, had wanted all PROs to be using the UCDS by 1993. By 1992, however, it had decided to completely overhaul the program, launching the Health Care Quality Improvement Initiative (HCQII).

The HCQII was outlined in an influential article in the *Journal of the American Medical Association* by Stephen F. Jencks, the key methodologist at the HCFA, and Gail R. Wilensky, the HCFA administrator in the Bush administration.[86] Citing the importance of variations research such as that completed by Wennberg, Chassin, Hannan, Williams, and others, as well as some of the present authors' writing on the importance of quality improvement and Total Quality Management in medical care, Jencks and Wilensky suggested that the PROs would move from policing individual providers to supplying information on quality.

In particular, the PROs would use nationally uniform criteria to examine patterns of care, rather than having clinicians apply essentially intuitive local criteria to look for problems. Second, the PROs would emphasize persistent differences between observed and achievable care and de-emphasize occasional, unusual deficiencies. Third, the PROs would work with providers, demonstrating problems with care and allowing the individual providers to conduct detailed reviews. Clearly then, the HCQII program intended to take advantage of Continuous Quality Improvement strategies and forgo the inquisitional focus that had informed the PRO and PSRO programs.

Jencks and Wilensky suggested that two data systems could provide the backbone for the HCQII. The first was the National Claims History File, which contained information on all financial claims paid by the HCFA. This file was composed of more than one billion line items per year. It would be supplemented by a slightly scaled-down version of the UCDS. The UCDS itself was to be converted from its former use as a screen for physician reviews to a data base for monitoring care and the risk-adjusted outcomes (as discussed in Chapter Three). In this way, the UCDS would support the Patient Care Algorithm System (PCAS), which was designed to apply decision rules to certain methods of care and to monitor compliance with algorithms. In 1992, Jencks and Wilensky disclosed that an American Medical Association work group had been reviewing these algorithms for clinical validity. The PCAS, based on the UCDS and supplemented by outcomes as measured through the National Claims History File, would make the HCQII a reality, not a mere acronymic nightmare.

The grand scheme involved development of completely new skills for the PROs through a series of pilot projects and a formal curriculum. Most important, the PROs were to formulate projects with local hospitals and train the hospitals' medical staffs in pattern analysis. This may strike the reader as very similar to the activities planned by the JCAHO, and Jencks and Wilensky allow that "some synergy appears logical."[87]

To gain more detailed information, the HCFA had planned to concentrate on cardiovascular disease. A six-point plan was drawn up, providing for:

1. Careful abstraction of discharges

2. Development of risk-adjustment methods

3. Conversion of guidelines into PCAS algorithms

4. Analysis of patterns of care using risk-adjusted outcomes

5. Work with physician groups to understand the use of guidelines

6. Intervention projects for particular hospitals

These ambitious plans have only partly materialized, and we review them in detail not to suggest that they are a solution to PRO weaknesses but to indicate the shift in the way regulators are framing the questions.[88] The emphasis on working with hospitals and using data was new and in many ways revolutionary.

With the election of President Clinton, the departure of Wilensky, the appointment of Bruce Vladeck as head of the HCFA, and the emphasis on health care reform, some of the PRO projects have been lost in the shuffle. Nonetheless, in 1993, the HCFA proceeded with the fourth scope of work, in which attention was to shift from identification of individual problem cases to identification of patterns of concern. The number of full reviews was reduced, but more focused reviews were to occur. Cooperative ventures between the PROs and health care providers were encouraged, including development of joint action plans.

The evolution of the PRO program is quite interesting. There has been a recognition that the traditional activities of the PROs were wasteful and often inappropriate, and that the only rational course will be to develop hospital-specific data that can then be used by physicians to plan quality improvement strategies. However, it remains to be seen whether or not the PROs themselves can bring about the kind of cooperation necessary to improve the quality of care. Their efforts at collecting data, analyzing it, and feeding it back to institutions have not yet transformed them into an effective quality improvement resource. Indeed, the sanctioning functions of the PRO program are still its most important undertaking, and they work against its role as a promoter of better-quality hospital care.[89]

The federal government is clearly searching for new answers. Despite ongoing difficulties, the overall indications are favorable. The shift is toward something that looks like responsive regulation, with greater cooperation and emphasis on learning. Like the JCAHO, the PRO program administrators appear to have been influenced by the modern quality movement's suspicion of inspection and endorsement of teamwork. The PRO program's interest in systems of care is symptomatic of a new way of thinking about quality, one we can only hope will grow.

Tort Law and Medical Malpractice

In Chapter Two, we followed the progress of medical malpractice through the mid-1970s. From 1974 through 1994, rates of litigation varied sinusoidally, but average costs, or severity, of claims continued to rise. The past twenty years have been marked by slow but profound changes in the structure of the health care industry. However, the basic conceptual framework, that of individual physician responsibility for substandard care that leads to injury, has changed very little since the mid-1940s. Only the most recently suggested reform (enterprise liability) holds promise for integration with quality improvement efforts. However, as elsewhere, the potential promises of this regulation have been confused by increasing federal preemption of what have previously been state issues.

As noted in Chapter Two, although there was steady inflation of malpractice claims and premiums from the mid-1960s, neither individual practitioners nor the government showed much concern until the early 1970s. In 1972, the federal government performed a significant study of malpractice litigation that suggested there was little cause for concern about dislocation in the markets from medical liability insurance. But by the mid-1970s, claims rates were mounting.[90] The inability of actuaries to calculate reasonable premiums with this unpredicted increase in claims led many commercial insurers to leave the field. In several states, physicians were unable to obtain medical malpractice insurance, and states reacted by cobbling together so-called "joint underwriting associations," quasi-governmental sources of insurance against medical malpractice liability. One prevalent strategy was for large hospitals or groups of hospitals to self-insure. Another outgrowth of the 1970s crisis was the effort by a number of medical societies to set up their own physician-owned insurance companies, which are now affiliated in the Physician Insurance Association of America.

In short, the mid-1970s crisis provoked changes in the insurance markets that are still in effect today. In the mid-1990s, one finds in most jurisdictions that physicians are insured by physician-owned firms, and that hospitals are either purchasing insurance or self-insuring. These arrangements often lead to double representation in claims brought against physicians and hospitals.

In addition to this reorganization of the liability insurance industry, the crisis of the mid-1970s gave rise to the now well-established practice of physicians and their insurers seeking tort reform in state capitols. Although its somewhat neutral moniker would suggest otherwise, tort reform is chiefly an effort by chronic defendants to obtain changes in law that will make it more difficult for plaintiffs to bring claims. Tort reform intends to make claims less valuable for the plaintiff's attorney, the critical economic player in medical malpractice litigation.

Reform in the mid-1970s involved several strategies. The most direct method was simply to reduce attorney fees. For instance, in the 1975 California reforms that served as a model for other states for the next twenty years, attorney fees were fixed at 40 percent of the first $50,000 recovered; 33⅓ percent of the next $50,000; 25 percent of the next $500,000; and 15 percent of any amount beyond $600,000. Other populous states, such as New Jersey and New York in 1976, enacted similar reforms.[91]

Another rule having similar impact was the *collateral source offset*. The collateral source rule was a common law doctrine that prohibited defendants from submitting evidence regarding compensation or reimbursement to a patient for any costs associated with an injury. Some states simply overturned the collateral source rule; others, such as California, created a discretionary offset. Less populous states—for example, Alaska, Idaho, and Nebraska—held that any collateral benefits would be subtracted from judgments rendered.[92] Again, this decreases the income that can be drawn from a case by the plaintiff's attorney, as that income is determined by a percentage of the award to the injured patient.

One more variation on this theme was to require periodic payments. A plaintiff's attorney would normally expect to receive payment at the time that a claim is disposed, as all of his or her costs have occurred up to that point. Periodic payment postpones disbursement to the injured plaintiff, doling the money out as is necessary for future medical care, household production losses, lost earnings, and pain and suffering. The absence of a lump sum makes it much more difficult for the plaintiff's attorney to recover full cost. Again, California led the way in the mid-1970s, requiring mandatory periodic payment of future damages when the award was in excess of $50,000. A few other states followed suit.[93]

A number of other measures often accompanied these more important initiatives in tort reform.[94] As a result, as Paul Weiler has reported, claims rates and premiums leveled off in the late 1970s and early 1980s.[95] But tort reform does not necessarily promote better-quality care; just the opposite may be true. Insofar as these reforms reduced claims rates, they also reduced the deterrent effect associated with malpractice litigation, in theory thereby increasing the number of medical injuries due to substandard care.

Some might argue that to the extent that it reduces the anger and emotional suffering that characterize physician attitudes toward medical malpractice, tort reform may induce the profession to undertake more thoroughgoing quality improvement efforts. However, there is no empirical basis for this suggestion, and even the conceptual argument does not seem strong. Of course, there is also little empirical evidence of a deterrent effect associated with tort litigation. The theory of deterrence would have it that increased malpractice claims create economic incentives that in turn lead to reduced rates of medical injury. Most of the evidence on this issue derives from the Harvard Medical Practice Study. Though some publications from that study, including some coauthored by Troyen Brennan, have suggested that there may be a deterrent effect, in the final analysis, there is no statistically significant evidence of deterrence. Therefore the entire role of malpractice in the regulation of the quality of care must be assessed.

In any case, claims rates again began to rise in the mid-1980s. This led to greater proliferation of the tort reforms discussed above, as many more states enacted mandatory collateral source offsets, screening panels, mandatory periodic payment, and changes in attorney fees. More states also began simply to cap awards, again using California's example. In 1975, the California legislature had put a cap of $250,000 on noneconomic damages, a provision that was subsequently found to be constitutional. During the same year, Indiana limited recovery for any injury or death of a patient to $500,000.[96] These efforts to limit or cap total awards were little emulated until the crisis of the mid-1980s; between 1985 and 1987, another twenty-one states adopted such caps.[97]

Once in place in almost fifty states, various packages of tort reform had significant effect. Epidemiological studies have demonstrated that changes in liability rules are associated with deflation in claims rates and premiums.[98] At an aggregate level, claims rates across the country showed significant deflation, with overall claims per one hundred physicians per year decreasing from a high of nearly seventeen in 1987 to a low of eleven in 1991.[99]

The success of tort reform has been the dominant story in malpractice litigation over the past twenty years. It continues unabated in the mid-1990s. Indeed, a great deal of the debate in Washington over health care reform surrounds the role of the federal government in malpractice law. Since the late 1980s, physician organizations have sought to have restrictive tort reform along the lines of California's path-breaking 1975 legislation passed at the federal level. A federal bill would preempt more permissive state laws and give all physicians the presumed benefits now enjoyed by California physicians.[100] Reforms of this nature were included in nearly every major proposal considered by the 103rd Congress, with the Clinton administration advocating a slightly less restrictive package than Senate Republicans. Again in the 104th Congress, tort reform is being debated.

The commitment to tort reform, both at the state and at the federal level, is difficult to understand in light of the available empirical evidence on medical injury and malpractice litigation. Research studies suggest that medical injuries are very common, leading to extraordinary levels of disability and even death.[101] However, only one in seven of negligent medical injuries gives rise to a medical malpractice claim. Hence one can hardly make a case that there is overclaiming by injured patients. Though research reveals that many claims are brought in cases in which there is no negligence or injury, other evidence suggests that the medical malpractice system does a relatively good job of distinguishing meritorious and nonmeritorious claims.[102] With most of the enormous costs of injury now borne by health insurers and disability insurers, one could imagine that the country's reaction might be to increase malpractice litigation rather than restrict it.

But this conundrum simply emphasizes the fundamentally peculiar role that malpractice litigation plays in health care. Physicians are so emotionally devastated when they are sued that professional organizations tend to make reduction of malpractice litigation a primary policy goal. The suffering described by physicians, both in their responses to specific questions and in the language they use to describe the system of malpractice litigation,[103] is far out of proportion to any financial repercussions of a suit. The greater part of academic legal analysis of tort law focuses on financial incentives, but in malpractice cases, the emotional impact appears to be even greater.

In fact, most physicians do not understand malpractice litigation as part of the overall system of quality improvement or as a remedy for social concerns about prevalence of medical injuries. Instead, they continue to approach medical injury, and the much less frequent malpractice claim, as a random event, a "bolt of lightning." In most cases, risk management, or coping with claims after an injury has occurred, is distinguished both organizationally and conceptually from any efforts at quality assurance or quality improvement. Malpractice has been carefully fenced off from rational quality assurance that physicians or hospitals might undertake. That is why quality improvement and malpractice litigation, even in the academic literature, are so rarely mentioned in the same breath. It should therefore not be surprising that modern efforts at quality improvement have rarely infiltrated medical malpractice and risk management. Risk management continues to emphasize better communication and prevention of patient dissatisfaction.[104] But there are some signs that malpractice litigation, which quite clearly is a regulatory influence on the health care industry, may be able to accommodate Total Quality Management. To understand how, it is necessary to backtrack slightly to discuss one other area of doctrinal change in malpractice law.

Under traditional medical malpractice law, the physician was the sole target of liability. Doctrines of the fellow servant and of charitable immunity made it difficult to sue nurses and hospitals. These points of law, however, eventually fell into desuetude.[105] More important, the tort doctrines of *apparent* and *ostensible authority*, subsets of the more generic concept of *agency liability*, slowly made their way into malpractice litigation. In most of tort law, employers are liable for the negligence of their employees. As most physicians are independent contractors with hospitals, agency liability is not applicable. However, in cases of negligence by physicians who bear a closer relationship to the hospital—for instance, physicians employed in emergency departments or as radiologists, anesthesiologists, or pathologists—it is possible, through an apparent or ostensible authority doctrine, to hold the hospital liable.[106]

In holding a hospital liable, one begins to treat malpractice not as the individual moral fault of a particular physician but as a systemic issue to be addressed by the organization. Once the move is made from individual liability to organizational liability, the potential for use of modern methods of quality improvement is open. Presumably, for instance, a hospital would be able to evaluate its risk for medical injuries, an analysis that is radically different from an individual physician's inquiries into aspects of isolated cases. Tort litigation can be transformed into rational regulatory incentives when the frame of reference is deficiencies in repetitive processes of care. The shift is from individual instances to analysis of the system as a whole.

Unfortunately, ostensible or apparent authority only reaches certain areas of the hospital, such as the radiology suite and the emergency department. More important, it relies on the legal assumption that patients cannot distinguish the hospital itself from certain employees.[107] Hospitals could avoid liability if, for example, they made efforts to clearly identify emergency room physicians as independent contractors.

Another pathway to hospital liability is the principle of *corporate liability*. First enunciated—though perhaps as an aside by the court—in the case of *Darling v. Charleston Community Memorial Hospital*, corporate liability makes hospitals responsible for the actions of physicians it has credentialed.[108] It thus draws the hospital's credentialing responsibilities into the malpractice arena. The problem, however, from the point of view of increasing hospital liability and perhaps bringing about rational deterrence, is that the hospital is liable only insofar as it is negligent in the credentialing process. This is not always easy to prove, and in many cases, courts would prefer to have peer review information remain confidential.[109] As a result, pure hospital liability is rare. Indeed, only one court has moved beyond ostensible authority and corporate liability to find a nondelegable responsibility for practitioners on the part of hospitals, that being the Alaska Supreme Court in the case of *Jackson v. Power*, another emergency department case.[110]

The fact that the common law has tarried at the doorstep of hospital responsibility for medical injuries has not chilled the interest of some academic observers in full-blown *enterprise liability* in medical care. Enterprise liability would involve making hospitals or other institutions assume all the liability for medical malpractice. Independent physician liability would disappear, and physicians would pay surcharges to hospitals for the costs of defending and compensating claims. The theoretical advantages of enterprise liability for better quality of care have been noted by several commentators.[111] They rely on careful empirical research, such as that completed by Ann Barry Flood, that shows greater correlation between institutional characteristics and some soft measures of quality of care than found between those measures and individual practitioner characteristics.[112] This research allows us to hypothesize that the hospital enterprise, if charged with all payment of malpractice claims, would attempt to understand the risks for medical injury and address them rationally at a systemic level. More careful credentialing might be a simple answer for hospitals, but ideally, enterprise liability would move far beyond that response toward encouraging better management of processes and services.

Here the work of Laura Petersen and Anne O'Neil is pertinent. They have evaluated the incidence of medical injuries, and the proportion that are preventable, in the medical service of a single teaching hospital. Using epidemiological methods, they have shown that medical injuries are associated with coverage schedules of physicians: when the primary physician is out of the hospital, more preventable injuries tend to occur. By putting a new computer program into place to assist physicians in signing out their patients, Petersen and O'Neil have eliminated the risk associated with cross-coverage and have decreased the incidence of preventable medical injuries overall. Before this epidemiological study was done, there was no specific evidence that any of the individual medical injuries were preventable by a managerial intervention in a process of care. Petersen and O'Neil's research demonstrates a productive merger of epidemiology, Total Quality Management, and medical injury investigation. The focus is on processes of care and appropriate incentives, not on individual physician liability and mistakes.[113] Thus a form of non-value-added regulation, malpractice litigation, holds the promise of becoming something that really adds value: an incentive structure for quality improvement emphasizing systemic causes of medical injuries.[114]

But the promise of enterprise liability has been clouded by developments elsewhere in medical malpractice law. If one accepts that liability must be spread to the organizational level, then it makes sense to include in the definition of "organization" managed care organizations and independent utilization reviewers as well as hospitals. Indeed, unlike enterprise liability, which is completely theoretical at this point (except, perhaps, in Alaska), liability for utilization reviewers and managed care organizations has been explored on numerous occasions in the courts, which have proved to be quite uninterested in organizational liability.

The issue has been most fully developed in the area of utilization review. In the mid-1980s, Lois Wickline, who had suffered a vascular injury as a result of what she claimed was premature discharge from a hospital, sued the California Medical Assistance Program (MediCal) for failure to allow her to stay in the hospital an additional few days.[115] A jury found MediCal liable, but the California Court of Appeals reversed the decision. Nonetheless, the court's opinion allowed that liability might be found on a different set of facts, leading many commentators to believe that an impending tidal wave of litigation could overwhelm utilization reviewers.[116] However, no new cases were reported for four years, until the same California court published its decision in the case of *Wilson* v. *Blue Cross of Southern California*.[117] The plaintiff's psychiatrist had recommended a three-to-four-week stay in an inpatient facility, but utilization management refused to allow further payment after ten days. Wilson was discharged and subsequently committed suicide. His parents brought suit against the utilization management firm, the hospital, and the insurance company, but the trial court found none of the three liable under summary judgment. The California Court of Appeals reversed this ruling, indicating that there obviously was negligent utilization review. However, the court provided no clear standard for determining where provider responsibility ended and utilization reviewer liability might begin. Few other similar lawsuits have been reported.

The failure of other common law courts to follow the *Wickline* and *Wilson* cases seems to suggest that judges are at this point unwilling to move away from physician-centric liability and to consider the responsibility of various institutions in the quality of care. The interrelatedness of cost containment and quality of care cannot logically be overlooked, but the courts seem to be loath to encumber cost containment activities, in this case utilization review, with significant liability.[118] As will be shown in Chapter Five, the effect of federal law is making it even more difficult to reach utilization reviewers as defendants.

We have suggested that as the health care system matures, integrated health plans, including providers, hospitals, nursing homes, and to some extent insurance capitation payment, will become the rule. These organizations will be able to take risk for covered lives directly and offer a variety of managed care products, such as staff-model HMOs, preferred provider organizations, and point-of-service plans. The traditional troika of physician, hospital, and insurance company will be vertically integrated into a tight delivery system. We further expect that local markets will be oligopolistic, with a few such delivery systems providing most of the care. One might expect that these integrated delivery systems would become the target of malpractice suits. Indeed, some advocates of enterprise liability have already concluded that the managed care organization or the integrated delivery system should be the enterprise that assumes sole liability.[119] But in reality, organizational liability in managed care—predominantly liability of HMOs—remains rather thin, as courts have proved reluctant to assign liability outside the doctor-patient relationship.

Most of the suits that HMOs have faced concern indistinct plan terms. Patients sue when services they thought were covered turn out not to be part of the conditions of coverage. Often, prior approval is a critical issue.[120] Recently, this issue has been the subject of great publicity following the decision in *Fox v. Health Net*, where a jury awarded $12.1 million in compensatory damages and $77 million in punitive damages to Nelene Fox after Health Net of Woodlawn Hills, an HMO, refused to pay for an expensive therapy for Fox's breast cancer.[121] This therapy, bone marrow transplant with high-dose chemotherapy, had been the subject of litigation in the past, but in this case the jury found that Health Net's refusal constituted a breach of contract and resulted in reckless infliction of emotional distress. These kinds of cases have been greatly affected by the impact of preemption under the Employee Retirement Income Security Act (ERISA), a subject addressed in Chapter Five.[122]

HMO liability for the negligence of physicians or health care provision (as opposed to coverage decisions) turns on many of the same principles that were discussed in connection with the development of corporate negligence for hospitals.[123] Vicarious liability is most easily found in a staff-model HMO where physicians are under direct contract with the HMO.[124] Other courts have been willing to find an IPA-model HMO liable, especially if most services are provided to the subscriber on the HMO premises and the professional association is paid on a per capita fee basis as opposed to fee-for-service.[125] Courts have also used the notions of ostensible agency, holding that the HMO physicians are the ostensible agents of the HMO.[126] These cases depend to a large degree on marketing materials and referral practices that would provide evidence of ostensible agency. Yet another pathway for liability, again paralleling the hospital context, is the concept of negligent retention of physicians on an HMO panel.[127] Yet none of these situations has provided the grounds for a court to find absolute enterprise liability for an HMO.[128] And as will be shown, federal law threatens to immunize managed care organizations rather completely from the claims of state tort law. The integration of more modern notions of quality improvement with malpractice through enterprise liability thus remains a somewhat distant goal.

One place where there appears to be a glimmer of hope for the project of converting the medical malpractice threat into a quality-improving signal is in the movement toward practice guidelines, a subject discussed briefly in the last chapter. Practice guidelines are "systematically developed statements to assist practitioners in patient decisions about appropriate health care for specific clinical circumstances."[129] The federal government has been very actively promoting the use of practice guidelines in health care, largely because they are intended to address both poor-quality care and inappropriate care. As noted in Chapter Three, the guidelines movement has been given impetus by health services researchers like Jack Wennberg and Robert Brook, who have demonstrated that there are significant rates of inappropriate use of health care services.[130] First discussed only in the late 1980s, the development of practice guidelines has today become a major industry among clinical subspecialty societies, and the federal Agency for Health Care Policy Research is committed to the development and promulgation of literally dozens of practice guidelines through 1999.

Because they specify a standard of care, practice guidelines bear a natural relationship to malpractice litigation. This was quickly recognized by experts in health law, who predicted that practice guidelines would be used by malpractice litigants for evidentiary purposes.[131] In fact, one can argue that practice guidelines may help to rationalize malpractice litigation by providing courts with the kind of impartial evidence necessary to make determinations of negligence. Moreover, the incentive of avoiding malpractice litigation may lead more physicians to comply with practice guidelines.[132] Ideally, guidelines and malpractice litigation will be mutually reinforcing.

Recent empirical evidence suggests that guidelines are indeed being integrated into malpractice litigation and are influencing plaintiffs' attorneys.[133] An attorney is more likely to bring a suit if practice guidelines appear to have been violated, and less likely if the physician appears to have been in compliance. Because of this screening process, the primary use of practice guidelines in litigation has so far been for inculpatory purposes.

Some courts have already discussed the role of practice guidelines in malpractice litigation. For example, in *Washington v. Washington Hospital Center*, a patient had been injured in the operating room owing to a faulty endotracheal tube placement, with resulting hypoxic injury.[134] The plaintiff's expert cited the American Society of Anesthesiology Standards for Basic Intraoperative Monitoring, which were based on guidelines developed by anesthesiologists working with risk managers at the Massachusetts General Hospital. The court relied heavily on the guidelines in its finding of negligence, rejecting the defendant's assertions that the standards were only encouraged, not mandatory. This sort of case suggests that it may be wise for institutions to follow practice guidelines that have gained some broad use and respect. It also creates incentives for development of practice guidelines so that malpractice litigation may be avoided in the future. Because responsible guidelines will emerge largely from epidemiological data on processes of care, it follows that guideline-based litigation can have a positive effect on the quality of medical care, assuming sound methods of guideline development.

Of course, providers and hospital administrators will have to ensure that blind adherence to guidelines does not impair the quality of care. Today, many guidelines remain opinion-based, as scientific evidence is lacking on many important treatment and diagnostic issues. If quality improvement comes down to slavish reliance on poorly considered guidelines, it will be self-destructive. Modern methods of quality improvement emphasize a continual search for better designs and processes, and ideally guidelines will not work against this.

A number of states have recognized the potential for guidelines to contribute to improvement. The best known is Maine, which created the Liability Demonstration Project in 1990.[135] Physicians who agree in advance to follow certain practice guidelines in anesthesiology, obstetrics and gynecology, radiology, and emergency medicine are granted an affirmative defense if sued (they can move to have the case dismissed). Moreover, the plaintiff cannot introduce the guidelines to show departure from the standard of care.

From the viewpoint of the defendant, Maine's procedural use of guidelines is actually rather weak. But in Minnesota, a 1993 law authorized the commissioner of health to accept practice guidelines as an absolute defense in malpractice suits. Though some constitutional doubts remain about the absolute defense, Minnesota may afford a peek into the future.[136] Litigation encouraging the development of guidelines provides an example of synergy between what might be termed the "regulatory role" of the liability system and Continuous Quality Improvement.[137]

In summary, tort law has some potential to encourage better-quality care among providers. Unfortunately, however, malpractice doctrine insists that the central paradigm of litigation be the individual patient versus the individual doctor, pitting them against one another in an emotional battle that acquires moral overtones. Physicians cannot help but react in a defensive fashion, viewing the occurrence of medical injury as a random event over which they have little control. The emotional content of malpractice suits provides little basis for the "systems thinking" needed to achieve fundamental improvement.

The extent of physician opposition to medical malpractice has become increasingly clear over the past decade. Significant tort reforms have been put into place in nearly every state, reducing the claims rates dramatically. However, this has done little to decrease provider demand with regard to further tort reform. Consideration by the 104th Congress of federally mandated tort reform reflected the ongoing commitment of the medical profession to reducing the incidence of malpractice claims. The policy debate has barely been affected by the proposition that rational preventive techniques could reduce medical injuries, and hence malpractice litigation. The cultural and conceptual disconnection between quality improvement and malpractice litigation continues.

Nor do other legal developments encourage the idea of malpractice litigation as a quality-improving system. Federalization of malpractice law is leading to further restrictions on the plaintiff's ability to sue various institutional players, as will be shown in Chapter Five. It is growing more difficult to sue managed care organizations and utilization reviewers, even though these institutions play an increasingly prominent role in the delivery of health care. As more and more responsibility is taken from the doctor-patient relationship and placed in institutional structures, one would expect just the opposite set of trends. In fact, real gains in the quality of care may demand a radical reform of the way in which medical injuries are addressed.

Medical malpractice will never be a form of responsive regulation. Moving toward enterprise liability through integrated delivery systems could, however, convert the deterrence signal from malpractice into a quality-inducing influence. In Chapter Seven, we will discuss more radical change in medical injury compensation as an element in our proposed new rules.

Public Data Initiatives

The one initiative in public and private regulation that takes as its origin modern health services research and that also holds some promise for quality improvement is public data reporting. The gathering and sharing of information on health care practices is relatively recent in the history of regulation. The first steps in data reporting were taken by the federal government. Using discharge data tapes, the Health Care Financing Administration had long been able to calculate death rates for Medicare patients. In 1989, William Roper, the HCFA administrator, decided to make these death rates public for the first time. Since then, more than six thousand hospitals have had their death rates measured and published annually.

The HCFA has now ceased publication of mortality rates, which appear to have had little influence on medical care. After an initial storm of disapproval by the health care industry, it became clear that these death rates, even though they were adjusted for severity of illness, would have only a modest impact on patient choice or hospital reputation. Nor did hospitals find them very useful.[138] Public data reporting did not, however, die with the marginalization and cessation of the publication of Medicare death rates. Instead, it received new life in two states, New York and Pennsylvania, where public authorities concentrated on evaluating death rates and complications in specific procedure areas.

The New York story is in many ways the most compelling. Under David Axelrod, the New York State Department of Health determined in the late 1980s to risk-adjust mortality rates related to heart surgery.[139] In addition to ranking hospitals, New York rates individual heart surgeons on adjusted mortality rates. Initially, this information was shared only with hospitals, but *New York Newsday* filed several Freedom of Information Act requests, and eventually the New York State Supreme Court ordered disclosure.[140]

The Department of Health's initial insistence on confidentiality was sensible. Rather than engaging in a publicly divisive debate about whether a hospital appeared to be performing adequately, the department thought that it could lay the groundwork for quality improvement by sharing information with hospitals on a confidential basis. Not all agreed. Consumer advocates thought that patients should be able to make their own assessments of provider performance. In addition, many in the hospital industry perceived the risk-adjusted measures as inaccurate and in many cases inappropriate.

Even though many providers were outraged, the Department of Health did not terminate the program when courts ordered that names be published. It continued its data-gathering process and honed the risk-adjustment formula. It began to make explanatory booklets available to patients and continued to report the risk-adjusted death rates on a yearly basis. As is discussed in Chapter Six, providers slowly began to believe that the reports were relatively valid.[141]

Today, there is reason to believe that the Cardiac Surgery Reporting System (CSRS) is having a positive impact on the quality of care. Actual mortality rates decreased from 3.52 percent in 1989 to 2.78 percent in 1992. The risk-adjusted measures show an even greater decrease of 41 percent.[142] Though the Department of Health admits that reductions in overall mortality may be due to physician misrepresentation or referral of high-risk patients out of state, there is some evidence that hospitals are engaged in renewed efforts to reduce mortality rates from coronary artery bypass graft surgery (CABG). This would suggest that even though data reporting of specific criteria may be viewed initially in a very negative light by the medical profession, it may also constitute necessary groundwork for improvement efforts.

Although the efficacy of Pennsylvania's public data reporting has not been demonstrated, the state has pursued an even more conscientious regulatory path than that taken in New York. In New York, the CABG data reports were primarily an initiative of the Department of Health. In Pennsylvania, on the other hand, the data collection and dissemination are the product of state legislation. The Pennsylvania Health Care Cost Containment Act of 1986 explicitly states that its goal is to "promote the public interest by encouraging the development of competitive health care services in which health care costs are contained and to assure all citizens reasonable access to quality health care."[143] The statute created the Health Care Cost Containment Council, which was authorized to develop a computerized system for the collection and analysis of data, a dissemination strategy for data so collected, uniform claims and billing forms for the state, and a methodology for publishing data that reflects provider quality and provider service effectiveness.[144] The statute even specified in detail the data elements that were to be collected by the council. Moreover, the Pennsylvania legislation required that physician-specific information be made available to the public.[145]

Pennsylvania eventually adopted the UB-82 as a uniform billing data form. In addition, the Health Care Cost Containment Council contracted with MediQual Systems of Westboro, Massachusetts, to use the MedisGroups severity-of-illness system to standardize data and calculate expected morbidity and mortality rates. The first public report put together by the council was on coronary artery bypass grafting. Throughout 1992, the council received written comments on a methodological plan it had proposed for reporting. In late 1992, the council reported on 1989 data. The final reports contained the mean age of each practitioner's patient population, the percentages of patients with cardiogenic shock and congestive heart failure, the percentages in each of the five MedisGroups severity classifications, the number of women, and the occurrence of myocardial infarction. The reports were generally well accepted, although hospitals have complained bitterly about the costs of the data reporting requirements. Allegheny General Hospital in Pittsburgh, which has thirty thousand discharges annually, spends $400,000 a year to report its data to the council, using the Medis-Groups software.[146]

The CABG reports were only one example of the sorts of information envisioned by the Health Care Cost Containment Council. Pennsylvania planned to track, using the MedisGroups information, the patterns of patient improvement and deterioration during hospital stays. The council also continued to report cost information. Though the impact on the wider public was difficult to gauge, large companies and insurance carriers appeared to be making some purchasing decisions based on this information. There seems to be continued enthusiasm in the Pennsylvania State Legislature for the health council's reports, as enabling legislation was reenacted in 1993 with few changes.[147]

Available outcome measures are still quite crude. Their inaccuracies may be due to inadequate controls for severity of illness and to the poor quality of the reported data. The domains of care they address are rarely well defined. Nonetheless, the data-reporting systems in New York and Pennsylvania are encouraging, in that they reflect regulatory commitment to more outcome information, providers' willingness to supply that information, and the overall utility of such systems in a health marketplace.

Indeed, one can envision these reports as the basis for regulation in the future. The consumer/patient needs information on potential substandard care. Responsive regulation can set a baseline by publishing outcome information. Moreover, this information can provide appropriate benchmarking for hospitals interested in launching quality improvement strategies. We have advocated—and we think the point is widely accepted within the medical profession—that providers pay attention to data. Though in Pennsylvania and New

York there may be argument about the flaws of the data, these states have shown that outcome measures can be consistently improved and are thus a reasonable first step in regulating for general improvement in quality of care.

Another potential benefit of such programs is that the state plays a more passive role. Hospitals (or integrated delivery systems) can be prompted to produce their own improvement strategies. If successful, a hands-off system of regulation based on reports of outcomes could render obsolete the traditional JCAHO emphasis on the structures of health care and regulator-initiated sanctions against individual practitioners. The statistical basis of the outcome measures provides a foundation for an improvement strategy cycle.

There is every indication that state data reporting will become more widespread. Forty-two of the fifty states have either implemented or plan to implement some sort of system for collecting and disseminating health care data. A noteworthy example is Colorado's Health Data Commission, which is authorized to compile, correlate, analyze, and develop data and distribute it to health care providers, third-party payers, and the general public.[148] Colorado hospitals must now send the state inpatient and outpatient data. The commission computes severity-adjusted medical outcome rates, as well as comparative information on average charges and procedure rates. Health care purchasers are planning to use this information to decide where to do business.[149]

The Florida Agency for Health Care Administration has outlined plans for a new reporting system that will make use of a recently established data base. Georgia has a similar program and plans to disseminate non-patient-specific data to the public. The Michigan Department of Public Health is responsible for establishing a comprehensive health information system that will provide quality and utilization data on all providers.[150] The Department of Public Health will publish this information and make it available to agencies and individuals. The Vermont Health Care Authority has established a health care data base that will determine capacity and distribution of existing resources, identify health care needs, evaluate effectiveness of intervention programs in improving patient outcomes, and provide health care information to consumers and purchasers.[151] These states and many others demonstrate a growing commitment to public data initiatives.

Private regulators are just as eager to get into the outcome measurement and dissemination business. As discussed earlier, the JCAHO is developing an Indicator Measurement System. All 5,200 accredited hospitals have been invited to submit clinical data as an optional part of the accrediting process. Indicators are now available in several specialties, and many hospitals initially seemed quite interested in the IMSystem. Recently, however, enthusiasm has cooled, and many hospitals have dropped out of indicator programs. The NCQA has promoted its HEDIS criteria as a public data-reporting format.

Perhaps most important, purchasers of health care are banding together to request similar data from local health care providers. For instance, the Midwest Business Group on Health wants to use statewide data and their own cost analyses to examine care provided for patients undergoing coronary artery bypass grafting. Quaker Oats Company, as part of its Informed Choices Program, is using data from the Illinois Health Care Cost Containment Board to disseminate information for employees. In Cleveland, a coalition of purchasers has developed the Cleveland Health Quality Choice Program, which provides a full report on quality and utilization in hospitals.[152] They are now reporting on measures such as length of stay, mortality rates, and patient satisfaction. Moreover, many companies are now asking managed care organizations to produce information on quality of care before adding them to lists of health care insurance options for employees. Proactive health care institutions—for example, the Kaiser Permanente groups—are developing their own quality report cards. The Federal Employees Benefits Program and Metropolitan Life Insurance Company have also released report cards.[153]

In many ways, then, data reporting is taking on a life of its own, independent of state-based regulators. Hospitals faced with demands for data will have to confront in turn their own deficiencies. Ideally, this process will act as a driving force for quality improvement.

We have reached a critical juncture with regard to government oversight of data reporting. Not only are many states interested, but private groups are advocating report cards. It is not at all clear that government regulation of such reporting, rather than regulation generated by the marketplace, will be most appropriate. (In either case, the data are likely to be publicly available.) Certainly for the insured population, it is sensible to allow better-informed benefits administrators at large employers to make these decisions on behalf of employees. On the other hand, for those employed in small workplaces, for the self-employed, or for those without insurance, public information may prove to be more useful.

Of course, the costs associated with gathering quality information will have to be weighed against its potential benefits. The history of health care is one of similarly reasonable ideas that have turned out on broader analysis to be ineffective and very expensive. Further analysis of public data initiatives is obviously necessary, and we will return to this issue in Chapter Seven. But for now, we may conclude that the migration from inspection to specification of outcomes represents a step in the direction of responsive regulation that is immune from capture.

Health Care and Quality Oversight Today

Our review of the evolution of health care regulation since 1975 offers a somewhat mixed picture for those committed to improving quality of care through responsive regulation. Clearly, the major change in medical care has been the emergence of integrated care prompted by cost competition. The isolation of the doctor has ended. The triad of passive insurer, dominant physician, and independent hospital is now being replaced by the delivery system that accepts risks, employs doctors, and pays for care on a capitated basis. These changes will no doubt accelerate under the influence of federal law, the subject of Chapter Five.

It follows that the alternative delivery system provided by the managed care organization should be the focus of quality regulation in the future. There is some progress toward regulatory structures for alternative delivery systems, especially on the private side through the NCQA. Although weak regulations in most states, combined with the effort by providers to enact any-willing-provider laws, may derail some appropriate oversight of managed care organizations, there are rich opportunities in the mid-1990s to think innovatively about quality regulation in integrated organizations that manage care.

And such innovation is needed soon. The movement toward managed care—utilizing integrated delivery systems that compete sharply with one another on the basis of price—could affect quality quite negatively, especially if the average consumer (patient) can only partially judge quality. Thus a major target for new rules must be inappropriate cost/quality trade-offs.

Fortunately, there is some evidence that the old-line regulators, such as the JCAHO and the federal peer review programs, are moving in the direction of responsive regulation that is consistent with modern quality improvement techniques. These initiatives must still be cultivated and honed, but the foundation for new rules is already being laid.

Our review suggests one other theme. Though academics have been interested in trying to change the nature of tort liability so that more appropriate signals may give thrust to quality improvement, the enthusiasm for such ideas as enterprise liability is at best lukewarm. In addition, doctrinal barriers have helped to prevent tort law from reaching managed care organizations. Hence liability is not a significant factor in creating signals for quality improvement in the alternative delivery system. Without major changes in tort doctrine, we cannot hope for a more rational deterrence effect from medical malpractice than we have had in the past, and in this regard the past record has been nothing short of miserable.

In short, traditional quality regulators are thinking innovatively, though they have not been bold enough. The timing is right for major reform in regulation of quality, but the entire story has not been told. There are elements of today's health care environment that militate against such reform. To obtain a better understanding of those elements, we must examine the revolutionary changes brought about by federal law over the past twenty years. We do so in Chapter Five.

Notes

1. Unfortunately, we have insufficient space to discuss regulation of the long-term care/nursing home industry. Arguably, a number of quality lessons have been learned there, but we simply lack resources to explore them.

2. See, for example, T. A. Brennan, *Just Doctoring: Medical Ethics in the Liberal State* (Berkeley: University of California Press, 1991).

3. Brennan, *Just Doctoring*, 24.

4. 42 U.S.C.A. §300 E(b)(1)(A–V).

5. See 42 U.S.C.A. §300 E–10.

6. See 42 U.S.C.A. §300 E–9(c). Moreover, a $10,000 civil penalty could be levied against employers failing to comply for each thirty days of noncompliance.

7. See 42 U.S.C.A. §300 E–9(a)(1)(A–B).

8. 42 U.S.C.A. §300 E(c).

9. 42 U.S.C.A. §300 E–4(a).

10. The community rating obviously decreases the competitive advantage given to the HMOs. The act carefully defines the community rating system, authorizing variation in rates based on the number of persons in a family. The variation must not be more than 110 percent of the rate that would otherwise be fixed for the community for individuals and families. See 42 U.S.C.A. §300 E–1(8)(A)–(C).

11. See, for example, *Solorzano v. Superior Court*, 13 Cal. Rptr. 2d 161 (Cal. App. 2 Dist. 1992) (holding that the federal Health Maintenance Organization Act did not preempt the field when a court granted injunctive relief under state unfair trade and deceptive practice laws). See also *Physicians Health Plan, Inc., v. Citizens Insurance Company of America*, 673 F. Supp. 903 (W.D. Mich. 1984) (holding that the Michigan Insurance Code requiring no-fault insurers to offer coordinated benefits policies was not preempted by the federal Health Maintenance Organization Act or ERISA).

12. See generally, J. P. Weiner and G. de Lissovoy, "Razing a Tower of Babel: A Taxonomy for Managed Care and Health Insurance Plans," *Journal of Health Politics, Policy and Law* 18, no. 1 (1993): 75–103.

13. As Weiner and D'Lissovoy note, organizational terms included *network model plans*, *preferred provider organizations* (PPOs), *primary care networks* (PCNs), *competitive medical plans* (CMPs), *health insuring organizations* (HIOs), *triple option plans* (TOPs), *exclusive provider organizations* (EPOs), *open-ended HMOs* (O/HMOs), and *point of service plans* (Weiner and D'Lissovoy, 78).

14. Weiner and D'Lissovoy, 93.

15. See Ohio Gen. Stat. §1742.01 (1992).

16. See Md. Code Ann. §19–705.1. (1994)

17. See Md. Code Ann. §19–705.1.

18. See, for example, Md. Code Ann. §19–710 (g)(2).

19. See, for example, Md. Code Ann. §19–713 (b).

20. Mass. Gen. Laws, chap. 176i, §1.

21. See Texas Statutes, Art. 20A.13 (a)(d), 14, 29. This statutory construction makes it very difficult in Texas to hold managed care organizations liable under malpractice common law. See, for example, *Williams v. Good Health Plan, Inc.-HealthAmerica Corporation of Texas*, 743 S.W. 2d 373 (App. 4 Dist. 1987).

22. See J. Johnsson and M. Mitka, "Don't Mess with Texas: Lone Star Doctors Gear Up for Managed Care," *American Medical News*, April 4, 1994, 1, 7–9.

23. See 10 Cal. Stat. Ann. §1350. The survey can be conducted with only four weeks' notice; see 10 Cal. Code of Regs. §1300.80 (Medical Survey Procedures).

24. See, for example, Colo. Stat. Ann. §10–16–416.

25. See J. Johnsson, "Dad's Protests Lead to Record Fine Against California HMO," *American Medical News*, December 12, 1994, 1.

26. Physician Payment Review Commission, *Annual Report 1995: Monitoring Health Plan Performance and Quality* (Washington, D.C.: Physician Payment Review Commission, 1995), 348.

27. See E. Zablocki, "Is Accreditation in Your Future?" *HMO Magazine* (July/August 1992): 48–52.

28. See Zablocki, 49.

29. "Health Plan and Employer Data and Information Set," version 2.0, National Committee for Quality Assurance (1994).

30. See Physician Payment Review Commission, *Annual Report 1995*, chap. 15.

31. See "HEDIS Sets the Stage for Health Plan Report Cards: USQA Quality Monitor," *Journal of Health Care Performance Measurement and Improvement* 1 (May 1994): 8–9.

32. See *PPRC Annual Report 1995*, chap. 11, "Provider-Driven Integration."

33. See P. W. Philbin, "From the Ground Up: Planning the Seeds of Network Development," *Hospitals and Health Networks* 67 (June 5, 1993): 46.

34. See S. S. Mick and D. A. Conrad, "The Decision to Integrate Vertically in Health Care Organizations," *Hospital and Health Services Administration* 33 (fall 1988): 345. See also J. Kosterlitz, "All Together Now," *National Journal* 25 (1993): 2704.

35. See L. R. Burns and D. P. Thorpe, "Trends and Models in Physician-Hospital Organizations," *Health Care Management Review* 18 (fall 1993): 7–11.

36. The management services organization is a corporation that provides management services to physician groups. The management services organization can bond the physician groups to a hospital

through various contracts. In some situations, the management services organization may mark the initial effort of a hospital reaching out to affiliate more closely with physician groups. It can also be used as a vehicle for transferring capital from the hospital to physicians, allowing them to expand facilities.

37. These descriptions were originally developed by S. Sinclair and T. Walsh as part of a practicum course with the Massachusetts Attorney General's Office. See memorandum dated May 27, 1994, *Practicum Project Report* (on file with authors).

38. See J. Johnsson, "Medical Centers Lose Power in Twin Cities Market Shift," *American Medical News*, May 2, 1994, 1.

39. C. Lehman, "Shaping Integrated Health Care Delivery Systems: Innovative Practice and Inconsistence Laws," April 1994 (article on file with authors).

40. See D. B. Higgins, "IRS and HHS on Integrated Delivery: New Rules or Just Talk?" *Health Law Reporter* 2 (B.N.A.) (1993): 586–587.

41. See Lehman, 8.

42. Physician Payment Review Commission, *Annual Report 1995: Provider-Driven Integration* (Washington, D.C.: Physician Payment Review Commission, 1995), 254.

43. See Me. Rev. Stat. Ann., Tit. 24–A, §2672 (West 1993) ("Selective contracting does not cause unreasonable discrimination against or among providers."); Wis. Stat. §628.36 (1993): "No provider may be denied the opportunity to participate in a health care plan other than a limited service health organization [HMO], [or] a preferred provider plan."

44. See J. Johnsson, "Physician and Patient Protection: California Assembly Sends Sweeping Managed Care Law to Governor," *American Medical News*, September 19, 1994, 3.

45. Texas Administrative Code, Tit. 28, §3.3 703 (1994). If the "preferred" designation is withheld by the alternative delivery system, the managed care organization must then select three of its preferred physicians to review the application and recommend action.

Practice privileges cannot be used to deny preferred status to specialty practitioners. Managed care organizations are obliged to make "a good faith effort to have a mix of for-profit, not-for-profit, and tax-supported institutional providers under contract as preferred providers."

46. See Texas Administrative Code, Tit. 28, §3.3 704.

47. See Mich. Comp. Laws §550.53 (1994).

48. See Ind. Code Ann. §27–8–11–3 (West 1994).

49. See New Hampshire Rev. Stat. Ann. §420–C:5 (1993).

50. J. Somerville, "Doctors, HMO's Give Peace a Chance," *American Medical News*, April 3, 1995, 3.

51. See E. J. Emanuel and A. S. Brett, "Managed Competition and the Physician-Patient Relationship," *New England Journal of Medicine* 329 (1993): 879–882; M. Angell, "The Doctor as Double Agent," *Kennedy Institute of Ethics Journal* 3 (1993): 279–286; E. H. Morreim, *Balancing Act: The New Medical Ethics of Medicine's Economics* (Boston, Mass.: Kluwer, 1991); A. L. Hillman, "Financial Incentives for Physicians in HMOs: Is There a Conflict of Interest?" *New England Journal of Medicine* 317 (1987): 1743–48.

52. See P. Starr, "The Framework of Health Care Reform," *New England Journal of Medicine* 329 (1993): 1666–72; M. Angell, "The Beginning of Health Care Reform: The Clinton Plan," *New England Journal of Medicine* 329 (1993): 1569–70; A. M. Epstein, "Changes in the Delivery of Care Under Comprehensive Health Care Reform," *New England Journal of Medicine* 329 (1993): 1672–76.

53. See Brennan, *Just Doctoring*; S. J. Bernstein, E. A. McGlynn, A. L. Siu, C. P. Roth, M. J. Sherwood, J. W. Kersey, J. Kosecoff, M. R. Hicks, and R. H. Brook, "The Appropriateness of Hysterectomy: A Comparison of Care in Seven Health Plans," *Journal of the American Medical Association* 269 (1993): 2398–402; J. E. Wennberg, A. G. Mulley, D. Hanley, R. P. Timothy, F. J. Fowler, N. P. Roos, M. J. Barry, K. McPherson, E. R. Greenberg, D. Soule, T. Bubolz, E. Fisher, and D. Malenka, "An Assessment of Prostatectomy for Benign Urinary Tract Obstruction: Geographic Variations and the

Evaluation of Medical Care Outcomes," *Journal of the American Medical Association* 259 (1988): 3027–30; K. L. Kahn, E. B. Keeler, M. J. Sherwood, W. H. Rogers, D. Draper, S. S. Bentow, E. J. Reinisch, L. V. Rubenstein, J. Kosecoff, and R. H. Brook, "Comparing Outcomes of Care Before and After Implementation of the DRG-Based Prospective Payment System," *Journal of the American Medical Association* 264 (1990): 1984–88; H. R. Burstin, S. R. Lipsitz, and T. A. Brennan, "Socioeconomic Status and Risk for Substandard Medical Care," *Journal of the American Medical Association* 268 (1992): 2383–87; J. Z. Ayanian, B. A. Kohler, T. Abe, and A. M. Epstein, "The Relation Between Health Insurance Coverage and Clinical Outcomes Among Women with Breast Cancer," *New England Journal of Medicine* 329 (1993): 326–331.

54. See A. S. Relman, "Medical Practice Under the Clinton Reforms— Avoiding Domination by Business," *New England Journal of Medicine* 329 (1993): 1574–76.

55. Jacque Sokolov, presentation at Institute for Health Care Improvement Annual Meeting. San Diego, Calif., December 5, 1994.

56. See J. Katz, *The Silent World of Doctor and Patient* (New York: Free Press, 1984).

57. See E. J. Emanuel and L. L. Emanuel, "Four Models of the Physician-Patient Relationship," *Journal of the American Medical Association* 267 (1992): 2221–26.

58. The Patient Protection Act was introduced to both houses of Congress in the latter part of the debate on health care reform in 1994. See H. R. 4527, 103rd Cong., 2d sess., 1994; S. 2196, 103d Cong. 2d sess., 1994. Notably, the AMA was aligned with Senator Paul Wellstone, a prominent supporter of the single-payer health plan. Their alliance was based on their opposition to for-profit insurance companies, including the four largest: Aetna, Cigna, Metropolitan Life/Travelers, and Prudential, together known as the Alliance for Managed Competition.

59. See B. McCormick, "Hospital Loses over Economic Credentialing," *American Medical News,* March 28, 1994, 4 (Georgia radiologist wins $12.7 million award from hospital that terminated his services

because of poor economic performance). See also J. D. Blum, "Economic Credentialing: A New Twist in Hospital Appraisal Processes," *Journal of Legal Medicine* 12 (1991): 427–470.

60. A. S. Relman, "Medical Insurance and Health: What About Managed Care?" *New England Journal of Medicine* 331 (7) (1994): 471–472.

61. See A. Donabedian, "Evaluating the Quality of Medical Care," *Milbank Memorial Fund Quarterly* 44 (1966): 166–203.

62. See J. S. Roberts, J. G. Coale, and R. R. Redmond, "A History of the Joint Commission on Accreditation of Hospitals," *Journal of the American Medical Association* 258 (1987): 936–940.

63. See Roberts, Coale, and Redmond, 940.

64. M. D. Merry, "Can an External Quality Review System Avoid the Inspection Model?" *Quality Review Bulletin* 17 (1991): 315.

65. See D. S. O'Leary, "Accreditation in the Quality Improvement Mold—A Vision for Tomorrow," *Quality Review Bulletin* 17 (1991): 72–77.

66. See O'Leary, 74.

67. See O'Leary, 75.

68. For a long discussion of these issues, see D. S. O'Leary and M. R. O'Leary, "From Quality Assurance to Quality Improvement: The Joint Commission on Accreditation of Healthcare Organizations and Emergency Care," *Emergency Medicine Clinics of North America* 10 (3)(1992): 477–492.

69. See A. A. Skolnick, "Joint Commission Will Collect, Publicize Outcomes," *Journal of the American Medical Association* 270 (1993): 165, 168, 171.

70. See D. M. Nadzam, R. Turpin, L. S. Hanold, and R. E. White, "Data-Driven Performance Improvement in Health Care: The Joint Commission's Indicator Measurement System (IMSystem)," *Joint Commission Journal on Quality Improvement* 19 (1993): 492–500.

71. See D. S. O'Leary, "The Measurement Mandate: Report Card Day Is Coming," *Joint Commission Journal on Quality Improvement* 19 (1993): 487–491.

72. See R. Bergman, "Hospital Allied to Ask JCAHO to Reconsider Indicator Mandate," *Hospitals and Health Networks* 67 (July 5, 1993), 50.

73. See D. Burda, "JCAHO Hits a Wall with Plan on Indicators: Hospitals Balk at Costly and Inefficient Program to Measure Clinical Outcomes," *Modern Health Care*, March 14, 1994, 30–40.

74. Twenty-three percent of the 451 beta sites dropped out of the project from 1990 to 1993. More important, nearly half of the participating institutions decided to leave the program in 1994; see Burda, 32.

75. See L. Oberman, "Joint Commission Seeks Competitors in Hospital Review," *American Medical News*, March 27, 1995, 5.

76. Tax Equity and Fiscal Responsibility Act, PL 97–248 §143, 96 Stat. 324, 382 (1982).

77. See H.R. Conf. Rept. 760, 97th Cong., 2d sess., 1982, reprinted in *U.S. Code Congress and Administrative News* (1982), 1190, 1222–23.

78. Richard Mellette, "The Changing Focus of Peer Review Under Medicare," *University of Richmond Law Review* 20 (1986): 315; T. S. Jost, "Administrative Law Issues Involving the Medicare Utilization and Quality Control Peer Review Organization (PRO) Program: Analysis and Recommendations," *Ohio State Law Journal* 50 (1989): 1–60.

79. Jost, 2–3.

80. H.R. Conf. Rept. 47, 98th Cong., 1st sess., 1983, reprinted in *U.S. Code Congress and Administrative News* (1983), 487.

81. See P. E. Dans, J. P. Weiner, and S. E. Otter, "Peer Review Organizations: Promises and Potential Pitfalls," *New England Journal of Medicine* 313 (1985): 1131–37.

82. PL 99–509, 100 Stat. 2044 (1986).

83. See H.R. Conf. Rept. 1012, 99th Cong., 2d sess., 1986, reprinted in *U.S. Code Congress and Administrative News* (1986), 4005–6.

84. PL 100–93, 101 Stat. 691 (1987).

85. See, for example, *Lavapies v. Bowen*, 883 F. 2d 465, 466 (6th Cir. 1989); *Thorbus v. Bowen*, 848 F. 2d 901 (8th Cir. 1988); *Varandani*

v. *Bowen*, 824 F. 2d 307 (4th Cir. 1987); *Anderson v. Sullivan*, 959 F. 2d 690 (8th Cir. 1992).

86. S. F. Jencks and G. R. Wilensky, "The Health Care Quality Improvement Initiative: The New Approach to Quality Assurance in Medicare," *Journal of the American Medical Association* 268 (1992): 900–903.

87. See Jencks and Wilensky, 901.

88. See, for example, memorandum from Chief of Medical Review Branch, Division of Health Standards and Quality, Healthcare Financing Administration, to Region Nine PROs, December 13, 1993. The memorandum details the task of building a community of those committed to improving quality, monitoring access to quality of care, protecting beneficiaries, promoting informed choices, and developing an infrastructure. Each PRO was assigned certain activities that are specified under these major subheadings. For example, under "Monitoring Access to Quality of Care," the PRO was to analyze performance of HMOs and health plans, using a set of national performance standards; profile patterns of care using a nationally representative sample of hospital discharges; expand PRO monitoring of ambulatory surgery and disease prevention; and compare practice manners and quality of care across regions. More important, with regard to building a community of those committed to improving quality, the PRO was now to involve practitioners, providers, and accreditors in developing PRO agendas, programs, and projects and improving linkages to other nongovernmental activities such as surveyors line the JCAHO and managed care organizations. These changes would be revolutionary.

89. See H. Rubin, "Watching the Doctor-Watcher: How Well Do Peer Review Organizational Methods Detect Hospital Care Quality Problems," *Journal of the American Medical Association* 267 (1992): 2349–55. The difficulty for the PRO program of identifying valid quality problems is illustrated by recent research that suggests there is very poor agreement between PRO judgments and those made by Rand reviewers.

90. Weiler relates that total premiums had reached $370 million by 1970. See P. C. Weiler, *Medical Malpractice on Trial* (Cambridge,

Mass.: Harvard University Press, 1991), 26. See also U.S. Department of Health, Education, and Welfare, *Report of the Secretary's Commission on Medical Malpractice* (Washington, D.C.: U.S. Government Printing Office, 1973); G. O. Robinson, "The Medical Malpractice Crisis of the 1970's: A Retrospective," *Law and Contemporary Problems* 49 (1986): 5–20.

91. See California Business and Professions Code §6146 (West 1992); New Jersey Court Rules §1:21–7 (1976); N.Y. Jud. Law §474a (1976).

92. See Cal. Civ. Code §3333.1; Alaska Stat. §09.55.548; Neb. Rep. Stat. §44–2819.

93. Cal. Civ. Proc. §667.7; see, for example, Kan. Stat. Ann. §40–3403 and N.M. Stat. Ann. §41–5–7.

94. Many states have limited the ad damnum clause, which had allowed plaintiffs to state at the outset of the trial the amount of damages claimed. See, for example, Alaska Stat. §9.55.547; R.I. Gen. Law §9–1–30. Other states employed pretrial screening panels to hear the merits of particular cases before allowing them to go to court. These screening panels were based on the probably erroneous assumption that large numbers of claims are brought in cases without much merit. For examples of screening panel requirements, see Neb. Rev. Stat. §§44–2840 to 2841. See also Mass. Gen. Laws Ann., chap. 231, §60B; N.Y. Judiciary Law §148–a.

95. See Weiler, 27.

96. See Cal. Civ. Code §3333.2. The constitutionality of the limit on noneconomic damages was upheld in *Fein* v. *Permanente Medical Group*, 695 P. 2d 665 (Cal. 1985). See also Ind. Code §§16–9.5–2–2 (now codified at 27–12–14–3).

97. See American Medical Association, *AMA Tort Reform Compendium* (Chicago: American Medical Association, 1989).

98. There is formidable literature in this area. One of the best discussions is found in P. Danzon, *Medical Malpractice: Theory, Evidence, and Public Policy* (Cambridge, Mass.: Harvard University Press, 1985). For recent discussions of empirical assessments, see F. A. Sloan, "State Responses to the Malpractice Insurance Crisis of the

1970's: An Empirical Assessment," *Journal of Health Politics, Policy and Law* 9 (1985): 629–646; F. A. Sloan, P. M. Mergenhagen, and R. R. Bovbjerg, "Effects of Tort Reforms on the Value of Closed Medical Malpractice Claims: A Micro Analysis," *Journal of Health Politics, Policy and Law* 14 (1989): 663–689.

99. See P. C. Weiler, H. H. Hiatt, J. P. Newhouse, W. G. Johnson, T. A. Brennan, and L. L. Leape, *A Measure of Malpractice: Medical Injury, Malpractice Litigation, and Patient Compensation* (Cambridge, Mass.: Harvard University Press, 1993).

100. See T. A. Brennan, "Improving the Quality of Medical Care: A Critical Evaluation of the Major Proposals," *Yale Law and Policy Review* 10 (1992): 431–462.

101. See Weiler and others, 40–50.

102. See, for example, F. W. Cheney, K. Posner, R. A. Caplan, and R. J. Ward, "The Standard of Care and Anesthesia Liability," *Journal of the American Medical Association* 261 (1989): 1599–1601; H. S. Farber and M. J. White, "Medical Malpractice: An Empirical Examination of the Litigation Process," *RAND Journal of Economics* 22 (1991): 199–212; M. I. Taragin, L. R. Willett, A. P. Wilczek, R. Trout, and J. L. Carson, "The Influence of Standard of Care and Severity of Injury on the Resolution of Medical Malpractice Claims," *Annals of Internal Medicine* 117 (1992): 780–784.

103. See N. Hupert, A. Lawthers, T. A. Brennan, and L. P. Peterson, "Physicians' Perceptions of Medical Malpractice," *Social Science Medicine* (1995) (in press).

104. Some suggest that this is quite rational. See G. B. Hickson, E. Wright Clayton, S. S. Entman, and F. Sloan, "Obstetricians' Prior Malpractice Experience and Patient's Satisfaction with Care," *Journal of the American Medical Association* 272 (1994): 1583–87.

105. See, for example, K. S. Abraham and P. C. Weiler, "Enterprise Medical Liability and the Evolution of the American Health Care System," *Harvard Law Review* 108 (1994): 381–436; and *Bing* v. *Thunig,* 143 N.E. 2d 3 (N.Y. App. 1957).

106. See, in the emergency room context, *Jackson v. Power,* 743 P. 2d 1376 (Alaska 1987); *Albain v. Flower Hospital,* 553 N.E. 2d 1038 (Ohio 1990); and *Torrence v. Kusminsky,* 408 S.E. 2d 684 (W. Va. 1991).

107. See Abraham and Weiler, 390–400.

108. *Darling v. Charleston Community Memorial Hospital,* 211 N.E. 2d 253 (Ill. 1965).

109. See, for example, *Elam v. College Park Hospital,* 183 Cal. Rptr. 156 (Cal. App. 4th Dist. 1982); *Pedroza v. Bryant,* 677 P. 2d 166 (Wash. 1984).

110. *Jackson v. Power,* 743 P. 2d 1376 (Alaska 1987).

111. As discussed by Abraham and Weiler (see "Enterprise Medical Liability," 420–431), there would be several steps to full enterprise liability: 1) the hospital electing medical liability would be liable to its patients for malpractice by any affiliated providers; 2) patients would receive full notice of the hospital liability and physician immunity at the time of the admission; 3) health care providers would be relieved of all liability except if they showed reckless indifference for the welfare of the patient; 4) physicians would pay the hospital an annual surcharge; 5) the amount of the surcharge would be set by agreement between participating hospitals and affiliated care providers and overseen by the State Department of Insurance; 6) hospitals could choose to work with third-party payers to bring managed care organizations into the picture. The locus for enterprise liability is debated by the leading proponents of the concept. Compare Abraham and Weiler with W. M. Sage, K. E. Hastings, and R. A. Berenson, "Enterprise Liability for Medical Malpractice and Health Care Quality Improvement," *American Journal of Law and Medicine* 20 (1994): 1–28.

112. See H. R. Burstin, S. Lipsitz, S. Udvarhelyi, and T. A. Brennan, "The Effect of Hospital Financial Characteristics on Quality of Care," *Journal of the American Medical Association* 270 (1993): 845–849.

113. The initial evidence that an enterprise approach might lead to lower incidence of medical injury was provided by a Harvard study of anesthesia, in which claims data was used to provide the impetus

or new safety monitoring during anesthesia, leading to reduction in claims rates. See J. H. Eichhorn, "Prevention of Intraoperative Anesthesia Accidents and Related Severe Injury Through Safety Monitoring," *Anesthesiology* 70 (1989): 572–577; J. H. Eichhorn, J. B. Cooper, D. J. Cullen, W. D. Maier, J. H. Philip, and R. G. Seeman, "Standards for Patient Monitoring During Anesthesia at Harvard Medical School," *Journal of the American Medical Association* 256 (1986): 1017–20.

114. Some have argued that there must be deterrence value in the present tort system. However, these arguments are based simply on the costs of negligent claims, not the nature of the deterrence signal. See M. J. White, "The Value of Liability in Medical Malpractice," *Health Affairs* (fall 1994): 75–87.

115. *Wickline v. The State of California*, 239 Cal. Rptr. 810 (Cal. App. 2d Dist. 1986). Wickline suffered severe vascular compromise.

116. See, for example, J. D. Blum, "An Analysis of Legal Liability in Health Care Utilization Reviews and Case Management," *Houston Law Review* 26 (1989): 191–228.

117. *Wilson v. Blue Cross of Southern California*, 222 Cal. App. 3d 660, 271 Cal. Rptr. 876 (1990).

118. See E. Lu, "The Potential Effect of Managed Competition in Health Care on Provider Liability and Patient Autonomy," *Harvard Journal on Legislation* 30 (1993): 519–539; C. J. Hamborg, "Medical Utilization Review: The New Frontier for Medical Malpractice Claims?" *Drake Law Review* 41 (1992): 113–138; P. H. Mihaly, "Health Care Utilization Review: Potenal Exposures to Negligence Liability," *Ohio State Law Journal* 52 (1991): 1289–1308.

119. See Sage, Hastings, and Berenson, 9–12.

120. See, for example, *Loyola University of Chicago v. Humana Insurance Company*, 996 F. 2d 895 (7th Cir. 1993).

121. See M. A. Hiltzik, "Supreme Court Won't Allow State Suit in Death Case; Litigation: U.S. Court's Action Underscores the Limiting of Choices Available to Patients Unhappy with Insurers on Their Case," *Los Angeles Times*, May 16, 1995, D1.

122. See *Kuhl* v. *Lincoln National Health Plan of Kansas City, Inc.*, 999 F. 2d 298 (8th Cir. 1993).

123. See H. R. Parise, "The Proper Extension of Tort Liability Principles in the Managed Care Industry," *Temple Law Review* 64 (1991): 977–1005.

124. See, for example, *Sloan* v. *Metropolitan Health Council of Indianapolis, Inc.*, 516 N.E. 2d 1104 (Ind. App. 1st Dist. 1987), in which plaintiffs alleged a negligent failure to diagnose, and the Indiana Court of Appeals reversed a summary judgment in favor of the HMO.

125. See, for example, *Dunn* v. *Praiss*, 606 A. 2d 862 (N.J. 1992). This case can be compared to others in which vicarious liability is not found, especially where the HMO plays only an administrative role. See, for example, *Raglin* v. *HMO Illinois, Inc.*, 595 N.E. 2d 153 (Ill. App. 1st 1992) and *Chase* v. *Independent Practice Association, Inc.*, 583 N.E. 2d 251 (Mass. 1991).

126. See *Boyd* v. *Albert Einstein Medical Center*, 547 A. 2d 1229 (Pa. Super. Ct. 1988). This case involved the perforation of a patient's chest wall during a breast mass biopsy by a participating HMO specialist.

127. See *McClellan* v. *Health Maintenance Organization of Pennsylvania*, 604 A. 2d 1053 (Pa. Super. Ct. 1992).

128. For instance, in *McClellan*, the court explicitly refused to reach plaintiff's claim that corporate negligence could apply to IPA model HMOs.

129. See K. Hastings, "A View from the Agency for Health Care Policy and Research: The Use of Language in Clinical Practice Guidelines," *Joint Commission Journal of Quality Improvement* 19 (8) (1993): 335–341.

130. See T. A. Brennan, "Practice Guidelines and Malpractice Litigation: Collision or Cohesion?" *Journal of Health Politics, Policy and Law* 16 (1) (1991): 67–85.

131. See M. Hall, "The Defense Effects of Medical Practice Policies in Malpractice Litigation," *Law and Contemporary Problems* 54, no. 2 (1991): 119–145; C. Havighurst, "Practice Guidelines as Legal

Standards Governing Physician Liability," *Law and Contemporary Problems* 54, no. 2 (1991): 87–117; D. W. Garnick, A. M. Hendricks, and T. A. Brennan, "Can Practice Guidelines Reduce the Number and Costs of Malpractice Claims?" *Journal of the American Medical Association* 266 (1991): 2856–60.

132. See R. Grilli and J. Lomas, "Evaluating the Message: The Relationship Between Compliance Rate and the Subject of a Practice Guideline," Medical Care 32 (3): 202–213.

133. See A. L. Hyams, J. A. Brandenburg, S. R. Lipsitz, and T. A. Brennan, *Final Report to the Physician Payment Review Commission: Practice Guidelines in Malpractice Litigation* (Washington, D.C.: Physician Payment Review Commission, Grant No. 92–G04, 1994).

134. See *Washington* v. *Washington Hospital Center*, 579 A. 2d 177 (D.C. Ct. App. 1990).

135. See G. H. Smith, "A Case Study in Progress: Practice Guidelines and the Affirmative Defense in Maine," *Joint Commission Journal of Quality Improvement* 19 (8) (1993): 355–362.

136. See R. M. Sorian, A *New Deal for American Health Care* (Washington, D.C.: Health Care Information Center, 1993).

137. There are other examples of the manner medical malpractice law is being modified by changes in the health care system. For example, the Health Care Quality Improvement Act of 1986 created the National Practitioner Data Bank. See 42 U.S.C. §1101 *et seq.* The data bank was designed to provide a single source of information on physicians who might repeatedly provide poor care but escape detection by moving from state to state or hospital to hospital. Hospitals, malpractice insurers, health care entities, physicians, dentists, and other health care practitioners must report any payments made under malpractice insurance policies, any licensure actions, or any restrictions of clinical privileges. Moreover, hospitals must query the data bank whenever physicians are newly admitted to clinical staff or when clinical privileges are renewed every two or three years. Many are now charging that the reporting

requirements are making it more difficult to settle lawsuits for small amounts; physicians simply do not want to appear in the data bank, although in 1993, forty-six thousand practitioners were reported.

There is no public access to the data bank, but consumer advocates and some members of Congress have sought such access. If granted, it is likely to further alienate practicing physicians from the data bank concept. As previously noted, physicians display a negative, knee-jerk reaction to anything associated with malpractice litigation. In many ways, their negative attitude toward malpractice litigation tends to isolate them from significant quality improvement efforts surrounding medical injuries. Opening the data bank would only polarize the profession further. Moreover, since empirical research has demonstrated that the medical malpractice system works more like a lottery than a systematic method for uncovering and compensating medical injuries, physicians and hospitals may well question the utility of public access to the data bank. Access will not serve any important quality improvement efforts, and since it will create further polarization around medical malpractice, it could frustrate quality improvement.

The other significant area of federal influence in medical malpractice litigation is related to the Emergency Medical Treatment and Active Labor Act of 1986 (EMTALA). See Note, "The Evolution of a Federal Malpractice Law," *Stanford Law Review* 45 (1992): 263. The act was intended to end hospital dumping of indigent patients from one emergency room to another. It created specific standards and responsibilities for emergency room personnel regarding stabilization and transfer of patients. Those who violate the act face fines of up to $50,000 and treble damages. For an excellent discussion of EMTALA, see B. R. Furrow, "Quality Control in Health Care: Developments in the Law of Medical Malpractice," *Journal of Law, Medicine, and Ethics* 21 (1993): 173–192.

It appears that federal EMTALA will preempt state law. See U.S. Code §1395 dd(f). For example, state screening panels have been declared inapplicable to EMTALA claims even when they are required under state law. See *Reid v. Indianapolis Osteopathic Medical Hospital, Inc.*, 709 F. Supp. 853 (S.D. Ind. 1989). Congress did not intend to replace the state malpractice law with EMTALA, and in fact stated so explicitly. See U.S. Code 1395 dd(f): "The provisions of this Act do not preempt any state or local law requirement except, at the extent that the requirement directly conflicts with a requirement of this section." Nonetheless, several courts have found that the federal legislation itself creates a reasonableness standard. See, for example, *Burditt v. United States Department of Health and Human Services*, 934 F. 2d 1362 (5th Cir. 1991); *Deberry v. Sherman Hospital Association*, 741 F. Supp. 1302 (N.D. Ill. 1990).

Insofar as there is intermixing of EMTALA claims with malpractice litigation, the federal standard will tend to supplant state malpractice law. Because it addresses a true quality problem, that is, the injuries that might arise in a transfer of a patient from one emergency department to another, the federal law could have a healthy influence on medical malpractice. Moreover, its guidelines for appropriate transfer are specified fairly clearly. This too will tend to improve the signal sent by medical malpractice law, in that the criteria for transfer under EMTALA could be understood as quite similar to practice guidelines. But to the extent that EMTALA becomes viewed as just another part of a poorly functioning medical malpractice system, it could simply promote defensive practices without any real focus on quality. As with other areas of the federalization of malpractice law, the overall effect is not promising.

138. See D. M. Berwick and D. L. Wald, "Hospital Leaders' Opinions of the HCFA Mortality Data," *Journal of the American Medical Association* 263 (2) (1990): 247–249.

139. For a full discussion of the New York initiative, see D. Sharrott, "Provider-Specific Quality of Care Data: A Proposal for Limited Mandatory Disclosure," *Brooklyn Law Review* 58 (1992): 85–121.

140. See *Newsday Inc. v. New York State Department of Health*, 19 Media Law Report (BNA) 1477 (Sup. Ct. Albany County 1991).

141. See D. Zinman, "Access to Heart Doc Rating Debated," *Newsday*, December 15, 1992, 59.

142. See E. L. Hannan, H. Kailburn, M. Razz, E. Shields, and M. Chassin, "Improving the Outcomes of Coronary Artery Bypass Surgery in New York State," *Journal of the American Medical Association* 271 (1994): 761–766.

143. 35 Penn. Stat. §449.2.

144. 35 Penn. Stat. §449.5.

145. 35 Penn. Stat. §449.7. Only the CABG reporting data is physician-specific.

146. See E. Gardner, "Indicator System Accepting All Test Pilots," *Modern Health Care*, June 21, 1993, 32. In contrast, the JCAHO visits cost Allegheny Hospital less than $50,000 per year.

147. The legislature did insist, after consulting with the Hospital Association of Pennsylvania and the Pennsylvania Medical Society, that the council be given greater access to technical advice. See Senate Bill 1052 §1(f) (1993). In addition, the legislature wanted the council to develop and implement more and better outreach programs to make information understandable and usable to purchasers and providers.

148. Colo. Rev. Stat. §25–28–104 (1992).

149. See K. Pallarito, "Group Questions Reliability of Financial Data," *Modern Health Care*, February 5, 1990, 50.

150. See Mich. Comp. Laws §333.2616 (1992).

151. See Vt. Stat. Ann., Tit. 18, §9410(a) (1992 Supp.). In some ways, this may compete with the Hospital Data Council, which was created to review all hospital budgets and evaluate hospital costs in Vermont (Vt. Stat. Ann., Tit. 18, §9452).

152. See "CHQC: Revolutionizing Healthcare in Cleveland," *NCG News* 1, no. 2 (1994): 1, 4.

153. See L. Oberman, "Federal, MetLife Reports to Put Spotlight on Quality," *American Medical News*, September 26, 1994, 4.

5

The Federalization of
Health Care Oversight

Implications for Quality

Through the early 1970s, the regulatory signals facing hospitals and health care providers came primarily from the state or from within the health care industry itself. Accreditation by the Joint Commission for Accreditation of Health Care Organizations (JCAHO), medical malpractice litigation based on state common law, state licensing functions, and certificate-of-need programs were the major influences on the quality of medical care. The only aspect of regulation that was entirely federal was that found in the Medicare system, in the form of the Professional Standards Review Organizations (PSROs)—and later the Peer Review Organizations (PROs). Earlier chapters have shown how over the past two decades, these patterns of regulation have undergone significant changes, with greater and greater emphasis on measuring outcomes and less on the structure of quality oversight in hospitals or on the sanctioning of individual hospitals and doctors. These changes have begun a reformation of quality regulation in the United States.

But our story would be incomplete if we overlooked the subtle yet revolutionary effect of federal law in the health care field. We have already seen that the federal HMO Act of 1973 planted seeds of change that have led to growth in the managed care industry. However, with the passage of the Employee Retirement Income Security Act of 1974 (ERISA) and a decision in the Supreme Court in the case of *Goldfarb* v. *Virginia State Bar*, federalization of much of health care law was begun.[1] The subsequent rise of fraud and abuse provisions in Medicare law, the growth of importance of Medicaid funding, and changes in federal tax law posture added a vast new set of rules to health care provision.[2] Some of the laws accelerated the movement toward a market in medical care with emphasis on price competition. Others encouraged competition on quality, while still others affected significant existing rules on quality.

Our search for new rules to regulate for improvement would be hampered if we did not understand how federal law affects the actions of providers, hospitals, and integrated delivery systems (IDSs). Responsive regulation that integrates modern quality theory and enables rather than frustrates providers must be aligned, to the extent possible, with the themes of federal law. In addition, to the extent that federal law dictates a market in medical care, it will affect the potential cost/quality trade-offs we have identified as a target for new rules.

Antitrust Law

Antitrust litigation will play an important role in shaping health care in the next decade, but it is its effect on the ways in which we oversee quality of care that are our subject. Because antitrust law is most concerned with competition, it will inhibit collaborative efforts between institutions in the health care market that might be considered competitors. Because much of quality improvement arises from collaboration and commitment to patient good—which at least in part is independent of economic concerns—there is the potential for a clash between market efficiency and quality of care that will be mediated by antitrust law. But we will find that most antitrust law has been crafted by federal enforcers so as not to frustrate quality improvement, and we will see that increased competition might also mean increased quality competition.

Health care was generally unprepared for the incentives created by antitrust litigation. Before 1975, it was not at all clear that antitrust law could apply to the learned professions like medicine. Only with the decision of *Goldfarb* v. *Virginia State Bar* did lawyers and other members of learned professions become potentially liable for violations of the Sherman Act. As the Supreme Court noted, "The nature of an occupation's standing alone does not provide sanctuary from the Sherman Act . . . nor is the public service aspect of professional practice controlling in determining whether §1 includes professions."[3] It was clear that courts would now consider doctors and hospitals to be competitors in a marketplace, and that efforts to monopolize—or more generally, to reduce competition— would lead to stiff penalties.

The details of antitrust law are beyond the scope of this book, but in light of the impact that antitrust statutes could have on the enterprise of quality improvement, some background is appropriate, especially as most readers will be quite unfamiliar with the field. A number of federal statutes form the basis of antitrust law. The most important of these is the Sherman Antitrust Act, of which Section One prohibits contracts, combinations, or conspiracies that restrain trade, and Section Two prohibits monopolization or attempts to monopolize.[4] The Sherman Act and other federal antitrust statutes, including Section Seven of the Clayton Act that addresses mergers, overlap to a large extent, as does enforcement authority between the Department of Justice Antitrust Division and the Federal Trade Commission (FTC). Individual plaintiffs can bring suits under the Sherman Act and seek treble damages.

Given the multiple authority and overlapping statutes, most commentators prefer to analyze antitrust law in terms of the various restraints of trade the law is intended to prohibit. The Sherman Act's broad proscription of every combination, contract, or conspiracy that restrains trade would to some extent apply to almost any contract.[5] Therefore judges have had to mold a definition of unreasonable restraints of trade. In so doing, the courts have created certain pigeonhole definitions where there is unanimity that the effect of an agreement or activity is so plainly uncompetitive that it is unlawful per se.[6]

Per se violations include the division of markets into territories, tying arrangements between two products, horizontal and vertical price fixing, and group boycotts (including concerted refusals to deal). Although many restraints of trade do not fall into these pigeonholes, the categories are nonetheless very helpful in organizing an antitrust inquiry. If the case fits none of the per se definitions, the courts must apply a rule of reason, inquiring whether or not the activity would suppress or perhaps destroy competition.[7]

Applying the rule of reason is not always straightforward. The antitrust laws were designed not to protect a single competitor but competition generally.[8] The plaintiff can demonstrate an antitrust violation by showing that the defendant has sufficient market power to potentially restrain trade or have adverse effects on competition; the plaintiff need not prove actual detrimental effects. The defendant can counter by demonstrating the benefits or "redeeming virtues of a supposedly restraining activity."[9] The plaintiff then has one more opportunity to show that this particular virtue could be obtained by some other means that does not violate antitrust laws. As proof of these issues is burdensome for the plaintiff, the per se route is obviously more attractive.[10]

In health care, it is perhaps easiest to consider various types of restraints. Section One of the Sherman Act focuses on conspiracies or contracts between competitors. Section Two refers to cases where a single actor monopolizes a market. The former are much more common in the health care sphere. Section One defines three different types of violation: horizontal combinations, vertical combinations, and mergers that involve both vertical and horizontal restraints. Horizontal restraints involve firms at the same level of competition that agree to restrain trade. When firms operate on different levels in the chain of production and attempt to restrain trade, this is considered a vertical restraint. Examples of horizontal restraints include price fixing, market allocations, joint ventures, or group boycotts. Companies are prohibited from engaging in certain types of vertical integration, such as exclusive dealing arrangements, tying arrangements, territory and customer limitations, and boycotts.

As consolidation of the health care industry continues, there will be ample opportunity for analysis of the antitrust implications of new health care delivery systems. For our purposes, it is sufficient to consider several discrete categories of vertical and horizontal restraints that are found in the health care industry and have implications for quality of care. These include:

1. Horizontal integration through mergers, particularly of hospitals

2. Vertical integration of hospitals and exclusive contracts for medical staffs within hospitals, as well as changes in medical staff privileges that can potentially represent combinations of the hospital and the medical staff

3. The operation of horizontal networks of providers

4. Integrating efforts undertaken by managed care organizations and insurance companies

We will discuss each of these categories in turn and suggest how it can and does affect the potential for responsive regulation.

Generally, courts are asked to review mergers that cause concern about reduced competition resulting from the combination of market shares. This sort of effect on competition can occur when two hospitals merge. Especially in smaller geographical areas, where mergers can create entities that control a significant proportion of the marketplace, plaintiffs aggressively seek federal court intervention under the Sherman Act. Perhaps more important, both the Department of Justice Antitrust Division and the FTC oversee such mergers. Indeed, it would be imprudent for any hospitals to consider a merger without first consulting with federal authorities and obtaining a "hold harmless" letter.

The authority of federal enforcers to approve mergers underlines the fact that, at least in the abstract, antitrust litigation, like tort litigation, appears to be an "unresponsive" form of regulation. But this would be too simplistic. Federal authorities are willing to confer with hospitals that wish to merge. In health care, the authorities often issue policy statements and seek input from providers and the industry.

For example, in 1992, the Justice Department and the FTC analyzed five steps that would go into approval of a merger:

1. Definition of the appropriate product and geographical market (not exceeding certain concentration levels)

2. Potential adverse competitive effects

3. Evaluation of barriers to entry

4. Consideration of the efficiencies posed by the merger

5. The potential for firm failure

These considerations now provide the backbone for federal overview.[11] They were amended and expanded in joint guidelines issued in September 1993 and September 1994. Although the health care industry has complained that these guidelines are not specific enough, they are an indication of the government's willingness to listen to providers and to give them guidance on antitrust enforcement.

Defining the market is the most difficult part of the analysis of a hospital merger. This is especially true as more care is managed, demand for inpatient care dwindles, and hospitals move increasingly to provision of outpatient care. Moreover, with integration of medical staffs, affiliation with independent practice associations, and relationships with health maintenance organizations (HMOs), the borders of the hospital as a provider of particular services become less clear. Vertical integration makes it much more difficult to define the nature of the horizontal restraint on trade posed by mergers.

This is not a new problem. Courts have long had to struggle with the definitions of product markets.[12] Typically, the judge—or more rarely, the jury—must decide how reasonably interchangeable certain products are and how economically significant various products' submarkets are in the definition of a health care market. Of course, the health care system makes these product definitions particularly difficult. Patients are the ultimate consumers, but they are usually insensitive to cost—or at least were until copayments and deductibles increased sensitivity in recent years. Moreover, until recently, most patients lacked information on important dimensions of the quality of medical care services and the appropriateness of procedures. Indeed, a great deal of the demand for such services and procedures was generated by health care providers rather than patients. The Ninth Circuit Court has acknowledged all of these problems in a leading decision on health care:

> The health care industry, moreover, presents a particularly difficult area. The first step to understanding it is to recognize that not only is access to the medical profession very time consuming and expensive, both for the applicant and society generally, but also that numerous government subventions of the costs of medical care have created both a demand and supply function for medical services that is artificially high. The present supply and demand functions of medical services in no way approximate those which exist in a purely private competitive order. An accurate description of those functions, moreover, is not available. Thus, we lack baselines by which could be measured the distance between the present supply and demand functions and those which would exist under ideal competitive conditions.[13]

The government generally relies on a calculation known as the Herfindahl-Hirschmann Index to estimate the market-concentrating effects of a merger.[14] The calculation itself is very simple; but the effect of market concentration in health care remains quite murky.[15]

Once the court decides on a market definition and the degree of concentration, the real antitrust analysis of anticompetitive effects begins. Any merger has the potential for adverse economic effects.[16] Consider, for example, two hospitals in a large metropolitan area. Their competition gives patients a choice in products. Once a merger occurs, they may no longer have to compete to please patients. The merger thus reduces quality-based competition, restrains trade, and represents an antitrust violation.

On the other hand, merged institutions could cross-fertilize quality inpatient efforts, for example, through benchmarking used in common inpatient and ambulatory satisfaction forms. Sharing of information by the two hospitals could promote quality improvement by consolidating resources and providing mutual education. However, from a market standpoint, competition would be reduced. The critical insight is that the valuable impulse of providers engaged in quality improvement to cooperate with each other, a strategy promoted by mergers, can conflict with efforts to police the market and could be a violation of antitrust laws.

Fortunately, the government has recognized this problem. In both September 1993 and September 1994 guidelines, the Department of Justice explicitly demarcated a safety zone for quality and outcome information. The joint Department of Justice/FTC guidelines create a safety zone for exchanges of information among hospitals. Among other conditions, the safety zone must be managed by a third party and the data must be at least three months old and aggregated from at least five reporting hospitals.[17] Any outcome data on specific procedures that is provided by medical societies must be aggregated over all their members. The guidelines permit medical societies to develop practice parameters for patient management.[18] Thus antitrust regulation looks surprisingly responsive.

Another reason that merger scrutiny has not impeded quality improvement is that federal prosecutions are rare. During the 1980s, only eight hospital mergers were challenged.[19] Analysis of these seems to indicate that the federal authorities do selectively block those mergers that would create significant market concentration. Nonetheless, the 1992 Justice Department/FTC merger guidelines—and their progeny—do not predict well the mergers that will be challenged. Here, the industry's desire for more precise guidelines and predictability (responsiveness) does seem well-founded.[20]

In 1993 and 1994, the federal government continued to send mixed signals about what sorts of mergers might be allowed. For example, in January 1994, the Justice Department sanctioned the merger of the only two hospitals in Manchester, New Hampshire. Although the Justice Department did not comment on its decision, the state of New Hampshire approved the merger because of the promise of cost savings through efficiencies.[21] This case contrasts with the FTC's unanimous decision to oppose the merger of the only two hospitals in Pueblo, Colorado.[22] The FTC was convinced the merger would allow the new entity to raise prices and diminish quality.

Still later in 1994, the federal government and the state of Florida demonstrated a willingness to consider an innovative merger between dominant providers within a geographical region. The critical issue in *United States and State of Florida* v. *Morton Planned Health Systems, Inc., and Trustees of Mease Hospital, Inc.* was that merger of some parts of hospitals was deemed efficient, whereas that of other parts was ruled to be inefficiently monopolistic.[23] The Justice Department and the state of Florida, operating under the September 1993 guidelines, allowed the partial merger of Morton Planned Health Systems and Mease Hospital, creating an organization that would in many ways dominate care in northern Pinellas County. The decree ruled that certain parts of the two hospitals' operations, including outpatient services as well as laboratory, radiology, and mental health care for inpatients, could be merged. In addition, the partnership would operate all tertiary acute inpatient care, including most of the advanced technology units. But the partnership managers were not to discuss or exchange information concerning any independent services—in particular, managed care negotiation and contracting, marketing, and pricing. This sort of hybrid merger may be the hallmark of the future as the federal authorities strive to maintain competition in some areas but allow integration in others. They may also allow a great deal of quality partnering. In summary, the government's merger policy, at least from the perspective of quality of care, shows some degree of responsiveness.

As managed care drives down the demand for inpatient services, hospitals will be increasingly anxious about merger policy. Half-empty, financially strapped hospitals are not the best culture for quality improvement. But it appears that federal authorities understand this, and are adapting policy accordingly.

The second area where antitrust concerns might affect quality improvement is that of relationships between medical staffs and hospitals. Perhaps the greatest amount of antitrust litigation in health care arises from complaints by physicians who have been refused staff privileges. As was pointed out in Chapter Two, medical staffs traditionally have been independent of the hospital and have made their own determinations of who should receive staff membership and what criteria should be applied in professional discipline. This was primarily a quality issue, and as we have indicated, it was the major method of quality assurance and improvement undertaken by hospitals. A hospital's executive committees and board of trustees could influence medical staff decisions to some extent. The underlying rationale for this activity was quality of care, but there was certainly the possibility that "quality of care" provides an excuse for exclusion of economic competitors.

The leading case on the anticompetitive efforts of medical staff arose out of a dispute between members of the medical staff of a small hospital in Astoria, Oregon. The case of *Patrick* v. *Burget* illustrates the sharp conflict between market imperatives provided by antitrust law and efforts to improve quality of care through a traditional peer review by medical staff. The facts of this case are quite involved, but they center on a conflict between Timothy Patrick, a surgeon, and his former colleagues at the Astoria Clinic. Patrick's colleagues brought several charges of inappropriate or negligent care against him, and he in turn alleged that the complaints were economically motivated.[24]

Patrick eventually sued in federal district court, alleging that the Astoria Clinic had violated Sections One and Two of the Sherman Act in an effort to reduce competition. The clinic partners denied the charges, but in a subsequent jury trial, a verdict was lodged against all respondents on a Section Two claim and several respondents on a Section One claim. Damages of $650,000 were awarded to Patrick. The members of the Astoria Clinic appealed to the Federal Court of Appeals for the Ninth Circuit. This court subsequently reversed the district court decision,[25] ruling that despite the possibility that the Astoria Clinic physicians had used the peer review process to discriminate and disadvantage a competitor, such peer review proceedings were immune from antitrust scrutiny under the so-called state action doctrine. Because the peer review process was required by the state of Oregon and was ultimately overseen by the Board of Medical Examiners, there could be no antitrust violation.[26]

Patrick appealed to the Supreme Court. He argued that the activities of the Astoria Clinic were not motivated by concerns over the quality of care but rather by clinic doctors' own economic interests. He had effectively been removed as a competitor through the ruse of peer review. Moreover, he argued that the state of Oregon's supervision of the peer review process was insufficient to allow a finding under the state action doctrine. In a decision that surprised many observers, the Supreme Court agreed with Patrick, ruling that there was inadequate evidence that the state of Oregon had actively supervised the peer review process. Moreover, in the Court's view of the facts, the anticompetitive activities had been patent. The Court was aware of the policy arguments elaborated by the supporters of the Astoria Clinic: "The policy argument of this effective peer review is essential to the provision of quality medical care and that any threat of antitrust liability will prevent physicians from participating openly and actively in peer review proceedings essentially challenges the wisdom of applying antitrust laws to the sphere of medical care and as such is properly directed to Congress.[27]

Patrick v. *Burget* thus starkly contrasts the notion of collaborative quality improvement efforts by a medical staff with market incentives to create a more competitive environment. As we have seen, the idea of collaborative activity by organized professionals to bring about continuous quality improvement is dependent on cooperation and, if you like, combination. Insofar as physicians are defined as the critical economic actors in the health care sphere, many concerted efforts, including those aimed at improving the quality of care, can be seen as antitrust violations.

The Supreme Court realized that Congress had already addressed this issue. In 1986, prompted by Representative Wyden, who was concerned about the ongoing *Patrick* v. *Burget* litigation in Oregon, Congress passed the Health Care Quality Improvement Act (HCQIA).[28] The government was anxious about rising rates of medical malpractice and attempted to promote better-quality care by protecting peer review participants from litigation. The HCQIA was thus intended to decrease the threat of antitrust litigation and improve care. It also laid the foundation for the National Practitioner Data Bank, which was to receive computerized reports on all instances of physician incompetence.[29]

Clearly, the framers of the HCQIA faced a very difficult task. On the one hand, they wanted to promote better-quality care by allowing peer review committees to do their work free of unnecessary or frivolous litigation. On the other hand, especially in cases like *Patrick*, it is clear that peer review committees can wield their power for the purpose of decreasing competition, which in turn probably increases health care costs. Moreover, competition could presumably improve quality while at the same time creating incentives for cost-effective care.[30] Although, as Representative Wyden stated, "doctors are in the best position to do something about malpractice because they see it happening around them,"[31] it is not at all clear that unlimited immunity from antitrust litigation is the most desirable public policy. Therefore Congress qualified HCQIA protection when certain conditions were present.[32] Many commentators believe that although the HCQIA's intent was to protect peer review considerations, the legislation itself afforded little such protection. Subsequent litigation has borne this out.[33]

The *Patrick* case involved exclusion of a present staff member. Other litigation involves staff candidates who have been excluded altogether. The plaintiffs typically complain that staff privileges have been denied for anticompetitive reasons rather than for true concerns about credentials or expertise. For example, in the well-known case of *Weiss* v. *York Hospital*,[34] the plaintiff, an osteopath, claimed that the medical staff had discriminated against him because he was an osteopath and would not provide him privileges at the York Hospital, which controlled many of the major invasive procedures in the York, Pennsylvania, metropolitan statistical area. The *Weiss* case documented that the Medical Affairs Committee of the hospital's board of directors had taken apparently special steps to review Weiss's application and had based its determination on very little hearsay evidence.

The court's analysis focused on the Section One Sherman Act claims, and in particular on the possibility of a medical staff acting as a combination of doctors, or in combination with the hospital. The court concluded that a conspiracy of the latter type was not possible as the hospital and medical staff were not competitors. On the other hand, the court was willing to find the medical staff to be made up of a multiplicity of competitors, rather than a single cohesive group incapable of constituting a combination. Therefore the Circuit Court of Appeals found the plaintiff's characterization of the medical staff's activity as a traditional boycott to be appropriate. Although other courts have ruled that medical staffs are incapable of such conspiracies, there continue to be some cases that find antitrust violations in similar circumstances.[35]

This kind of decision further frustrates the traditional role of the medical staff as the arbiter of quality within a health care institution. It suggests that the move to a competitive market, which is in some ways the major theme of federal influence on health care since the mid-1980s, will require new understanding of the sources of quality improvement. But again one must question if it is appropriate in a maturing health care system to think of individual doctors as competitors. Consider the improbable parallel of treating commercial airline pilots as competitors in the airline industry.

But both the *Patrick* and *Weiss* cases may be somewhat anachronistic in a health care delivery system dominated by IDSs with physicians tightly bound to hospitals. More important may be those cases involving exclusive contracts between hospitals and physicians. The leading case in this area for a long time was the 1984 decision *Jefferson Parish Hospital* v. *Hyde*, in which an anesthesiologist brought a tying claim against the hospital and the anesthesia group with which the hospital had executed an exclusive contract.[36]

The plaintiff's claim was that the hospital, in signing the exclusive contract, had illegally tied the provision of hospital services to one anesthesiology group, thereby inhibiting competition. He alleged that there were two separate markets, one for anesthesiology services and the other for medical care generally. In a somewhat tortured decision, the Supreme Court found that the per se rule against tying did not apply to the arrangement in question. The Court thought that patients could still make decisions about anesthesiology services if they so wished, and that the fact that they had to accept a certain set of anesthesiology services within Jefferson Parish Hospital did not restrain trade.

For our purposes, the central issue is again the definition of patient demand. In *Jefferson Parish*, both the Circuit Court and the Supreme Court were well aware that patients had few incentives to compare the costs, and insufficient information to compare the quality of care, of different anesthesiologists. Nonetheless, the courts accepted the fiction of the discriminating patient and delved into

.the intricacies of attempting to define the appropriate markets and the nature of the tying.

We have suggested that the mid-1990s are a quite different health care setting from the mid-1980s, at least in some jurisdictions. Patients are better informed about the quality of care and will become even more informed as data-reporting requirements develop. In addition, a great deal of health care reform is oriented toward increasing patients' economic incentives to select cost-effective care. Hence, much of the reasoning behind the decision in *Jefferson Parish* might not be repeated today, although it is still not a given that patients would want to select their own anesthesiologists.

The critical insight, however, is that the "tying" of hospital and physician staff is what vertical integration is all about. Physician services must be "tied" to other services if vertical integration is to occur. And to a large extent, cross-functional quality improvement efforts, like those reviewed in Chapter Six, are often quite dependent on collaborative efforts among various specialists and institutions. The mandates of antitrust law could inhibit such activities.[37]

Thus far, it does not appear that fears of antitrust actions are inhibiting the integration of hospitals with physician staff. The Supreme Court's decision in *Copperweld Corporation* v. *Independence Tube Corporation*[38] (parallelling the *Weiss* decision) states that a parent and its subsidiary are not distinct entities. Therefore physician-hospital organizations are not capable of "combining" or "conspiring." Moreover, even if the hospital has a relationship with a distinct physician organization, the Justice Department/FTC guidelines make it clear that so long as the members of a multiprovider network share substantial risk (through capitation or sharp incentives), there is no antitrust violation. Another method of avoiding antitrust scrutiny is through the so-called *messenger model,* in which an agent (the messenger) represents individual providers to purchasers, with no direct provider-purchaser contact. This technique was explicitly approved by the Justice Department in 1993.[39]

Although *Patrick, York Hospital,* and *Hyde* may all in some ways suggest that quality improvement efforts could be frustrated by antitrust litigation, the evolution of health care delivery has to some extent made these decisions moot. Providers are able to work together under capitated risk, which is the likely dominant mode of the future. Thus this aspect of antitrust, though not necessarily responsive, is not corrosive either.

Concerns about vertical integration of hospitals and providers lead naturally to concerns about horizontal integration of providers, the third area of antitrust litigation we survey. The government remains suspicious of provider-dominated networks, evincing its traditional fear of horizontal price-fixing first enunciated in *Arizona* v. *Maricopa County Medical Society*.[40] In that case, the Medical Society of Maricopa County had attempted to negotiate maximum fee schedules with third-party payers. The medical society was also willing to analyze the appropriateness of procedures. The Supreme Court found that the society could not be considered a single firm and instead represented a horizontal price-fixing arrangement, albeit at maximum prices.

In the dozen-odd years since *Maricopa County*, groups of physicians have chafed under antitrust requirements that they not control managed care organizations. Courts ruling on these issues have continued to reiterate the stance of the Supreme Court in *Maricopa County*.[41] In order to avoid restraint of trade, physicians in managed care organizations have to share in the risk of the enterprise, defined by one court as risk of nonpayment between 15 and 25 percent.[42] Moreover, the FTC has discussed the parameters of per se illegality and stated that "a substantial financial contribution to support the establishment or operation of the plan" is necessary to avoid an antitrust violation.[43] The federal authorities wish to avoid sham preferred provider organizations or other types of managed care organizations in which physicians would simply be fixing prices. The FTC has gone so far as to suggest that distribution of relative value scales for payment by the American Society of Internal Medicine might be an antitrust violation.[44]

The Justice Department has indicated that health care joint ventures would be in a *safe harbor* if they controlled less than 35 percent of a market.[45] Both sets of joint guidelines issued by the Justice Department and the FTC suggest that the physicians in a managed care venture must not only share substantial financial risk but must also constitute no more than 20 percent of the physicians practicing in a particular specialty in a geographical market.[46] This effectively prohibits physicians from establishing dominant managed care organizations within geographical areas.

The American Medical Association has argued that these rules must be changed to allow physician involvement in the establishment of managed care organizations.[47] The AMA advocated the passage of the Health Care Antitrust Improvement Bill of 1993, sponsored by Senators Orrin Hatch and Strom Thurmond. The first tier of this rather complicated bill, dealing with safe harbors, defines certain types of joint ventures and joint purchasing arrangements that would be allowed under the antitrust laws without further analysis. Most important, provider networks that account for less than 20 percent of provider type or specialty would be allowed.

The second tier of the bill is more controversial. Joint ventures that do not fall into one of the safe harbors could have their exemption from antitrust law provided by the attorney general in a specific *certificate of review*, which would have to be provided within ninety days. The point of certificates of review is to give potential joint ventures a relatively prompt green light from the federal authorities.

The third and most controversial tier is an exemption that protects all health care joint ventures, whether or not they fall into safe harbors or receive a certificate of review. So long as a joint venture disclosed its cooperative activities, it would automatically receive limited protection from antitrust prosecution. In addition, damages would no longer be trebled, and there could be no punitive damages. The aim of this portion of the act is to allow physicians to play a much larger role in joint ventures, with minimal fear of retribution under the antitrust laws. For example, so long as a network is

nonexclusive (providers may join competing networks), the network could contain up to 50 percent of the providers or specialists of
any type in its geographical area. This would be a much greater concentration than is presently allowed under the antitrust law.

In part, the AMA's case is that a physician-directed integrated
delivery system can provide higher-quality care. The argument is
that such networks are more likely to be sensitive to individual
patient need and can deal more adequately with the potential conflicts between cost-effectiveness and quality that were discussed in
Chapter Four.[48] The opponents of the AMA bills suggest, of course,
that physician-dominated independent practice associations or
alternative delivery systems would simply be cartels, with associated
price-fixing and inefficiencies. The activities of nascent physician
"unions" give credibility to the concerns of those who oppose physician control over managed care organizations.[49]

The limits of the government's flexibility are illustrated in several advisory opinions of recent years. For example, the FTC will
allow a large group of networked radiologists to provide readings of
files throughout California so long as the preferred provider uses a
"messenger" model and remains nonexclusive.[50] It will also allow 22
percent of the cardiologists in Denver to form a joint venture and
market capitated services to health plans.[51] But two questions linger:
might provider-dominated networks offer better-quality care? and
secondarily, does the probability of better care outweigh that of
higher cost due to decreased competition? As yet, there is insufficient information available to answer these questions, but federal
authorities may be open to responsive resolution of cases.

The fourth area of antitrust friction with health care concerns
the business of insurance. Antitrust doctrine has yet to catch up
with the reorganization of health care insurance. Traditionally,
courts presumed that insurance issues were beyond the reach of
antitrust analysis. The McCarran-Ferguson Act had granted insurers protection from antitrust laws, largely because it was thought
best to allow states to regulate insurance and because some collu-

sion between insurance companies was necessary to allow appropriate actuarial rating.[52]

Beginning with the decision of *Group Life and Health Insurance Co. v. Royal Drug, Inc.*, the Supreme Court began to narrow the definition of *business of insurance*.[53] In this case, the Court held that contracts between insurers and participating pharmacists did not involve the business of insurance under the McCarran-Ferguson Act. The subsequent decision of *Union Labor Life* v. *Pireno*, concerning the use of panels of chiropractors in benefit decisions by insurance companies, continued this trend of interpreting the nature of insurance narrowly. These cases opened the door to antitrust analysis of managed care organizations and other entities that bear risk in the financing markets for health care.[54] The growth of self-insured plans (discussed later in this chapter) administered by third-party administrators has further reduced the importance of the McCarran-Ferguson Act in antitrust issues pertaining to health care financing.[55]

But the courts have not been able to define the market for health care underwriting. As recently as 1993, the First Circuit Court of Appeals—the federal appeals court with arguably the greatest experience in health care antitrust issues—struggled to define the nature of the market, in a suit brought by an independent practice association model HMO. The HMO had claimed that the exclusive dealing clause in contracts between its competitor and participating physicians was a restraint of trade.[56] In this case, the options for an appropriate product market were 1) the demand for health care financing by consumers, and 2) the demand for physician services as purchased by an IPA.

Arguably, the appropriate market was physician services, but the court simplistically focused on the demand for health care financing. Clearly, physicians do not have an unlimited market for their services; one purchaser can dominate the market for physician services in a given geographical market. This suggests that there needs to be a broad rethinking of federal antitrust precedent to keep up with the evolving marketplace.

That the federal courts are awakening to the monopolization of contracts with providers by managed care organizations is revealed by the recent *Marshfield Clinic* decision.[57] In this case, Judge John C. Shabaz awarded Blue Cross & Blue Shield United of Wisconsin $10.5 million as compensation for the clinic's monopolistic behavior. The court found that the clinic, by forbidding its affiliated physicians to contract with other HMOs, had sought to monopolize health care and control prices. When a single insurer controls a market by sweeping up all the providers, quality may suffer. Courts should prohibit such monopolies, but they will continue to struggle with the definition of the market.

Antitrust law has the potential to be a source of responsive regulation and to develop the market context for other forms of responsive regulation. In health care, there is a rapidly evolving marketplace, with vertical and horizontal integration and many new forms of health care organization. The driving forces behind these trends are cost consciousness and management of health care, but quality improvement will tend to be one of the concerns of the new structures. Overall, the score card suggests that antitrust enforcers are showing some tendencies toward responsiveness, and this should be encouraged.

The Employee Retirement Income Security Act of 1974

The Employee Retirement Income Security Act (ERISA) has perhaps an even greater influence than antitrust law on the design of new rules for health care quality.[58] Poorly understood and little noticed, ERISA has severely hampered states' efforts to address the interrelated problems of health care cost and quality. ERISA's prominence in health care has grown over the past few years, as the Supreme Court has broadly construed its preemption provisions. In effect, federal district and circuit courts, following the Supreme Court's decisions, have prohibited almost any state legislation designed to ameliorate the current health care crisis. Remarkably, in the ongoing debate regarding health care reform, little attention has been paid to this very real and virtually insurmountable barrier to change.[59] Most of the discussions of ERISA overlook perhaps the most important aspect of ERISA preemption: the manner in which it blocks any sort of structural reform of health insurance by states. The reformation of ERISA will therefore be critical to any effort to regulate for improvement.

ERISA was enacted by Congress in 1974, at least in part in an effort to protect participants in employee pension and benefit plans and their beneficiaries from abuses by those who manage such plans. Employee welfare benefit plans as defined by the statute include benefit plans that, "through the purchase of insurance or otherwise," provide medical, surgical, or hospital care or benefits in the event of sickness, accident, disability, or death.[60] It is apparent that no one foresaw the wide-ranging implications that ERISA would have for health care.

Congress appears to have perceived ERISA as a form of redress for specific kinds of problems that it thought could best be remedied through uniform (that is, federal) standards. Legislators were particularly cognizant of the need for "equitable standards of plan administration; . . . minimum standards of plan design [and] of fiscal responsibility," as well as the importance of insuring the vested portion of unfunded liabilities against premature plan termination and of expanding and increasing participation in private retirement plans.[61]

Although promulgated for the purpose of protecting employees, ERISA is favored by employers—especially interstate employers—because of its preemption of state law. Section 1144(a) of ERISA states that it "shall supersede any and all State laws insofar as they may now or hereafter relate to any employee benefit plan" described in Section 1003(a). State law includes "all laws, decisions, rules, regulations, or other state action having the effect of law."[62]

Despite this broad jurisdiction, ERISA imposes virtually no

substantive requirements on employee benefit plans. Moreover, the Department of Labor, charged with administering ERISA, has not promulgated any meaningful regulations pertaining to the substance of employee benefit plans and has focused instead on pension plans, thereby perpetuating the situation that had inspired Congress to enact ERISA in the first place.[63]

A three-part analysis is used to determine whether ERISA preempts state law. First, preemption is presumed if the state law "relate[s] to any employee benefit plan." ERISA's preemption provision was originally drafted to cover state laws that "related to" the subject matters regulated by ERISA.[64] Thus only laws pertaining primarily to funding and disclosure requirements would face preemption. The broader language of relating to "any employee benefit plan" was intended by ERISA's principal sponsors to avert "the threat of conflicting or inconsistent state and local regulation of employee benefit plans."[65] The "relate to" requirement had originally been construed as *not* preempting laws having only a remote or tangential impact on ERISA plans.[66] Yet recently, most courts have placed a growing emphasis on the expansion of the "relate to" clause during the statute's drafting process as indicative of congressional intent that ERISA preempt any state law having any impact on an ERISA-qualified plan, no matter how attenuated the impact.[67] Under this extremely inclusive interpretation, even state laws that are consistent with ERISA have been preempted.[68]

Second, a state law relating to an employee benefit plan may be saved from preemption if it "regulates insurance, banking, or securities."[69] Under conventional preemption analysis, a federal statute will be presumed not to preempt areas traditionally left to state legislation unless there is an express or implied indication of congressional intent to occupy the field to the exclusion of state regulation.[70] ERISA's preemption clause explicitly provides that it does not supersede any state law that "regulates insurance."[71] Such regulation is "saved" by this clause. As discussed in the previous section, what qualifies as "the business of insurance" amenable to state regulation by virtue of the savings clause has been the focus of ongoing and ever-intensifying judicial inquiry.[72]

The third step of the ERISA preemption analysis concerns the *deemer clause*. State insurance regulation may be saved only to the extent that it regulates genuine insurance companies or insurance contracts. As a result, a state may not "deem" an employee benefit plan to be an insurance plan in an effort to avoid preemption if the benefit plan would not otherwise qualify as an insurance company or contract. The deemer clause therefore limits the application of the savings clause to conventionally insured employee benefit plans.

A self-insured plan does not carry on the "business of insurance" because the policyholder does not transfer risk or spread risk across a pool larger than the policyholder itself. Self-insured plans frequently contract with insurance companies for administrative services. In this context, the insurance company acts only as a third-party administrator. It does not act as an insurer because it neither assumes nor pools risk. Thus a state law cannot simply deem a self-funded plan to be insurance for the purpose of saving it from ERISA preemption.

Through the intricate three-step dance of the "relate to," "savings," and "deemer" clauses, ERISA permits states to regulate insurance plans but preempts any regulation of self-insured or uninsured plans.[73] Perhaps the Supreme Court's most compelling ground for adhering to this interpretation of the interaction of these provisions is that, at least since the 1985 case of *Metropolitan Life Insurance Co. v. Massachusetts,* Congress has been aware of the distinction, or "disuniformity," between insured and self-insured plans and, whether through design or neglect, has not amended the statute to alter its preemptive effect.[74] However, this may simply be a function of congressional gridlock or a measure of the success of various employer-sponsored interest groups in resisting state regulation, rather than a reflection of legislative intent or approval.[75]

Initially, only organizations with relatively large and healthy employee populations opted for self-funding, as their large size facilitated risk-spreading. However, as ERISA preemption has been used to provide an ever-expanding shield from state regulation, self-funding is growing in popularity among employers of all sizes.[76] It currently accounts for approximately 65 percent of all ERISA-qualified employee health benefit plans.[77]

In the absence of any meaningful federal effort over the past decade, states have formed the vanguard in trying to reform health care financing and quality improvement. Many of these efforts are now vulnerable to ERISA-based challenges. Consider the case of employer mandates to provide certain kinds or levels of benefits to employees.[78] In *Metropolitan Life*, a Massachusetts statute required "insured" employee benefit plans to provide coverage for mental health services. This requirement was designed in part to reduce the problem of adverse selection in mental health insurance. *Adverse selection* has many definitions, but in this context, it referred to the situation in which healthy individuals, who are less likely to need services, do not purchase insurance coverage. Thus the remaining pool consists of high-risk individuals more likely to use services and file claims. Adverse selection results in the inability to distribute risk over a heterogeneous pool and therefore drives up the cost of coverage for the sick.

Noting that a majority of states use mandated-benefit statutes to regulate the substantive content of insurance contracts, the Court ruled in *Metropolitan Life* that such laws are saved from preemption to the extent that they qualify as permissible state regulation of the "business of insurance" under the McCarran-Ferguson criteria.[79] The Court's ruling came only after an exhaustive analysis of the relationship between the savings and deemer clauses, and their relationship to the insured/self-insured distinction. It is worth noting the inhibitory impact of ERISA preemption in this case. What really saved the Massachusetts legislation was the state's decision not even to attempt to enforce that portion of the statute that imposed the same employer mandate on self-insured plans.[80] *Metropolitan Life* essentially frees the self-insured plan from state oversight.

Because ERISA does not mandate that benefit plans be provided or maintained at any particular level, an employer can revise such a plan without the consent of the employee. ERISA only requires that a plan amendment not discriminate against participants or interfere with or retaliate for a participant's exercise of rights under the plan.[81] Absent a contract of assurance that benefits will continue, an employer is free to increase or reduce benefits without notice to or the consent of the employee.[82]

Thus in *Vasseur* v. *Halliburton Co.*, an employer was allowed to modify a benefit plan so as to limit inpatient coverage to licensed hospitals as opposed to rehabilitation facilities. Similarly, in *McGann* v. *H & H Music Co.*, an employer was permitted to reduce lifetime medical benefits of $1 million per participant to $5,000 for AIDS-related claims after learning that one of its employees had AIDS.[83] Because the reduced coverage would pertain to any employee who developed AIDS, not just the HIV-infected plaintiff, the modification was ruled not unlawfully discriminatory under ERISA. *McGann*, recently affirmed by the Supreme Court without comment, could be logically extended to permit after-the-fact termination or reduction of benefits for other high-ticket health problems, such as cancer.[84] States would be powerless to halt such activities.

With the growing awareness of the extent of ERISA preemption, employee benefit plans are now asserting their right to be completely free of state regulation of health care financing. State attempts to redress adverse selection by cross-subsidizing uncompensated care and high-risk pools are being challenged and overturned. In *Bricklayers Local No. 1 Welfare Fund* v. *Louisiana Health Insurance Association*, ERISA preempted a Louisiana statute that had created a state health insurance association to fund and administer a catastrophic health insurance program.[85] New York's hospital rate-setting scheme was struck down for similar reasons in *Travelers Insurance Co.* v. *Cuomo*, although the Supreme Court subsequently reversed this decision.[86] The New York statute imposed a series of surcharges over the basic DRG (diagnostic related group) rate that

were based on the patient's particular kind of coverage. The surcharges were intended to reduce hospital rate disparities between
commercial insurers and Blue Cross and Blue Shield plans and
thereby preserve the economic viability of "the Blues."

New Jersey provides another example. The state's rate-setting
legislation was deemed to be unenforceable by the trial court in
United Wire, Metal & Machine Health & Welfare Fund v. *Morristown
Memorial Hospital,* which employed a rationale quite similar to that
of the *Travelers* court.[87] The New Jersey law granted discounts to
certain payers but included charges in the DRG rate to subsidize
uncompensated care and inadequate Medicare reimbursement.
Although this rate-setting legislation was the oldest of its kind and
did not explicitly regulate the terms or conditions of ERISA benefit plans, the trial court still found it to be preempted for "relating
to" such plans. Because the law did not purport to regulate insurance, the trial court further decided that it could not be saved from
preemption. Subsequently, the New Jersey legislature passed new
legislation that abandoned rate setting.[88]

As damaging as the Supreme Court's preemption analysis has
been to state efforts in the area of health care financing, the Court's
disposition of several still unresolved questions concerning health
care quality will carry the potential for even greater harm. At present, it is not clear whether state regulation of health maintenance
or preferred provider organizations will be undermined by ERISA
preemption; whether permissible state insurance regulation will
include the ability to regulate relations between insurers and
providers; or whether state challenges to determinations arising
from utilization reviews will be preempted. New rules to improve
health care quality may speak to all of these issues, especially insofar as such rules address cost/quality trade-offs in the emerging
health care system.

Decisions from lower courts indicate that ERISA's influence will
grow. ERISA preemption was recently invoked—albeit unsuccessfully, in the final analysis—to block Virginia's efforts to regulate pre-

ferred provider organizations. *Stuart Circle Hospital Corp.* v. *Aetna Health Management* involved Aetna's challenge of a number of any-willing-provider clauses in a state statute that governed contracts between insurers and preferred providers.[89] The trial court found that the statute "related to" ERISA employee benefit plans because it regulated insurer-established preferred provider organizations that served as vehicles for delivering health care services to employees covered by such plans. The statute could not be saved from preemption, as it did not regulate "the business of insurance." The trial court reasoned that instead of regulating the insurer's relationship with the insured, the statute focused on the relationship between the insurer and providers. The case thus provides an interesting footnote to the controversial any-willing-provider statutes discussed in Chapter Four.

The *Stuart Circle* decision was later reversed on appeal.[90] The Fourth Circuit Court characterized the any-willing-provider statute as the kind of insurance regulation properly saved from preemption because it was part of Virginia's overall insurance code and also regulated "the business of insurance." In this regard, the court reasoned that though the statute did focus on the insurer-provider relationship, it indirectly regulated the insurer-insured relationship. Moreover, because the law sought to protect an insured's choice of providers, it affected how the insured's "risk" would be spread over the risk pool and thus deserved to be saved from preemption as the business of insurance.

Currently, Virginia is one of twenty-eight states regulating preferred provider organizations and one of more than twenty with specific any-willing-provider clauses.[91] Although Virginia's preferred provider legislation has managed to survive preemption so far, the Supreme Court's continuing predilection for giving ERISA an exceedingly broad jurisdiction could portend the eventual overturn of *Stuart Circle* and jeopardize each of the twenty-seven other state regulations. The appellate rationale that saved the Virginia statute from preemption in *Stuart Circle* is by no means airtight. Other jurisdictions could find, as did the trial courts in *Stuart Circle* and *HCA Health Services of Virginia, Inc., v. Aetna Life Insurance Co.*, that state regulation of insurers' dealings with providers does not satisfy the McCarran-Ferguson definition of "the business of insurance" upheld in *Metropolitan Life*.[92] Although the *Stuart Circle* appellate court rejected an assertion by Aetna that preferred provider contracts do not transfer risk but merely facilitate the exchange of goods and services, other courts may be more receptive, as this distinction has proved critical to defining "the business of insurance" in the antitrust context.[93] In addition, should other courts—and eventually, the Supreme Court—prefer the *Stuart Circle* interpretation of the "relate to" requirement, HMO regulation will also be at risk.

As the Supreme Court has not resolved the insurer status of HMOs, preferred provider organizations, and other managed care entities, lower courts will continue to reach conflicting decisions about whether such entities are insurers subject to the ERISA preemption savings clause. Some courts have found that because an HMO actually provides health care, it does not qualify as an insurer, which typically reimburses either the patient or third-party provider.[94] But at least one court has ruled that HMO regulation can be saved from ERISA preemption because HMOs "assume the financial risk of providing benefits to their members and are therefore insurers for purposes of the savings clause."[95] The uncertainty surrounding ERISA preemption of HMOs is further evidenced by two decisions that ERISA preemption is not a defense for an HMO acting as a provider (as opposed to a payer and possible insurer).[96] Nevertheless, a 1993 conference hosted by the Group Health Association of America (GHAA) advised managed care groups, particularly HMOs, to structure themselves so as to take full advantage of the "bonus" of ERISA preemption from state regulation.[97]

The GHAA view is reinforced by the decision in *Elsesser v. Hospital of Philadelphia College*, in which the federal district court found that ERISA preempted a negligence claim against an HMO that had incorrectly instructed a physician about payment for an ambulatory cardiac monitor.[98] Although the court left standing an ostensible agency theory, the plaintiff's case was nonetheless greatly weakened by the ERISA preemption. If the reach of ERISA continues to expand, it may well be that HMO liability will decline and that any-willing-provider laws at the state level will be invalidated. This in turn will mean that liability for medical negligence will continue to attach to the individual practitioner, that managed care organizations and utilization reviewers will be essentially immune from liability, and that these parties will be allowed to contract narrowly with providers. ERISA thus retards the development of the sort of liability that could rationally give rise to improvements in the health care system as a whole. Once again, the federalization of health law is preventing what might be considered a salutary development: the diffusion of liability into the entire structure of health care.[99]

The same phenomenon occurs in utilization review generally. ERISA has preempted an employee's ability to challenge a utilization review decision in *Corcoran* v. *United Health Care, Inc.*[100] The plaintiff in *Corcoran* was covered by a self-funded employee benefit plan that required participants to obtain precertification from United Health Care (UHC), an independent utilization review organization hired by the plan to provide such services. UHC denied precertification of hospitalization for the plaintiff's high-risk pregnancy despite her history of similar problems, her obstetrician's vigorous recommendation of hospitalization, and its own independently retained expert's opinion that hospitalization was necessary to permit constant fetal monitoring. Instead, UHC authorized in-home nursing care for ten hours per day. At a time when no nurse was on duty, the fetus became distressed and died. The plaintiff attempted to assert claims against UHC under state common law, arguing that UHC's medical decision in denying hospitalization was negligent.[101]

There was no attempt to sue the self-funded plan itself. Nevertheless, the tort action was deemed preempted by ERISA because the state law that might have permitted such a claim "related to" ERISA benefit plans.[102] Acknowledging that utilization review determinations were, in fact, "medical decisions," the court found that such decisions were not actionable because they were made in the context of determining the availability of benefits under self-funded plans. In the court's view, permitting such decisions to be challenged through state tort remedies would undermine the uniform regulation of benefit plans that Congress intended to secure through ERISA preemption.

The *Corcoran* court was obviously disturbed by its decision, which left the plaintiff with "no remedy, state or federal, for what may have been a serious mistake." As interpreted by that court, ERISA preemption immunizes utilization review determinations from generally applicable liability rules, thereby fostering decision making that may lead to substandard care and decreasing a benefit plan's incentives to "seek out the [utilization review] companies that can deliver both high quality services and reasonable prices."[103] Feeling constrained by the congressional goal of uniform regulation to rule as it did, the court did not overlook the irony of applying a statute designed to safeguard workers in a manner so obviously detrimental to the plaintiff employee.

In a sense, the *Corcoran* decision promotes an artificial distinction between cost containment and quality improvement—a distinction that bodes ill for quality regulation in any case in which cost containment and improvement efforts come into conflict. *Corcoran* is not an isolated case. Several other courts have now decided that utilization management liability is preempted by ERISA.[104] One can take little comfort in the fact that utilization review is now the object of somewhat lax self-regulation.[105] Insofar as ERISA prohibits suits against utilization managers, it eliminates the institutional liability that enterprise liability would promote. The resolution of this conflict between federal law and state efforts to ensure good care will in part determine whether or not malpractice litigation will provide a strong regulatory basis for quality improvement.

In 1993, the court in *Kuhl v. Lincoln National Health Plan of Kansas City, Inc.*, held that an employee's group health plan could not be sued for state common law claims arising from the plan's pre-certification review because such claims "related to," and thus were preempted by, ERISA.[106] After an employee was diagnosed as needing immediate surgery for ischemic heart disease, the plan sought a second opinion. The second physician agreed with the first and stated that the employee was at high risk of sudden death. Following numerous delays extending over several months, the plan ultimately precertified the recommended surgery. By that time, however, Kuhl's heart had deteriorated to the point where the originally recommended surgery was no longer feasible. He died of the precise ailments first diagnosed seven months earlier. At the time, he was awaiting a heart transplant, which the plan had refused to precertify.

Responding to the health plan's contention that ERISA preempts state claims relating to the administration of plan benefits, the employee's estate also sought monetary damages for breach of ERISA-imposed fiduciary duties.[107] This claim failed because damages do not qualify as "equitable relief" available under ERISA. In leaving the Kuhls without a remedy, the court echoed the *Corcoran* decision, observing that Congress may not have foreseen ERISA's impact on utilization review "when it enacted a preemption clause so broad that it relieves ERISA-regulated plans of most tort liability." Still, it concluded, "modification of ERISA in light of questionable modern insurance practices must be the job of Congress, not the courts."[108]

It is difficult to predict how broad the ERISA preemption doctrine will grow. In 1995, the United States Supreme Court overturned the First Circuit's decision in the *Travelers* case.[109] However, the importance of the Supreme Court decision is undermined somewhat by a peculiar footnote that suggests the ruling does not apply to self-insured plans.

The *Travelers* decision offers some hope that the Supreme Court has recognized the imbalance between regulators and regulated that ERISA has created. Unless, as Braithwaite has noted, regulators have *some* leverage over industry, responsive regulation cannot occur. Cooperation can take place only when the two sides come to the table, but pre-*Travelers* ERISA takes away the regulator seat.

Fraud and Abuse Law

Reviewing antitrust and ERISA, one might conclude that federalization accelerates the changes toward a market environment.[110] Just the opposite is the case with other federal influences, especially federal fraud and abuse law. Under the Medicare program, there are severe penalties for defrauding the federal government. Although the antifraud provision has long been a part of the Medicare statute, it was amended significantly in 1977, when the crime was upgraded from a misdemeanor to a felony.[111] In addition, Congress broadened the definition of *kickbacks*, or cash payments to encourage referral of work, to create a brighter line for prosecutors. For example, even if a physician had performed some service, kickbacks for referrals were found to be illegal.[112] Kickbacks could include any false statements about services, as well as "remuneration" from referrals or purchases.[113]

In the mid-1980s, prosecution of the fraud and abuse statutes received a significant boost from the Third Circuit Court of Appeals decision in *United States* v. *Greber*.[114] In this case, the defendant was the president of Cardio-Med, Inc., an organization that provided Holter monitor services. Cardio-Med billed Medicare for these services and once payment was received, forwarded a portion to the referring physician. The federal government charged that this was a kickback. In its decision, the court repudiated the theory that the prosecution had to show intent. It ruled that the statute prohibited *any* "remuneration" and did not require analysis of the defendant's state of mind. In so ruling, the court diverged from a previous decision by the Fifth Circuit Court of Appeals that had required a finding of intent before the defendant could be successfully prosecuted. *Greber* significantly reduced the threshold for fraud and abuse pros-

ecution.[115] The "no intent" ruling has subsequently been endorsed
by other federal appeals courts.

A broader definition of fraud and abuse and the lower threshold
for prosecution that it brings tend to interfere with the development
of a market in health care. Although pure kickbacks should be illegal, the market often requires a variety of financial incentives if it
is to operate appropriately and efficiently. The extension and expansion of the Medicare definition of fraud and abuse brings into question many activities that are critical in the evolution of competing
vertically integrated plans. Federal prosecution now proceeds on the
assumption that doctors should not participate in any arrangements
in the marketplace that would lead to financial inurement, even if
such activities produce greater efficiency.

Physicians and investors in health care markets have pushed
the federal government to delineate the activities that are appropriate under the fraud and abuse provisions of the Medicare law.
The Department of Health and Human Services (DHHS) has
responded by promulgating ever more expansive safe harbor regulations. First offered in draft form in 1989, safe harbors have now
been incorporated into federal regulations.[116] They are intended to
assure investors that certain arrangements will not be subject to
federal scrutiny. For example, investments are legal if there is no
relationship between participation and the volume of referrals. The
safe harbor rules also go into detail about appropriate space and
equipment rentals, personal services, and warranties. As in antitrust, the safe harbors represent at least a step toward responsive
regulation.

But existing safe harbors have not clarified the most important
issue, which is the nature of economic relationships that can exist
between partners in a joint venture. As discussed earlier, joint ventures are becoming a critical element in the revolution of the
health care delivery system. Insofar as some providers are involved
in joint ventures and enjoy certain economic incentives within the
venture, there is the potential for the appearance of a kickback or

"remuneration." The same might be true if certain kinds of induce-ments were paid for high-quality care.

These issues have been widely discussed in the *Hanlester Net-work* case.[117] The Hanlester Network consisted of three limited part-nerships of physicians. Each of the partnerships contracted with Smith Kline Beckman laboratories to perform laboratory tests. Physicians invested at least $1,500 in one of the partnerships, referred all patients who needed laboratory tests to the partnership, and eventually received a return on investment proportionate to their ownership. Most received a 50 percent return on investment. The government charged that the arrangement was a violation of the Medicare/Medicaid fraud and abuse statute and prosecuted the limited partnerships. The Appeals Board of the DHHS eventually agreed with the federal government that prosecution was appropri-ate. Several more rounds of litigation occurred, with the govern-ment prevailing on its Greber theory until the Ninth Circuit Court of Appeals overturned the District Court in April 1995.[118] This case and others like it have only increased industry demand for clarifi-cation, as many aspects of the Hanlester referral system are critical to successfully integrated delivery systems.[119]

Yet there is little congressional or executive interest in restrain-ing fraud and abuse prosecution. In some ways, the prosecutions of the Medicare and Medicaid programs by the federal government can be seen as efforts to make the market work more efficiently by eliminating abuses. On the other hand, the antifraud statutes tend to frustrate what might otherwise be seen as fairly reasonable in-ducements for developing joint ventures. For instance, fraud and abuse prosecution has gone so far as to prohibit any sorts of rent waivers or parking privileges for physicians with whom hospitals are attempting to develop a close working relationship.[120] It is quite unclear how this contributes to quality in an increasingly market-driven environment.

Today, many arrangements between an IDS and physicians being recruited to join it could be construed as violations of Medicare fraud and abuse provisions. Any additional benefit or payment to induce referrals is illegal, yet that is what an IDS arrangement is intended to do. Future referrals are a dominant reason for the purchase of practices, but the promise of such referrals is prohibited. Collectively, much of the health care industry is averting its gaze from legally marginal arrangements. Aversion of gaze may be appropriate. If the IDS or physician-hospital organization is a means of improving quality, then the fraud statutes stand in the way of better medical care. Should the fear of kickbacks, rooted in a much different and simpler health care setting, frustrate integration?

Simply put, the fraud and abuse statutes forbid any physician profit from joint ventures. Though this proposition is conceptually aligned with the traditional notion that the physician is paid only for care of the patient, it is quite out of step with the modern health care market. Many of us might wish to bring an end to physician profiteering in health care ventures, largely because we fear that conflict of interest may harm the quality of patient care. However, this stance clearly conflicts with and frustrates the quality improvement that can be produced by integration.[121] If the federal government begins to aggressively prosecute "any remuneration" arising out of joint ventures, the growth of the market in medical care and the hope for quality-based competition will be dampened, perhaps significantly.[122]

Even more relevant to physician participation in the marketplace is the legislation referred to as "Stark I and II." Representative Fortney Stark has long been concerned with physician self-referral—in particular, physician referral of patients to laboratories or other medical practices owned by the physicians themselves. This has also been a concern of medical ethicists, who have long deplored such schemes. The American Medical Association has also prohibited patient referrals to physician-owned facilities.[123]

But there is no unanimity on the value of self-referrals. Perhaps unsurprisingly, the FTC has defended these arrangements as procompetitive and potentially conducive to cost reduction and quality improvement. The FTC and others have argued that physicians are uniquely positioned to ensure quality of care and to provide greater access.[124] Indeed, from the market viewpoint, physician profit from such entities is not inappropriate as long as it does not lead to inefficiencies.

Existing evidence suggests that inefficiencies have been common. For instance, physician investors utilizing their own outpatient diagnostic imaging centers tend to refer much more frequently than do physicians who are not investors. The same is true in workers' compensation programs.[125] However, one could imagine that with the maturing of the health care market and greater use of capitation, the incentives to overrefer would begin to evaporate. Furthermore, overutilization and poor outcomes might soon be part of reporting systems, and poor performance will further decrease the competitiveness of physicians who abuse self-referring relationships.

None of these possibilities have diminished Representative Stark's vigorous campaign to end self-referral. In December 1989, his Ethics in Patient Referrals Act was passed, becoming effective on January 1, 1992.[126] Known as Stark I, the act prohibited physicians from referring patients to clinical laboratories in which they had a financial interest. It was extended in so-called Stark II, part of the Omnibus Budget Reconciliation Act of 1993, which went into effect at the beginning of 1995. The latter statute goes beyond clinical laboratories to end self-referrals to nine other categories of ancillary medical services. Moreover, it applies not only to Medicare but also to Medicaid. Enforcement of Stark II, however, was suspended early in 1995.[127]

Stark II recognizes that the prohibition against self-referral could retard vertical integration. Therefore the statute creates relatively broad exceptions for physician ownership in hospitals, for physician services within the same group practices, for purchase of physician practices, and for services furnished under prepaid plans.[128] The legislation does, however, appear to be hostile to joint ventures other than physician-hospital plans, as there is no clear Stark exception for these quite prevalent arrangements. Moreover, Stark exceptions apply only to "ownership or investment interests," not to mere "compensation arrangements."[129]

Stark-style economic regulation is very much at odds with the shift toward markets in medical care.[130] If physicians can invest in a variety of services to which they refer patients, and if this provides the foundation for efficient, high-quality medical care, why should this not be allowed, even encouraged? One could imagine that the attraction of greater profit would lead physicians to provide higher-quality care, and they might do this by owning and supervising the organizations through which care is provided. As capitation creates fundamental incentives to minimize utilization, the argument for investment becomes more compelling.

To some extent, Stark I and II can be seen as reiterations of the pervasive federal suspicion that physicians will take advantage of any health care marketplace. In antitrust, this prejudice was apparent in the ongoing definition of the physician as the primary economic actor and in the hostility to physician domination of managed care organizations. In Stark I and II, as well as in much of the fraud and abuse litigation, the underlying motivation is the fear of physician profit at the expense of the patient (moral hazard) and the potential for poor care that this arrangement implies. If capitated payment, outcome measures, and Total Quality Management become part of the health care delivery system, there may be less need for these federal regulations. More important, as the focus in quality assurance shifts from the individual doctor's commitment to the individual patient to a strategy based on industrial quality improvement, the need for bans on self-referrals in particular becomes less urgent.

Fraud and abuse policy has not produced responsive rules. Much of what we see in Stark I and II represents federal command and control of the market and hostility toward anything other than the traditional physician commitment to the patient as a basis for quality. Nor does fraud and abuse law address the critical problems of cost/quality trade-offs in a managed care environment. Its emphasis on prohibition of referral mechanisms is skew to the real quality problems raised by managed care.

Tax Policy

Tax policy is less easily characterized from the viewpoint of new rules. Because an overwhelming proportion of the hospital industry has nonprofit status, the government has always had significant power to dictate institutions' behavior. The loss of the right to accept tax-exempt donations and the threat of liability to pay federal and state income tax have made most hospitals acutely aware of the need to adhere to Internal Revenue Service (IRS) rulings. The nature of the quid pro quo for the exempt status is not a new issue. A community benefit standard was established by the IRS in 1969 to ensure that hospitals appropriately acted as charities and provided care for those without insurance.[131]

Some propose that tax-exempt status be lifted from much of the health care delivery system. Over ten years ago, Robert Clark incisively argued that the nonprofit status of hospitals was simply acting as a barrier to the development of a purely competitive market. His views on the subject were quite influential in the eventual decision by the Utah Supreme Court to lift the state tax-exempt status of an Intermountain Health Care facility.[132] Subsequently, other states have begun to scrutinize the public charity status of health care institutions.[133] On the other hand, some states have taken a very liberal approach to property tax exemption.[134]

In 1990, several United States congresspersons asked the IRS to impose strict rules of compliance with the community benefits standard.[135] The impetus for this request was a General Accounting Office report revealing a poor correlation between hospitals' nonprofit status and the uncompensated care they provided. The IRS has responded by issuing new guidelines and beginning to engage in stricter scrutiny of the nonprofit status of various alternative delivery systems.

Such delivery systems present significant problems to the IRS. Nonprofit hospitals and previously nonprofit physician groups may come together to form HMOs or management service organizations, as discussed in Chapter Four. When this occurs, the IRS typically inquires as to whether or not the new organization is an integral part of the existing health care institutions. In the case of *Geisinger Health Plan v. Commissioner of Internal Review*,[136] the Tax Court ruled that the Geisinger Health Plan, an HMO developed by the Geisinger Clinic, did not perform an essential service for its charitable affiliates or their patients. Though the plaintiff argued that it was a "natural extension of the Geisinger system, enabling us to reach more people in its service area and to control the quality of health care delivered to the community," the IRS found the HMO subscription service to be an unrelated business. As with fraud and abuse provisions, the denial of not-for-profit status to the HMO complicates the relationships within the various units of an alternative delivery system and so will in some ways act as an obstacle to integration.

The IRS now clearly intends to scrutinize tax-exempt status for integrated delivery systems.[137] In the so-called Billings and Facey letters, the IRS granted nonprofit status to medical foundations that was contingent on certain factors establishing community benefit. There were four major categories of standards: traditional community benefit, community control, access to provider, and antikickback regulation. These are defined in some detail and offer evidence that the IRS is at least aware of the effort to integrate health care and is willing to consider this in its decisions regarding tax-exempt status. The most controversial aspect of the IRS's determinations has been that tax-exempt status is granted only on the condition that an IDS not violate federal antikickback regulations.[138] The Inspector General of the DHHS has been very concerned that inflated purchase prices were being paid for physician practices, largely to pay the vendors for future referrals to IDS hospitals and clinics. Making tax-exempt status contingent on careful compliance with antikickback rules reinforces the fraud and abuse statutes.

Another new area of tax law scrutiny concerns recruitment and retention of staff. The Hermann Hospital in Houston, Texas, recently disclosed voluntarily that it may have broken IRS rules when rewarding physicians with a variety of incentives. In October 1994, the hospital and the IRS entered into an agreement in which the hospital admitted guilt and paid a large fine. The closing agreement was widely read as a bridge between fraud and abuse prosecution and tax code violations.[139] The link between tax policy and fraud provisions was made explicit in proposed rules issued by the IRS in 1995.[140]

Tax law also regulates the participation of practicing physicians in vertically integrated organizations. If an IDS wishes to retain tax-exempt status, physician representation on the board is generally limited to 20 percent. The IRS has made it clear that PHOs cannot be tax-exempt organizations; indeed, participating hospitals must be careful not to lose their own tax-exempt status. Fair market value for service, appropriate capital contribution by physicians, and control over the board of the PHO must all be assured. Even taxable PHOs may face limits on the proportion of board members who can be physicians. Thus, the IRS—like the DHHS and the Justice Department—continues to apply pressure to keep physicians from dominating integrated plans.

The IRS rulings are not clearly at odds with the evolution of the market. In fact, they may push the industry toward a for-profit stance, which may be the natural evolution of health care. Of course, many will be concerned that quality might suffer in such an environment, whereas others will point to the benefit of quality competition.

Thus tax laws and fraud and abuse regulations, though ever more closely linked in enforcement, have different consequences. The latter complicates and retards the evolution toward the market; it is the kind of regulation that provides the foundation for providers' charges that regulation is obstructive. Tax policy simply pushes toward a for-profit footing for medical care. It might serve as the foundation for new rules in the future.

Medicaid

The last federal policy that provides the context for new rules is the Medicaid program. Medicaid is the federal-state cooperative program that provides medical care to the *deserving poor*. The deserving poor are defined by their qualification for a number of federal categories.[141] Succinctly put, the *categorically needy* are those who qualify for the federal Supplemental Security Income program (SSI) or families eligible for benefits under the Aid to Families with Dependent Children program (AFDC).[142] States are free to choose whether they participate in the Medicaid program, but if they do so, they must cover the categorically needy. States may also choose to provide coverage under a number of optional programs and may finance care for the so-called *medically needy*—those who would be categorically eligible but whose income exceeds eligibility levels.

The result of this patchwork is that states vary in the proportions of their populations to whom Medicaid benefits are provided. In 1988, for example, the maximum AFDC income eligibility level for a family of three ranged from $9,140 a year in Alaska to $1,416 a year in Mississippi.[143] Disparities have grown wider as some states have dramatically increased their Medicaid budgets, largely because much of the increase is paid for by the federal government. From 1987 to 1991, New York State's Medicaid service expense increased from $9 billion dollars to $17.4 billion dollars.[144] This explosive growth was driven by a policy of maximizing the use of outside (federal) resources. For example, the Office of Mental Health of the State of New York has aggressively shifted patients from state developmental psychiatric centers into cheaper, less structured community-based programs for which Medicaid reimbursement is available. Other states have followed suit.

The availability of significant federal subsidies has not, however, created a perception of Medicaid as "cost-free pork." Indeed, most states complain that they are being bankrupted by increasing Medicaid expenditures. In many states, Medicaid is the single largest budgetary item and continues to grow well beyond the rate of general inflation. This has led to ever-intensifying demands for changes in the Medicaid program generally—and especially for states to exert more control.

State control and experimentation with new forms of delivery under Medicaid are allowed under the *waiver process*. There are essentially two types of waivers available for states: demonstration and programmatic. Section 1115 of the Social Security Act allows states to conduct demonstration programs such as primary care case-management programs, to plan new methods of cost-effective medical care, to restrict the pool of providers from whom individuals may seek services, and to act as central brokers for assisting individuals.[145] Demonstrations are intended to be research-oriented and must be carefully evaluated by states. Programmatic waivers, on the other hand, are intended to allow states more flexibility in administration; they do not support new demonstration projects.[146]

Interest in Medicaid waivers has waxed and waned over the past decade. In the early 1980s, a number of states initiated demonstration waivers, many of which included experiments with managed care concepts.[147] From 1980 to 1990, there were 172 demonstration waivers, most of them initiated in 1980, 1981, and 1982. Included among these were the rate-setting measures in Maryland, Massachusetts, New Jersey, and New York that were discussed in Chapter Two. During the mid-1980s, programmatic waivers became more prevalent.[148]

But the latest wave of demonstration waivers is perhaps the most important. The Clinton administration reopened the demonstration waiver process and allowed a series of more sweeping changes in Medicaid. The most highly publicized example is the Oregon effort to ration services for Medicaid recipients.[149] In 1989, Oregon first applied for a Section 1115 demonstration waiver that would allow the state to put into place a list of eight hundred medical procedures or treatments that were rank-ordered according to cost-effectiveness. The Bush administration first refused to grant the waiver, but the Department of Health and Human Services under the Clinton administration subsequently relented, especially after concerns about possible discrimination against the disabled were addressed.[150]

Other demonstration waivers have subsequently been granted for more conventional but nonetheless sweeping reforms of Medicaid programs. For example, Hawaii's Health QUEST was implemented in April 1994. The QUEST program privatizes three state programs and creates a single purchasing pool through which managed care organizations bid for contracts on a fully capitated basis for more than eighty-eight thousand public clients. A five-year evaluation is planned. Part of the legislation is intended to spur the growth of managed care organizations. It is also meant to reduce administrative costs and improve the quality of care. With regard to the latter, there are plans to conduct on-site quality reviews and to survey beneficiaries.

A more disturbing scenario has played out in Tennessee. Tennessee's Medicaid expenditures tripled from less than $1 billion in 1987 to $2.8 billion in 1993. To bring costs under control, Tennessee has instituted the TENNcare program, through which the state's 900,000 Medicaid enrollees are pooled with 600,000 Medicaid-eligible, uninsured, and medically uninsurable individuals. TENNcare enrollees choose either an HMO or a preferred provider plan, and an individual primary care manager within the managed care organization through which they receive all their health services. The state is subdivided among twelve community health agencies, each of which contains at least two managed care organizations. The TENNcare benefits are more generous than traditional Medicaid benefit packages, encompassing prescription drugs, medical supplies, and home health care.

Each managed care organization is paid on a capitated monthly basis for services, subject to a 10 percent penalty for noncompliance with TENNcare rules. Uniform capitation rates were set for each community health agency. The 1994 base capitation rate was set at $1,230 per patient, which was 25 percent less than the

$1,641 actuarial rate that was established in a waiver application. Managed care organizations estimated in 1994 that they would have to achieve cost reductions of 35 percent from current medical service rates in order to meet this new bottom line.

Given the expedited capitation process and the relatively underfunded capitation rate, TENNcare was bound to engage in significant trade-offs between cost and quality. The program's reputation was sullied by hasty implementation in January 1994 after only eight months of planning. Moreover, only 6 percent of Tennessee residents had been enrolled in managed care organizations before the introduction of TENNcare; there simply was not a mature managed care industry ready to accept capitation. A number of managed care organizations used questionable marketing techniques, including offering cash, credit, and food as enrollment incentives. A large number of patients were administratively reassigned to new providers without consultation. To make matters worse, Tennessee received permission to eliminate Medicaid payments to hospitals serving a disproportionately large share of Medicaid and other low-income patients. This will probably impoverish hospitals already serving the poor in Tennessee.

Not surprisingly, Tennessee physicians sued the state in connection with TENNcare. The Tennessee Medical Association, which represents 6,700 of the state's 10,000 physicians, filed a suit on December 30, 1993, in an effort to force the state of Tennessee to disclose the capitation methodology. The suit was eventually dismissed by Tennessee courts, but other litigation brought by providers still persisted at the time of this writing.[151]

TENNcare demonstrates the federal government's willingness to allow state Medicaid programs to engage in sweeping managed care reforms. However, it also indicates that finances, not quality, may drive such state reforms. Whereas Hawaii's QUEST program has significant quality oversight features, TENNcare is obviously focused on costs. The result may be inferior care for recipients of Medicaid in Tennessee.

Remarkably, when reviewing changes in Medicaid financing, the federal government requires very little analysis of potential effects on health care outcomes. For instance, in Massachusetts, the Medicaid programmatic waiver to initiate managed care was the subject of a yearlong study costing less than $50,000.[152] With such a small study, it is impossible to fully evaluate the outcomes of the system or even to make reasonable guesses about the potential impact on health care. One could certainly argue that moving patients from established relationships with primary care providers to the new managed care providers under the Tennessee or Massachusetts program represents a dislocation for the poor that could affect their health. However, waiver studies have rarely addressed these issues.[153]

The approach of the federal government here is paradoxical in light of the effect of other federal initiatives. Compared to the shackles placed on state regulation by ERISA, and to some extent by antitrust law, Medicaid waivers give states significant leeway to experiment. The quality issues will differ between states as they struggle to reduce Medicaid budgets.[154] The waiver process is therefore a perfect target for responsive regulation as HCFA works with states to define new Medicaid programs. The potential for cost/quality trade-offs should call for new rules that regulators from the federal level and leaders of state Medicaid programs can work out collaboratively.

The other major policy development in the Medicaid program also involves a trade-off between cost and quality, the issue that dominates health policy as we approach the year 2000, but appears less apt to lead to responsive regulation. The litigation around the so-called Boren Amendment, Section 1902 of the Social Security Act, may provide a window onto the future if the federal influence in health care continues to grow and as friction between cost containment and quality improvement becomes more acute. Section 1902 sets forth the structure for rates of reimbursement for providers.[155] States participating in Medicaid must follow these rules in their payment of physicians, hospitals, and long-term care facilities.

Before 1980, the federal government simply required that providers be reimbursed on a *reasonable cost basis*—essentially the same "pass through" of costs that was the rule in Medicare and that fueled the inflation of the cost of care through the 1970s. States had some flexibility in defining reasonable cost reimbursement, but these definitions were subject to approval by the secretary of health, education, and welfare.[156]

To help states moderate the costs of Medicaid, Congress enacted the Boren Amendment, which empowered states to formulate new reimbursement methods. These reimbursement methods had to be "reasonable and adequate to meet the costs which must be incurred by efficient and economical facilities in order to provide care and services in conforming with applicable state and federal laws, regulations and standards."[157] Henceforth, states could develop their own programs for reimbursement and begin to gain some control over the costs of Medicaid. By 1981, the Boren Amendment had been extended to hospital services. At much the same time, and at the behest of the Reagan administration, Congress was reducing the federal contribution to the Medicaid program, creating additional state concerns about cost containment.[158]

Congress did not ignore the quality implications of such cost reductions. As the House committee overseeing the Boren Amendment noted, "The flexibility given the states is not intended to encourage arbitrary reductions in payment that would adversely affect the quality of care."[159] The reimbursement under the new state programs had to be sufficient to allow all Medicaid recipients to receive high-quality care. In many ways, this language is striking, given the calm assertions today that a great deal of money can be saved in both Medicare and Medicaid without reducing the quality of care.

The states moved quickly to reduce Medicaid costs.[160] Providers in a number of states began to feel the pinch of these reduced reimbursement levels and sought relief in federal courts. A variety of suits were filed under a federal statute known as Section 1983, which has long been used by civil rights activists to force states to comply with the requirements of federal law.[161] Faced with litigation in a number of circuits, the Supreme Court granted *certiorari* to review the reach of the Boren Amendment and ruled strongly in favor of providers in the decision of *Wilder* v. *Virginia Hospital Association*.[162] In short, the *Wilder* decision states that Congress intended health care providers to be the beneficiaries of the Boren Amendment and that as a result they could bring suits pursuant to 42 U.S.C., Section 1983, in order to enforce the provisions of the amendment. The Supreme Court did not define exactly what standards states had to meet in their reimbursement levels. Though "efficient and economical facilities" was treated by the Court as an objective benchmark, the opinion did not go into detail on "efficient and economical," nor did it define "reasonable and adequate" rates. Subsequent cases have found the courts attempting to ensure that states comply carefully with the procedural requirements of the amendment. In many cases, the states have had to undertake empirical analyses of the effects of new changes in reimbursement.

Compliance with *Wilder* represents a significant break with the past. In the period before *Wilder*, many states were changing their Medicaid reimbursement policies without any analysis of the impact on providers or, more important, on the quality of care. As the Fifth Circuit Court noted in the case of *Abbeville General Hospital* v. *Ramsey*, "[T]he [new] findings requirement is not a mere formality that can be satisfied simply by having a state officer think a bit about hospital costs and then copy out the statutory language on a piece of paper, put the heading 'assurances' on that piece of paper and sending it to HCFA."[163] Boilerplate assurances would no longer be acceptable.

The Boren Amendment primarily concerns reimbursement, but the federal government has sought to protect the welfare of Medicaid beneficiaries by ensuring that the state system of calculating reimbursement is appropriately cognizant of the quality of health care. Boren Amendment litigation is being brought by providers who are concerned mostly about the economic health of their institutions, but the litigation can also be understood as a means for providers to seek payment for better-quality care by enforcing federal laws against the states.

The critical issue in Medicaid will continue to be financing. How much will be cut out of the program by a hard-pressed federal government? And as these cuts occur, how will the program be redesigned to ensure quality? Using waivers as a vehicle for responsive regulation may be an important answer. Litigation over reimbursement patterns has far less potential to yield new rules that can guarantee quality in a cost-constrained environment.

Summary

The areas of federal law we have reviewed—in particular, antitrust litigation, the impact of ERISA, enforcement of fraud and abuse and bans on self-referral, tax laws, and the operation of Medicaid programs—provide a variety of lessons about the potential for emergence of new rules in our ever more complex health care environment. Federal policy is haphazard and somewhat inconsistent. Certain influences demonstrate a commitment to markets in medical care; others seem more oriented toward command-and-control regulation of providers, especially doctors. In the midst of such contradictory forces, the search for a rational strategy—even when it is undertaken with the best of intentions—is fraught with difficulty.

Yet certain lessons are clear. Antitrust is not a major impediment to quality improvement. In fact, antitrust enforcers have shown some responsive impulses; and they have certainly granted leeway for the sharing of quality information. Antitrust does not obstruct quality improvement at present.

On the other hand, ERISA and federal fraud and abuse laws do obstruct. The ERISA prohibition of state regulation prevents states from promulgating innovative solutions, and it destroys potential for collaboration. Fraud and abuse prosecution has the same ultimate effect, largely because it is based on an antiquated view of the health care market. Tax law and Medicaid policy simply reveal that federal law offers other opportunities for development of new rules—and other obstacles.

As far as the design of those rules is concerned, federal policy defines the architecture of the health care system and presents challenges. The confusing vectors of federalization must be understood, and where possible, used to the advantage of regulation for improvement.

Notes

1. See 29 U.S.C. §§1001–1461 (1988); *Goldfarb* v. *Virginia State Bar*, 421 U.S. 773 (1975).

2. See J. Blumstein and F. Sloan, "Redefining Government's Role in Health Care: Is a Dose of Competition What the Doctor Should Order?" *Vanderbilt Law Review* 34 (1981): 849–870; R. Bovbjerg, "Competition Versus Regulation: An Overdrawn Dichotomy?" *Vanderbilt Law Review* 34 (1981): 965–1002.

3. 421 U.S. 773 (1975), 787.

4. 15 U.S.C. §§1–7 (1988). This account follows, in general form, an excellent review of these issues presented by R. Goeke in a Harvard Law School paper, "The Effects of Health Care Reform on Antitrust Enforcement in the Health Care Field," June 15, 1994.

   The Clayton Act supplements the Sherman Act. §2 prohibits price discrimination, §3 proscribes corporate mergers that lessen competition or create monopolies in any line of commerce. See 15 U.S.C. §§13, 14, 18 (1988). In addition, the Federal Trade Commission protects consumers against unfair competition and unfair deceptive acts. See 15 U.S.C. §§41, 45(a)(1).

5. See, for example, *Standard Oil Company* v. *United States*, 221 U.S. 1 (1911).

6. See *National Society for Professional Engineers* v. *United States*, 435 U.S. 679, 692 (1978).

7. See J. H. Sneed and D. Marx, Jr., *Antitrust: Challenge of the Health Care Field* (Washington, D.C.: National Health Lawyers

Association, 1990); *Chicago Board of Trade v. United States*, 246 U.S. 231, 238 (1918).

8. See, for example, *Brunswick Corporation v. Pueblo Bowl-O-Mat, Inc.*, 429 U.S. 477, 489 (1977).

9. See P. Areeda, *Antitrust Law*, (Boston: Little, Brown, 1986), para. 1502. See generally, T. M. Jorde and D. J. Teece, "The Rule of Reason Analysis of Horizontal Agreements: Agreements Designed to Advance Innovation and Commercialized Technology," *Antitrust Law Journal* 61 (1993): 579, 602–603.

10. See F. H. Miller, "Vertical Restraints and Powerful Health Insurers: Exclusionary Conduct Masquerading as Managed Care?" *Law and Contemporary Problems* 51 (spring 1988): 195.

11. Mergers can be challenged under §7 of the Clayton Act or §1 of the Sherman Act. The latter requires a demonstration that there is an actual effect of restraining trade. §7 of the Clayton Act, however, proscribes mergers that will have anticompetitive effects in the future. See D. L. Glaser, "Clayton Act Scrutiny of Non-Profit Hospital Mergers: The Wrong Rx for Ailing Institutions," *Washington Law Review* 66 (1991): 1041–42. The Clayton Act's effect is preventive. The only potential problem with using the Clayton Act in the health care setting is that at least one court has suggested that the §7 claims brought by the Department of Justice are not valid when the merging institutions are nonprofit hospitals. See *U.S. v. Carilion Health System*, 707 F. Supp. 840 (W.D. Va. 1989), *affirmed* in an unpublished opinion, 892 F. 2d 1042 (4th Cir. 1989). However, other federal courts have allowed §7 claims to proceed against nonprofits. See *U.S. v. Rockford Memorial Hospital*, 898 F. 2d 1278 (7th Cir. 1990); *Federal Trade Commission v. University Health, Inc.*, 938 F. 2d 1206 (11th Cir. 1991).

12. As the First Circuit Court of Appeals has stated in a case concerning health care, "There is no subject in antitrust law more confusing than market definition. One reason is that the concept even in the pristine formulation of economists, is deliberately an attempt to oversimplify . . . for working purposes . . . the very complex economic interactions between a number of differently situated buyers

and sellers each of whom in reality has different costs, needs, and substitutes." [Citations omitted] *U.S. HealthCare, Inc.* v. *Health-Source, Inc.*, 986 F. 2d 589, 598 (1st Cir. 1993).

For example, in the case of *United States* v. *E. I. Du Pont de Nemours and Company*, 351 U.S. 377, 76 L.Ed. 1264 (1956), the Supreme Court had to decide whether or not Du Pont was attempting to monopolize interstate commerce in cellophane. To do so, the Court had to understand the relative product market. The Court concluded that purchasers of cellophane and other flexible wraps use these products interchangeably, so the product market had to extend beyond cellophane to other materials. The critical elements in the determination were the differences in character between the commodities and the lengths to which any one buyer would go to substitute one commodity for another. See *Du Pont*, 351 U.S., 393.

In another classic case, one that is even closer to today's health care context, the Supreme Court had to evaluate the anticompetitive effects of a merger between two shoe manufacturers. See *Brown Shoe Company* v. *United States*, 370 U.S. 294 (1962). In this case, each manufacturer also had a set of retail stores that sold the product. Thus there were both horizontal and vertical characteristics to the merger. The manufacturers argued that there were differences in quality, price, and grade of material between their two companies and that these matters should be taken into consideration. Instead, the Supreme Court found that the relevant market was much simpler—that is, men's, women's, and children's shoes. However, the Court did allow that there could be relevant submarkets that would constitute independent product markets for antitrust purposes. See *Brown Shoe*, 370 U.S. at 325.

13. *Arizona* v. *Maricopa County Medical Society*, 643 F. 2d 553, 556 (9th Cir. 1980), *reversed*, 457 U.S. 332 (1982).

14. In the decision of the *United States* v. *Carilion Health Systems*, 707 F. Supp. 840 (W.D. Va. 1989), the Western District of Virginia Federal District Court found no unreasonable restraint of trade in the merger of two hospitals in Roanoke, Virginia, primarily because the definition of hospital market based on inpatient procedures seemed

inadequate to the court. Since it appeared to the court that inpatient and outpatient services were reasonably interchangeable—a view that must be considered anachronistic given the emphasis on the continuum of care that is the hallmark of managed care organizations and insurers—the court could not find concentration and monopolization within a relevant geographical market.

Contrast this decision with that in *United States v. Rockford Memorial Corporation*, 717 F. Supp. 1251 (N.D. Ill. 1989), *affirmed* 898 F. 2d 1278 (7th Cir. 1990). Here, the court held that inpatient services were sufficiently distinct from outpatient services to qualify as independent markets. Since they were so distinct, the court held that "acute inpatient hospital care is the economically significant submarket of the healthcare industry that should be analyzed for purposes of determining the competitive effect of . . . consolidation" (*Rockford Memorial*, 1260–61). Reviewing the case, the Seventh Circuit Court of Appeals agreed that while a merger might not create problems in outpatient care, it would be proscribed by the Clayton Act if it led to a monopoly for inpatient services; see *United States v. Rockford Memorial Corporation*, 898 F. 2d 1278, 1284 (7th Cir. 1990).

15. The Herfindahl-Hirschmann Index (HHI) of market concentration, which is used also by the Federal Trade Commission and the Department of Justice, is based on a computation of the square of market percentages of each competitor. When a merger falls below 1,000 on the HHI, mergers are unlikely to have adverse competitive effects. When the postmerger HHI is above 1,800, however, the market is considered to be highly concentrated. See generally, J. B. Baker, "The Antitrust Analysis of Hospital Mergers and the Transformation of the Hospital Industry," *Law and Contemporary Problems* 51 (1988): 93, 149. Courts also tend to use the pure market share threshold of 60 percent for finding potential antitrust violations. For a discussion of the effects of market concentration, see G. J. Bazzoli, D. Marx, R. J. Arnould, and L. Manheim, "Federal Antitrust Merger Enforcement Standards: A Good Fit for the Hospital Industry?" *Journal of Health Politics, Policy and Law* 20 (1995): 137–169.

16. See Baker, 155.

17. Health Care Industry Policies, 4 Trade Reg. Rep. ¶13,150 at pg. 20,762.

18. For a good summary of the effects of the 1993 and 1994 policy statements on joint purchasing arrangements, physician joint ventures, and safety zones for hospital specialty care, see Physician Payment Review Commission, *Annual Report 1995: Physician Networks and Antitrust Law* (Washington, D.C.: Physician Payment Review Commission, 1995), chap. 13.

19. See Bazzoli, Marx, Arnould, and Manheim, 154.

20. See J. Zwanziger, "The Need for an Antitrust Policy for a Health Care Industry in Transition," *Journal of Health Politics, Policy and Law* 20 (1995): 171–177.

21. See O. S. Mudge and A. Gibofsky, "The Developing Application of Antitrust Laws to Hospital Mergers," *Journal of Legal Medicine* 15 (1994): 355–384, 382. States have been generally more willing to allow cooperative agreements between providers, including hospitals. A trenchant discussion of state cooperative agreements under the *Parker* v. *Brown* doctrine is contained in J. F. Blumstein, "Health Care Reform and Competing Visions of Medical Care: Antitrust and State Provider Cooperation Legislation," Cornell Law Review 1459 (1994).

22. See D. J. Marx and C. M. Murphy, "Antitrust Enforcement Encourages Health Care Providers to Cooperate Procompetitively," *Annals of Health Law* 3 (1994): 1–27.

23. *United States and State of Florida* v. *Morton Planned Health Systems, Inc., and Trustees of Mease Hospital, Inc.*, 94–748–CIV–T–23E 1994WL 655199 (M.D. Fla. 1994).

24. *Patrick* v. *Burget*, 486 U.S. 94 (1988). Patrick was recruited by the staff of the Astoria Clinic in 1972. The clinic was a private group practice that dominated the only hospital in Astoria, Columbia Memorial. Patrick was a general surgeon and did well at the clinic. However, after a year, he decided that it was financially more attractive to become an independent practitioner, and he left the clinic

staff. Once he established his private practice, he received no further referrals from the clinic. Instead, according to the Court, clinic doctors would refer patients to surgeons as far as fifty miles away.

In 1979, one of the partners in the clinic, Gary Boelling, lodged a complaint with the Columbia Memorial medical staff about a patient incident that involved Patrick. The executive committee of the hospital decided to report the case to the State Board of Medical Examiners, and in a hearing by a board committee, Patrick's care of the patient was criticized. The committee chairperson was Franklin Russell, another partner at the Astoria clinic. The Board of Medical Examiners issued a letter of reprimand to Patrick, but subsequently retracted it.

The battle between Patrick and the members of the medical staff at Columbia Memorial continued to brew. The executive committee of the medical staff terminated Patrick's privileges because it believed that the care he was providing was below the standard expected by the hospital. Patrick attempted to have the members of the committee reveal their personal bias against him, but they refused to do so and he resigned from the medical staff.

25. *Patrick v. Burget*, 800 F. 2d 1498 (9th Cir. 1986).

26. The Supreme Court elaborated the prohibition against finding a state liable under antitrust scrutiny in the case of *Parker v. Brown*, 317 U.S. 341 (1943). The Court ruled that a state could not be liable for anticompetitive effects.

27. *Patrick v. Burget*, 486 U.S. 94 at 94.

28. 42 U.S.C. §§11101–52 (1988), *amended* December 19, 1989, PL 10–239, 103 Stat. 2208 (1989).

29. See 42 U.S.C. §§11131–37. The best discussion of the Health Care Quality Improvement Act is contained in C. Scott, "Medical Peer Review, Antitrust, and the Effect of Statutory Reform," *Maryland Law Review* 50 (1991): 316–407.

30. See W. J. Curran, "Legal Immunity for Medical Peer Review Programs: New Policies Explored," *New England Journal of Medicine* 320 (1989): 233–235.

31. House Committee on Energy and Commerce, Subcommittee on Health and Environment, *Hearings on H.R. 5110*, 99th Cong., 2d sess., July 5, 1986, 192.

32. Among these conditions: 1) there is reason to believe that the action was in furtherance of quality health care; 2) there has been a reasonable effort to obtain the facts of the matter; 3) adequate notice and hearing procedures for the physician involved have occurred; 4) there is reason to believe that the action was warranted by the facts known after such reasonable effort to obtain facts. See Scott, 329. Thus the protections under the act were limited.

33. For example, in the case of *Manion v. Evans*, 986 F. 2d 1036 (6th Cir. 1993), the Sixth Circuit Court of Appeals faced a case in which peer reviewers at Lima Memorial Hospital had suspended the privileges of a pathologist in light of allegations of incompetence. The plaintiff eventually sued the hospital for alleged antitrust violations. The defendants moved for summary judgment under the HCQIA. The court reviewed the legislative history of the act in some detail and concluded that it was not possible to grant summary judgment on the part of defendants. While this result would not be surprising to many commentators (see Scott, 385), it nonetheless underlines the fact that courts will continue to scrutinize potential antitrust violations. See also *Bolt v. Halifax Hospital Medical Center*, 891 F. 2d 810 (11th Cir.), *cert. denied* 495 U.S. 924 (1990).

34. *Weiss v. York Hospital*, 745 F. 2d 786 (3rd Cir. 1984).

35. See, for example, *Boczar v. Manatee Hospitals and Health Systems, Inc.*, 993 F. 2d 1514 (11th Cir. 1993).

36. *Jefferson Parish Hospital v. Hyde*, 466 U.S. 2 (1984). The *Jefferson Parish* case is a matter of a nonprice vertical restraint. In that regard, it is similar to *Ball Memorial Hospital v. Mutual Hospital Insurance*, 784 F. 2d 1325 (7th Cir. 1986), in which the plaintiff hospital challenged Blue Shield's refusal to admit certain hospitals to its preferred provider network.

37. The other significant issue in *Jefferson Parish* (and in a comparable case that eventually did find an antitrust violation in a similar tying arrangement between hospital and anesthetist: *Oltz v. St. Peter's*

Community Hospital, 861 F. 2d 1440 [9th Cir. 1988]) was that the
Court accepted the fiction that patients choose anesthesiologists.
Generally, most patients are not true consumers of anesthesia services. The Seventh Circuit Court of Appeals allowed as much in
the decision of *Dos Santos v. Columbus Cuneo-Cabrini Medical Center*, 684 F. 2d 1346 (7th Cir. 1982). The court recognized that anesthesiology services are packaged with a variety of other physician
services in the hospital stay and the eventual hospital bill. In many
ways, then, the hospital is the contractor with or purchaser of anesthesiology services and is thus responsible for the quality of such services. In a sense, this sort of decision turns the antitrust analysis,
and the definition of the market, from patients' purchasing of physician services to health care organizations' purchasing of ancillary
services. In many ways, it represents a more accurate view of the
health care market, but it is not a paradigm that has dominated in
antitrust analysis.

38. 467 U.S. 752 (1984).

39. See Marx and Murphy, 21, describing the intent of the Department
of Justice with regard to the proposal by Case Western Reserve University and University Hospitals of Cleveland.

40. *Arizona v. Maricopa Medical Society*, 457 U.S. 332 (1982).

41. See, for example, *Capital Imaging Associates, P.C. v. Mohawk Valley
Medical Associates, Inc.*, 996 F. 2d. 537, 1993–1 Trade Cases
¶70,270 (2nd. Cir. 1993), *cert. denied*, 114 S. Ct. 388 (1993) (court
rules that the members of an independent practice association had
separate economic interests and so could conspire against one
another).

42. See *Hassan v. Independent Practice Associates, P.C.*, 698 F. Supp.
679, 689 (E.D. Mich. 1988).

43. See FTC enforcement policy with respect to physician agreements
to control medical prepayment plans, 46 Fed. Reg. 48, 982 (1981).

44. See American Society of Internal Medicine, Advisory Opinion, 105
FTC 505 (1985). Some of the interest of federal authorities in the
financial risks shared by members of a joint venture may be blunted

by the growth of capitation. The Department of Justice/FTC joint guidelines have suggested that payment on a capitated basis is evidence of substantial financial risk. If capitation continues to grow, the concern about financial risk could decrease. See Health Care Industry Policies, 4 Trade Reg. Rep. ¶13,150, at pg 20,764.

45. See Antitrust Division Business Review letter, *North America Shippers Association, Number 88–2* (March 16, 1988), cited in Goeke, "The Effects of Health Care Reform," 98.

46. See *Health Care Industry Policies*, 4 Trade Reg. Rep. ¶13,150, ¶20,764.

47. See Senate Committee on Finance, *Hearings on Health Care Reform* 103rd Cong., 2nd sess., May 12, 1994, statement of R. F. Corlin, M.D. (on file with authors).

48. See Senate Committee on Finance, *Hearings on Health Care Reform*, statement of R. F. Corlin, 8.

49. See H. Meyer and B. McCormick, "Florida Doctor's Union Tests Bargaining Limits," *American Medical News*, December 5, 1994, 1.

50. "California Managed Imaging Medical Group, Inc.—Staff Advisory Opinion, sec. 5, FTC Act., Nov. 17, 1993," Trade Regulation Reporter 5: ¶23, 581, pg. 23, 244 (Chicago: Commerce Clearing House, 1994.)

51. "Proposed Venture for Cardiologist Network Appears to Pass Muster Within Safety Zone," *BNA's Antitrust & Trade Regulation Report* 67: 366–367 (1994). Washington, D.C.: Bureau of National Affairs.

52. 15 U.S.C. §§1011–1015 (1989).

53. *Group Life and Health Insurance Co.* v. *Royal Drug Co.* 440 U.S. 205 (1979).

54. For a prescient discussion of these issues, see S. Law and S. Ensminger, "Negotiating Physicians Fees: Individual Patients of Society? (A Case Study in Federalism)," *New York University Law Review* 61 (1986): 1–84.

55. See *Reazin* v. *Blue Cross and Blue Shield of Kansas, Inc.*, *affirmed* 899 F. 2d 951 (10th Cir. 1990) *cert. denied*, 497 U.S. 1005 (1990).

56. See *U.S. HealthCare, Inc.* v. *Health Source, Inc.*, 986 F. 2d 589 (1st Cir. 1993).

57. *Blue Cross & Blue Shield of Wisconsin* v. *Marshfield Clinic*, 94–C–137–S 1995 WL 237451 (D. Wis. 1995) (damages awarded January 4, 1995). See also B. G. Clary and M. A. LaFond, "Antitrust and Integrated Delivery Systems: *Blue Cross and Blue Shield United of Wisconsin and Compcare Health Services Insurance Corporation* v. *The Marshfield Clinic and Security Health Plan of Wisconsin, Inc.*," *Health Law Digest* 23(2) (1995): 3–9.

58. Part of this section was published previously as M. A. Chirba-Martin and T. A. Brennan, "The Critical Role of ERISA in State Health Reform," *Health Affairs* 13 (1994): 142–156. See Employee Retirement Income Security Act of 1974, 29 U.S.C. §§1001–1461, §1144.

59. See W. K. Mariner, "Problems with Employer-Provided Health Insurance—The Employee Retirement Income Security Act and Health Care Reform," *New England Journal of Medicine* 327 (1992): 1682–85; L. O. Gostin and A. I. Widiss, "What's Wrong with the ERISA Vacuum?" *Journal of the American Medical Association* 269 (1993): 2527–32.

60. 29 U.S.C. §1002(1)(A).

61. House Education and Labor Committee, 93rd Cong., 2d sess., H.R. Rept. 93–533, reprinted in *U.S. Code Congress and Administrative News* (1974), 4640.

62. 29 U.S.C. §1144(c). Congress's preoccupation with ensuring uniformity of regulation from state to state was obviously intended to protect interstate employee benefit plans. See House Education and Labor Committee, H.R. Rept. 93–533, *U.S. Code Congress and Administrative News* (1974), 4650. Yet ERISA preemption does not distinguish between inter- and intrastate plans and protects both from state regulation.

63. 29 U.S.C. §1031(c). See generally, 29 C.F.R. §§2509–89 (1990).

64. §29 U.S.C. §1144(a); House Education and Labor Committee, H.R. Rept. 93–533, *U.S. Code Congress and Administrative News* (1974),

4655; accord S. Rept. 93–127, *U.S. Code Congress and Administrative News* (1974), 4871.

65. Remarks of Sen. Williams (Aug. 22, 1974), 120 Cong. Rec. S15737, reprinted in *U.S. Code Congress and Administrative News* (1974), 5177–90, 5188–89; *accord* Remarks of Rep. Dent (Aug. 20, 1974), 120 Cong. Rec. 29197, reprinted in Subcommittee on Labor of the Senate Committee on Labor and Public Welfare, *Legislative History of the Employee Retirement Income Security Act of 1974* (1976), 3:4670–71.

66. See *Shaw v. Delta Air Lines, Inc.*, 463 U.S. 85, 100 n. 21 (1983).

67. See, for example, *District of Columbia v. Greater Washington Board of Trade*, 113 S. Ct. 580, 583 (1992); *Ingersoll-Rand Co. v. McClendon*, 498 U.S. 133, 139 (1990); *Pilot Life Insurance Co. v. Dedeaux*, 481 U.S. 41, 45 (1987).

68. See *Metropolitan Life Insurance Co. v. Massachusetts*, 471 U.S. 724, 739 (1985). *Accord Mackey v. Lanier*, 486 U.S. 825 (1988).

69. 29 U.S.C. §1144(b)(2)(A).

70. See *Metropolitan Life Insurance Co. v. Massachusetts*, 741–745.

71. 29 U.S.C. §1144(b)(2)(a).

72. In *Union Labor Life Insurance Co. v. Pireno*, 458 U.S. 119 (1982), the Supreme Court outlined the reach of state insurance law in a manner that broadly affects ERISA. Interpreting the McCarran-Ferguson Act's impact on antitrust claims, the Court suggested that a particular business practice would qualify as the "business of insurance" depending on answers to the following questions: "*First*, whether the practice has the effect of transferring or spreading a policyholder's risk; *second*, whether the practice is an integral part of the policy relationship between the insurer and the insured; and *third*, whether the practice is limited to entities within the insurance industry" (*Union Labor Life Insurance Co. v. Pireno*, 129; emphasis in original.)

73. See *Metropolitan Life Insurance Co. v. Massachusetts*, 746–747.

74. See *Metropolitan Life Insurance Co. v. Massachusetts*, 724; see also *FMC Corporation v. Holiday* 498 U.S., 52, 62(1990).

75. Our discussions with various representatives of both business and
organized labor indicate that support for ERISA within these con-
stituencies is deep and broad. See also D. M. Foz and D. C. Schaffer,
"Health Policy and ERISA: Interest Groups and Semipreemption,"
Journal of Health Politics, Policy and Law 14 (1989): 239.

That the Supreme Court will remain undaunted in its expansive
reading of ERISA's preemption provisions is apparent from its decision in *District of Columbia* v. *Greater Washington Board of Trade*,
113 S. Ct. 580 (1992). In the District of Columbia, workers' compensation legislation required employers who provided health
insurance for their employees to provide equivalent coverage for
injury. The state law did not regulate the ERISA plan itself or
impose any standards for the way those plans should be administered or what such plans should provide. It simply said that
employers providing benefits through ERISA plans must make
equivalent benefits available to workers' compensation claimants.
Nevertheless, ERISA preempted this as "related to" an ERISA
employee benefit plan that was not otherwise "saved" from preemption. In reaffirming its broad application of ERISA preemption, the
Court stated: "ERISA preempts any state law that refers to or has a
connection with any covered benefit plans (and that does not fall
within a [savings clause] exception) 'even if the law is not specifically designed to affect such plans, or the effect is only indirect
[citations omitted],' and even if the law is consistent with ERISA's
substantive requirements." (*District of Columbia* v. *Greater Washington Board of Trade*, 583).

Consequently, the state law was overturned because it expressly tied
the mandated workers' compensation benefits to employer-provided
health insurance coverage—even if it did so simply to give the
employer a straightforward index for calculating benefits or to
ensure parity of treatment for both work-related and non-work-
related health problems. Thus, any attempt by states to rationalize
various employment-related benefits seems destined to fail by virtue
of ERISA preemption, regardless of how beneficial to the employee
such efforts might be.

76. See E. Felsenthal, "Health Plans Are Self-Insured by More Firms," *Wall Street Journal,* November 11, 1992, B1.

77. See, for example, R. A. Padgug and G. M. Oppenheimer, "AIDS, Health Insurance, and the Crisis of Community," *Notre Dame Journal of Law, Ethics, and Public Policy* 5 (1990): 35–57.

78. See R. J. Blendon, "Making the Critical Choices," *Journal of the American Medical Association* 267 (1992): 2509–20.

79. *Metropolitan Life Insurance Co.* v. *Massachusetts,* 743.

80. *Metropolitan Life Insurance Co.* v. *Massachusetts,* 735 n. 14.

81. 29 U.S.C. §1140.

82. See *Shaw* v. *Delta Air Lines, Inc.;* also L. Francis, "Consumer Expectation and Access to Health Care," *University of Pennsylvania Law Review* 140 (1992): 1881.

83. *Vasseur* v. *Halliburton Co.,* 950 F. 2d 1002 (5th Cir. 1992); *McGann* v. *H & H Music Co.,* 946 F. 2d 401 (5th Cir. 1991) *cert. denied sub nom Greenberg* v. *H & H Music Co.,* U.S. 113 S. Ct. 482 (1992). See also *Westhoven* v. *Lincoln FoodService Products, Inc.,* 616 N.E. 2d 778 (Ind. Ct. App. 1993) (employer's reduction of health benefits for employees with AIDS was not actionable under state antidiscrimination law, owing to ERISA preemption).

84. Like other elements of health policy, ERISA has been evaluated through the lens of AIDS, but its impact is really much broader. The *McGann* case has been relatively widely discussed in the health policy literature. Remarkably, however, none of these recent articles even mentions the case law discussed in this section. This is yet another indication of how underappreciated the impact of ERISA is.

85. *Bricklayers Local No. 1 Welfare Fund* v. *Louisiana Health Insurance Association* 771 F. Supp. 771 (E.D. La. 1991).

86. *Travelers Insurance Co.* v. *Cuomo* 813 F. Supp. 996 (S.D. N.Y. 1993), *affirmed in part, reversed in part,* 14 F.3d 708 (2nd Cir. 1993), *cert. granted,* 115 S. Ct. 305 (1994), *reversed,* 115 S. Ct. 1671 (1995).

87. *United Wire, Metal & Machine Health & Welfare Fund* v. *Morristown Memorial Hospital* 793 F. Supp. 524 (D. N.J. 1992), *reversed and remanded*, 995 F. 2d 1179 (3d Cir. 1993), *cert. denied*, 114 S.Ct. 382 (1993).

88. In a remarkable departure from the clear trend of previous ERISA preemption cases, however, the Third Circuit Court of Appeals reversed the lower court's preemption decision and found that the rate-setting legislation did not "relate to" ERISA plans. See *United Wire, Metal & Machine Health & Welfare Fund* v. *Morristown Memorial Hospital*, 995 F. 2d 1179 (3d. Cir. 1993). While purporting to rely on recent Supreme Court rulings (for example, *FMC Corporation* v. *Holliday*, the appeals court effectively articulated a *new* definition of what satisfies the "relate to" criterion of ERISA preemption. It found that a state statute "relates to" an ERISA benefit plan if it 1) is specifically designed to affect such plans; 2) singles out such plans for special treatment; or 3) creates rights or restrictions predicated on the existence of such plans.

89. *Stuart Circle Hospital Corp.* v. *Aetna Health Management*, 800 F. Supp. 328 (E.D. Va. 1992).

90. *Stuart Circle Hospital Corp.* v. *Aetna Health Management*, 995 F. 2d 500 (4th Cir. 1993). *cert. denied*, 114S. Ct. 579 (1993); *Blue Cross & Blue Shield* v. *St. Mary's Hospital of Richmond, Inc.*, 245 Va. 24 426 S.E. 2d 117 (1993) (Supreme Court of Virginia also finds preferred provider statute to be saved from preemption).

91. American Managed Care and Review Association, Washington, D.C., as cited in *BNA Health Law Reporter* 1 (1992): 195.

92. *HCA Health Services of Virginia, Inc.* v. *Aetna Life Insurance Co.*, 803 F. Supp. 1132 (E.D. Va. 1992). This case involved a similar challenge under the same statute, and reached a result analogous to the *Stuart Circle* trial decision.

93. *Group Life & Health Insurance Co.* v. *Royal Drug Co.*, 440 U.S. 205, 214 (1979).

94. For example, *Travelers Insurance Co.* v. *Cuomo*, 813 F. Supp. at 1007 *citing O'Reilly* v. *Ceuleers*, 912 F. 2d 1383, 1389 (11th Cir. 1990).

95. *Physicians Health Plan* v. *Citizens Insurance Co.*, 673 F. Supp. 903, 907–908 (W.D. Mich. 1987).

96. *Elsesser* v. *Hospital of Philadelphia College*, 802 F. Supp. 1286 (E.D. Pa. 1992) (no ERISA preemption of claims against an HMO where principles of professional malpractice rather than obligations under HMO's benefit plans were involved); *accord Independence HMO, Inc.* v. *Smith*, 733 F. Supp. 983 (E.D. Pa. 1990).

97. *BNA Health Law Reporter* 2 (1993): 860–961.

98. See note 96 above.

99. Other courts considering these issues and making a similar determination (that is, that ostensible agency survives an ERISA preemption challenge) include *Kohn* v. *Delaware Valley HMO, Inc.*, 91–2745, 1992 WL 22241 (E.D. Pa. 1992), and *Raglin* v. *HMO Illinois, Inc.* 595 N.E. 2d 153 (Ill. 1992). One court has been willing to preempt all medical negligence claims: *Altiere* v. *Cigna Dental Health, Inc.* 753 F. Supp. 61 (D. Conn. 1990).

100. *Corcoran* v. *United HealthCare, Inc.*, 965 F. 2d 1321 (5th Cir. 1992), *cert. denied*, 113 S. Ct. 812 (1992).

101. *Corcoran* v. *United HealthCare, Inc.*, 965 F. 2d 1324–25.

102. Article 2315 of the Louisiana Civil Code gives parents a cause of action for the wrongful death of an unborn child. The state courts had not decided whether the statute permitted a negligence suit against a third-party provider of utilization review services. *Corcoran* v. *United Health Care, Inc.*, 965 F. 2d 1327.

103. *Corcoran* v. *United Health Care, Inc.*, 965 F. 2d 1338.

104. See *Dukes* v. *United States Health Care Systems of Pennsylvania*, 848 F. Supp. 39 (E.D. Pa. 1994); *Spain* v. *Aetna Life Insurance Co.*, 11 F. 3d 129 (9th Cir. 1993).

105. For a discussion of the utilization review accreditation commission established by the American Managed Care and Review Association, see M. E. O'Kane, "Outside Accreditation of Managed Care Plans," in *Managed Health Care Handbook*, ed. Peter R. Kongstvedt (Gaithersburg, Md.: Aspen Publishers, 1993), 231–260.

106. *Kuhl v. Lincoln National Health Plan of Kansas City, Inc.*, 99 F. 2d. 298 (8th Cir. 1993), *cert. denied*, 114 S.Ct. 694.

107. This claim was asserted under 29 U.S.C. §1132(a)(3)(B)(i).

108. *Kuhl v. Lincoln National Health Plan of Kansas City, Inc.*, 304.

109. See *NYS Conference of Blue Cross/Blue Shield plans et al* v. *The Travelers Company et al*, 115 S.Ct. 1671 (1995).

110. Of course, another federal influence is the peer review organizations under Medicare. In addition, there are Medicare's financing initiatives—in particular, the Prospective Payment System and the Resource-Based Relative Value Scale for paying hospitals and doctors, respectively.

111. 42 USC §1320a–76.

112. See generally, D. Frankford, "Creating and Defining the Fruits of Collective Economic Activity: Referrals Among Health Care Providers," *Columbia Law Review* 89 (1989): 1861–1938.

113. See 42 U.S.C. §1320a–7b.

114. *United States v. Greber*, 760 F. 2d 68; *cert. denied* 474 U.S. 988 (1985).

115. See *United States v. Porter*, 591 F. 2d 1048 (5th Cir. 1979). There was a further extension of the reach of the fraud and abuse provisions of the Medicare Act in the decision of *United States v. Kats*, 871 F. 2d 105 (9th Cir. 1989). *Kats* endorsed the *Greber* interpretation and indicated that most federal courts would begin to enforce the fraud and abuse statute without reference to intent.

116. See proposed rules: Part 1001-Program Integrity: Medicare, 54 Fed. Reg. 3088 (January 23, 1989). Also 42 CFR, chap. 5, §1001.952.

117. See *Inspector General v. Hanlester Network*, New Developments: Medicare and Medicaid Guide (Commerce Clearing House), para. 39094 (March 1, 1991).

118. See *Hanlester Network et al.* v. *Shalala*, 51 F. 3d 1390 (9th Cir. 1995).

119. See *United States v. Cogiannattasio*, 979 F. 2nd 98 (7th Cir. 1992).

120. J. Johnsson, "Fraud Settlement Reached: Other Physician Recruitment Deals May Face Federal Scrutiny," *American Medical News*, October 25, 1993, 2.

121. See D. F. Thompson, "Understanding Financial Conflicts of Interest," *New England Journal of Medicine* 329 (1993): 573–576; see also T. A. Brennan, "Buying Editorials," *New England Journal of Medicine* 331 (1994): 673–675.

122. See *U.S. v. Siddiqi*, 959 F. 2d 1167 (2nd Cir. 1992) (physician accused of double billing when he billed for supervision of treatment performed by hospital); *U.S. v. Kensington Hospital*, Civ. A. 90–5430, 1993 WL 21446 (E.D. Pa. 1993) (conflicts litigation involving hospital, laboratory, satellite clinic, seven physicians, four administrators, and a host of joined parties).

123. See, for example, A. S. Relman, "Self-Referral—What's at Stake," *New England Journal of Medicine* 327 (1992): 1522–23; also Council on Ethical and Judicial Affairs, American Medical Association, "Conflicts of Interest: Physician Ownership of Medical Facilities," *Journal of the American Medical Association* 267 (1992): 2366–69.

124. See T. McDowell, "Physician Self-Referral Arrangements: Legitimate Business or Unethical Entrepreneurialism?" *American Journal of Law and Medicine* 15 (1989): 61–109.

125. See B. Hillman, G. Olson, P. Griffith, J. Sunshine, C. Joseph, S. Kennedy, W. Nelson, and L. Bernhardt, "Physicians' Utilization and Charges for Outpatient Diagnostic Imaging in a Medicare Population," *Journal of the American Medical Association* 255 (1992): 2048–51; A. Swedlow, G. Johnson, N. Smithline, and A. Milstein, "Increased Costs and Rates of Use in the California Workers' Compensation System as a Result of Self-Referral by Physicians," *New England Journal of Medicine* 327 (1992): 1502–06.

126. 42 USCA § 1395nn.

127. See 42 U.S.C. §1395 nn (West 1995).

128. 42 U.S.C.A. §1395 nn (h)(4)(A), nn (b)(3) (West 1995).

129. See J. Steiner, "Update on Hospital Physician Relationships Under Stark II," *Health Care Financial Management* 47 (December 1993): 66.

130. Stark II will apply to clinical laboratory services, physical therapy, occupational therapy, radiology and other diagnostic services, radiation therapy, durable medical equipment, nutrition, supplies, prosthetics, home health services, outpatient drugs, and outpatient hospital services. See 42 U.S.C. §1395 nn (a)(2)(C).

131. See generally, T. A. Brennan, *Just Doctoring: Medical Ethics in the Liberal State* (Berkeley: University of California Press, 1991), chap. 8.

132. See Brennan, *Just Doctoring*, chap. 8.

133. See, for example, *School District* v. *Hamot Medical Center*, 144 Pa. Cmwlth 668, 602 A. 2d 407 (Pa. Commonw. Ct. 1992); *Care Initiatives* v. *Board of Review of Wapello County*, 488 N.W. 2d 460 (Iowa Court App. 1992).

134. See, for example, *Rideout Hospital Foundation* v. *County of Yuba*, 10 Cal. Rptr. 2d 141 (Cal. Ct. App. 1992).

135. See D. Moskowitz, "Perspectives. Strapped Governments Eye Nonprofit Hospitals," *Faulkner and Gray's: Medicine and Health* 47(31) (Suppl.) (August 1, 1993): 4 p.

136. *Geisinger Health Plan* v. *Commissioner of Internal Review*, 100 T.C. 394 (1993).

137. Health care providers receiving favorable tax exemption determination letters include Facey Medical Foundation (March 31, 1993), Billings Clinic (Dec. 21, 1993), Harriman Jones Medical Foundation (Feb. 3, 1994), and Rockford Memorial Health Service (April 4, 1994). See M. Peregrine and B. Broccolo, "New Resources for Integrated Delivery System Tax Planning," *Exempt Organization Tax Review* 9 (1994): 789 (summarized in *Tax Notes* 63 (1994): 901–903).

138. See 42 U.S.C. §1320 a–7(b)(1).

139. See R. T. Greenwalt, "Hermann Hospital Closing Agreement: The View from Ground Zero," *Health Law Digest* 22(11): 3–9 (1994).

140. See J. Johnsson, "IRS Issues Rules on Physician Recruiting; First Time in 20 Years," *American Medical News*, April 3, 1995, 1, 7–8.

141. For a detailed discussion of the Medicaid program, see Brennan, *Just Doctoring*, chap. 8.

142. See 42 U.S.C.A. §1396a (a)(10)(A).

143. See B. R. Furrow, S. H. Johnson, T. S. Jost, and R. L. Schwartz, *Health Law: Cases, Materials, and Problems*, 2d ed. (St. Paul, Minn.: West Publishing Company, 1991), 570.

144. See J. W. Fossett, "Medicaid and Health Reform: The Case of New York," *Health Affairs* 12 (fall 1993): 81–94.

145. See 42 U.S.C. §1396(n)(b) (1983).

146. See A. Dobson, D. Moran, and G. Young, "The Role of Federal Waivers in the Health Policy Process," *Health Affairs* 11 (winter 1992): 77.

147. See Dobson, Moran, and Young, 78–79.

148. See Dobson, Moran, and Young, 74–77.

149. See generally, L. D. Brown, "The National Politics of Oregon's Rationing Plan," *Health Affairs* 10 (summer 1991): 42.

150. See W. J. Thomas, "The Oregon Medicaid Proposal: Ethical Paralysis, Tragic Democracy, and the Fate of the Utilitarian Health Care Program," *Oregon Law Review* 72 (1993): 47–156.

151. See J. Somerville, "TENNcare Suit Dismissed, State Need Not Notify Doctors," *American Medical News*, August 29, 1994, 4.

152. The program is now being evaluated much more extensively by NCQS. Personal communication, M. O'Kane, July 11, 1993.

153. The interests of states in programmatic waivers may increase as new requirements for evaluation of demonstration waivers take effect. In late 1994, the DHHS announced new rules for evaluation of demonstration proposals under §1115. See Department of Health and Human Services, Health Care Financing Administration, Medicaid Program, *Demonstration Proposals Pursuant to*

§1115(a) of the Social Security Act: Policies and Procedures, 59 Fed. Reg. 49249 (1994).

154. See J. Somerville, "Doctors Treating the Poor Hit Hard by Kentucky Cuts," *American Medical News,* December 12, 1994, 3.

155. 42 U.S.C. §1366(a)(13)(A) (1993 Supp.).

156. See S. Rept. 471, 96th Cong., 1st sess., 1979, pt. C., 28; H. Rept. 158, 97th Cong., 1st sess., 1981, chap. 11, 287.

157. See S. Rept. 471, 96th Cong., 1st sess., 1979, pt. C., 29.

158. See S. Rept. 139, 96th Cong., 1979, 1st sess., Title VII, 431, 472–474.

159. See S. Rept. 471, 96th Cong., 1st sess., 1979, pt. C., 29.

160. See generally, M. D. Daneker, "Medicaid, State Cost Containment Measures, and §1983 Provider Actions Under *Wilder* v. *Virginia Hospital Association,*" *Vanderbilt Law Review* 45 (1992): 487, 489.

161. See *Amisub (PSL), Inc.* v. *Colorado Department of Social Services,* 879 F. 2d 789 (10th Cir. 1989) *cert. denied,* 496 U.S. 935(1990); *Coos Bay Care Center* v. *Oregon Department of Human Resources,* 803 F. 2d 1060 (9th Cir. 1986), *vacated as moot* 484 U.S. 806 (1987); *Nebraska Health Care Association* v. *Dunning,* 778 F. 2d 1291 (8th Cir. 1985), *cert. denied* 479 U.S. 1063 (1987).

162. *Wilder* v. *Virginia Hospital Association,* 496 U.S. 498, (1990).

163. *Abbeville General Hospital* v. *Ramsey,* 3 F. 3d 797, 805 (5th Cir. 1993). Nonetheless, the courts have not been entirely clear about what further steps are needed. The *Abbeville* court, for instance, requested merely "an objective analysis, evaluation or some type of factfinding process" (*Abbeville,* 3 F. 3d, 805). Other courts have been slightly more specific. For instance, in the case of *Temple University* v. *White,* 941 F. 2d 201 (3rd Cir. 1991), *cert. denied,* 502 U.S. 1032, (1992), 140 hospitals charged the Pennsylvania Department of Public Welfare with failure to comply with the procedural and substantive requirements of the Boren Amendment. The Third Circuit Court agreed, and then ordered the Department of

Public Welfare to collect empirical data on hospital costs in Pennsylvania, calculate what an efficient and economical hospital operation would entail, determine what rates would be reasonable and adequate to meet such a hospital's need, and calculate rates that would guarantee reasonable access for Medicaid patients.

6

Regulation and Quality Improvement in Health Care Today

Regulation at both state and federal levels has changed significantly over the last two decades, and some evidence of responsiveness is available. Meanwhile, approaches to quality improvement have changed rapidly over the last ten years as they have been influenced by notions of Continuous Quality Improvement imported from other industries. Ideas about quality in medical care possess a new dynamism and urgency, and government regulation is struggling to shake its reputation as obstructionist. Looming over developments in both quality improvement and regulation has been the increasing influence of market incentives. As a result of market-inspired innovations, the health care industry has become much more complicated in the past decade. New organizational structures and the growth of managed care have transformed the traditional relationships between physicians, hospitals, and insurance companies. The emergence of third-party administrators and self-insured plans, concerns about the antitrust implications of networks, and the issue of profitability under capitated payment schemes all raise questions that simply did not exist in health care management in 1980. In short, there is an ongoing conceptual transformation of health care organizations. The new institutional structures, together with widespread innovation in quality measurement and improvement techniques, have set the stage for further radical change.

Our discussion so far has been of a general nature: we have

traced historical trends and sketched organizational rearrangements. However, health care involves living and breathing individuals: patients, providers, and regulators. Our analysis would be incomplete if we did not hear from those who are struggling on a daily basis to improve the quality of care in the rapidly changing health care—and regulatory—environment. Analytical approaches to health care organization have value only insofar as they ultimately affect individual behavior. We must know how real providers view regulation. Do they see it as confounding quality improvement? Do they have suggestions on how regulation can be improved? And do they sense a need to address the potential impact of cost constraints on quality?

To understand what is happening "on the ground" in health care institutions, we conducted a series of structured interviews from mid-1993 through mid-1994. We chose institutions that we believed were guided by a commitment to quality improvement, as opposed to mere quality assurance. We were interested in the perceptions of opinion leaders and administrators concerning the influence of regulation, which we defined broadly. Our investigation produced some surprises and many new insights, all of which tend to confirm the challenge of designing new rules to improve quality.

The Institutional Survey

Our research methodology was deliberately simple. We were most interested in the influence of regulation on quality improvement efforts within institutions. We recognize that the views of the regulators themselves, the perceptions of individual doctors and nurses, and the effects of institutional efforts on patient attitudes are all important as well. However, many of these various opinions and responses manifest themselves in the activities of the health care institution. Moreover, the institution is the primary target of regulation. We therefore thought it most important to understand the organizational environment of hospitals and managed care.

Within organizations, we desired a broad range of views. We therefore conducted structured interviews with staff at many levels, from leaders of quality improvement teams to chief executive officers. As it takes many blind men to describe the elephant, so too it seemed to us to require many different stories to understand how a health care institution was coping with external regulatory influences.

Our sample of institutions is not a random one, but is enriched with institutions that we believe demonstrate some level of commitment to modern approaches to quality improvement. We maintain that new rules must be designed to accommodate and promote Continuous Quality Improvement, so we visited institutions already engaged in such efforts, as their views of present regulation were most likely to be informative. The sample is also intended to represent the variety of institutions that provide health care today. Our original focus was on hospitals, but we soon realized that changes in the structure of health care were making the concept of free-standing hospitals anachronistic. Our sites therefore range from small, freestanding hospitals in relatively modest urban areas to large teaching hospitals in major metropolitan areas. We also evaluated hospitals in extended partnerships, hospitals that had set up their own health maintenance organizations (HMOs) and health plans, group practices that had merged with hospitals, and a traditional staff-model HMO. Surprisingly, however different the locations, the same themes often emerged.

At one end of our sample is the Sharp Health Care System, a community-based, not-for-profit organization that is now San Diego County's largest and most comprehensive health care delivery system. The Sharp network grew out of the Sharp Memorial Hospital, which was founded in 1955 at what was then the fringe of San Diego. The hospital grew steadily in the mid-1970s, but in the latter part of that decade made a specific decision to concentrate in certain areas, including women's care, cardiovascular medicine, critical care, and rehabilitation. In 1980, Sharp Memorial began to acquire other hospitals. In 1985, in an even bolder move, it merged with the Rees-Stealy Medical Group Practice, which then became the foundation for a network. In 1994, the Sharp Health Care network controlled six hospitals in San Diego, and nearly a quarter of San Diego residents seek care at Sharp.

The organization itself is the kind of hybrid that many believe represents the future of health care. The six hospitals in the network range from a tertiary care center to community hospitals. More than 1,300 physicians practice in affiliated group practices. These practices are integrated in varying degrees, with the Rees-Stealy group still the foundational unit. The system also maintains Sharp Health Plan, which is an IPA-model HMO with fourteen thousand members. Several rehabilitation facilities and six skilled nursing facilities complete the picture. Sharp has all the attributes of a fully vertically integrated system, with relatively tight relationships between admitting physicians and a chain of partner hospitals. The system is also developing experience with risk assumption through its HMO and is quite prepared to accept capitated payment for patients.

The organization has been committed to Continuous Quality Improvement for some time. Much of the leadership in this effort comes from the chief executive officer, Peter Ellsworth, who in the late 1980s discovered the potential of a core strategy for quality improvement. Sharp Health Care maintains a quality mission, headed by Jan Cetti at central headquarters. Cetti's office works directly with the hospitals and physician group practices to bring about quality improvement efforts, with a strong emphasis on teamwork. Each hospital monitors regulatory compliance independently but looks to the central office for leadership on improvement. The systemwide Quality Council is chaired by Ellsworth and is made up of equal numbers of physicians and administrators with a particular interest in quality.[1]

At the other end of our organizational spectrum is the Parkview Episcopal Medical Center. This hospital, which in 1993 had 305 beds and employed 915 people, is located in Pueblo, Colorado, an urban area of 300,000 people. Parkview is a not-for-profit entity owned by the Episcopal Church, but it is managed by Quorum, a for-profit hospital management firm previously associated with the Hospital Corporation of America (HCA). The hospital has a number of cooperative relationships with Corwin-St. Mary's, the other major hospital in Pueblo, which is owned by the Sisters of Charity. At the time of our initial visit in June 1993, Parkview was considering a merger with Corwin-St. Mary's, but the venture was subsequently prohibited by the Federal Trade Commission.

Parkview offers a full range of services but at the time of our visit did not have any partnership relationship with other health centers. It has recently developed a preferred provider organization. For the last decade, the hospital has also dealt with a large managed care organizations. Even though in some ways its warm and friendly ambience mirrors the small-town environment of Pueblo, it is very much a part of the larger, changing world of health care.

Although Parkview's institutional structure was quite different from that of Sharp Health Care, its introduction to Continuous Quality Improvement has been quite similar. In the late 1980s, Michael Pugh, chief executive officer of Parkview, attended several seminars given by W. Edwards Deming, the pioneer of Total Quality Management, and sought to apply TQM principles to the hospital's operations. Emphasizing systems of care, his leadership team identified seven focus points, many of which were in budgetary and support areas. Over time, a series of "pop-up teams" came to life to deal with specific issues around the medical center. A total of 148 teams had been put into place by June 1993.[2] These do not require approval by central management. All of the major cross-functional efforts were approved by the Quality Improvement Council, which Pugh himself heads. The hospital uses a series of vision statements and criteria to evaluate potential quality improvement efforts and adheres to a methodology created by the HCA Quality Resource Group. Only in 1992 did the institutional quality effort move into clinical care, with the improvement council approving teams on such diverse issues as pneumonia care, catheterization, and laminectomy. The commitment to improving care pervades Parkview. We were treated to long discourses on the attributes of modern methods of quality improvement from the housekeeping and dietary departments, the cardiac catheterization lab, the critical care units, the pharmacy, and even the cook who prepared lunch. Customer orientation and responsiveness to feedback are the rule.

The other institutions we visited lie somewhere between the types represented by Sharp Health Care and Parkview Episcopal Medical Center. For example, Strong Memorial Hospital in Rochester, New York, is a large tertiary teaching institution. In 1992, the hospital had 722 beds with 33,000 discharges and 400,000 outpatient visits. It is owned by the University of Rochester. Like the rest of New York, Rochester has been rapidly swept into the managed care environment, drawing more than 70 percent of its payment for employed patients from managed plans.[3] Maintaining a strong teaching program, Strong Memorial provides high-technology care to the Rochester area.

Strong Memorial has played an important role in building the rather unique pattern of cooperation that exists between health care institutions in and around Rochester. Fifteen years ago, influenced by large local employers, including Eastman Kodak, area hospitals formed a consortium that developed voluntary efforts to reduce health care costs through global budgeting and prospective payment. The result has been significant moderation of health care costs. In the late 1980s, the institutions in Rochester initiated a collaboration that was oriented toward measuring and improving the quality of care. This motivated the Strong Memorial leadership to embrace innovative programs, which in turn led to the present emphasis on Continuous Quality Improvement.

In Indiana, we conducted interviews at Community Hospital East, the flagship of a three-hospital network in the suburbs of Indianapolis. At the time of our interviews in June 1993, Community Hospital was considering a further affiliation with St. Vincent's

Hospital, a large competitor in the metropolitan area. Together, the two hospitals would have controlled almost 40 percent of the hospital beds in Indianapolis. Community Hospital itself has 550 beds and offers a full range of clinical services, including open-heart surgery. The medical staff is quite independent; the hospital has not moved as quickly toward vertical integration as it has toward horizontal integration.

The interest in quality improvement at Community Hospital goes back to the late 1980s, at which time the hospital first sought an affiliation with Paul B. Batalden, the founder and head of the Quality Resource Group at HCA. Batalden and his group had branched out slightly beyond the boundaries of HCA to take on a few consulting clients, one of which was Community Hospital. William Corley, chief executive officer of the hospital, trained much of middle management in quality improvement and remains the main quality coach. The leadership at Community Hospital has found it a major challenge to convert the other affiliated institutions to a quality improvement philosophy.[4]

A completely different kind of health care organization is the Park Nicollet Medical Center in Minnesota. Park Nicollet began as the St. Louis Park Medical Center, which started out with twelve physicians, all of whom had trained together after going to medical school on the GI Bill. These physicians were interested in academic careers, but they also wanted to be able to practice medicine privately. They formed the St. Louis Park Medical Center on this philosophy. The medical center evolved into a multispecialty group practice, but in the 1970s, it began to add primary care practitioners. Park Nicollet experienced explosive growth between 1975 and 1985, going from 16,000 patients to more than 160,000.

However, there was a price for this growth. There had been tremendous esprit de corps and high morale from the 1950s through the 1970s, with very low turnover rates in both patients and physicians. In the mid-1980s, a price war among HMOs, together with relatively poor administration, changed the character of the organization, and by 1989, Park Nicollet's enrollment had fallen to 100,000.[5] In the early 1990s, buffeted by ongoing changes in the health care market in the Minneapolis-St. Paul area, the center sought a relationship with a freestanding hospital. In the past, the clinic had always offered a capitated system and had purchased hospital services. This changed in June 1993, when Park Nicollet merged with Methodist Hospital, creating Health Systems of Minnesota.

In contrast to other organizations, much of the commitment to Total Quality Management at Park Nicollet is on the clinical side. Prompted to some extent by a health care oversight organization founded by local business interests (Business Health Care Action Groups), the clinic and Health Systems of Minnesota as a whole are carefully scrutinizing care processes and developing teams to foster better care at lower cost through use of clinical guidelines. The Minnesota environment has thus spawned a unique practice model and now influences the evolution of that practice as well as its quality improvement efforts.

Although many of the institutions we visited are not profit-seeking, their problems and the challenges they face with respect to quality improvement are much the same as those found in the for-profit sector. Hospital Corporation of America owns West Paces Ferry Hospital in Atlanta, which has 294 beds and a budget of nearly $160 million. Most of the upper-level administrators are HCA employees, and the HCA sets the strategic tone.

West Paces Ferry faces strong competition in the Atlanta market, which is generally perceived as being overbedded.[6] Many hospitals are forming partnerships and attempting to integrate vertically and horizontally through networks. In 1992, West Paces Ferry bought sixteen primary care clinics that had originally been Humana Health Stops. However, West Paces Ferry lacks control over the physician staff, 80 percent of whom admit patients to another hospital, thereby inhibiting vertical cohesion.

West Paces Ferry and its former chief executive officer, Chip

Caldwell, adopted Continuous Quality Improvement methods as a result of contact with Batalden's Quality Resource Group at HCA. When we interviewed Caldwell in 1993, his office reflected this commitment, as it was filled with run charts and other statistical tools that are central to quality improvement. Caldwell and his leadership team emphasize the customer focus of Total Quality Management and the importance of critical outcome measures. The administration has not hesitated to call upon its doctors to partici- pate in teams. Clinical efforts are seen as especially important to winning capitated contracts with managed care organizations; the team methodology allows the administration to identify new ways to increase the effectiveness of care.

In Massachusetts, we interviewed the leadership at an HMO and an academic medical center that enjoy a close relationship with one another. Harvard Community Health Plan (HCHP) was originally founded as a staff-model HMO by individuals associated with Har- vard Medical School. In the mid-1970s, the medical school had rec- ognized the importance of providing community care and had organized the HMO to accomplish this. However, HCHP was incor- porated without structural ties to the medical school; it was given a separate board and tax status. The health plan has thrived over the past twenty years, absorbing several other smaller group prac- tices and HMOs in Massachusetts and merging in 1994 with Pil- grim Health Plan, an IPA-model HMO, to create an entity that insures more than 950,000 enrollees in New England (including a 36 percent share of all insured individuals in Massachusetts alone).

HCHP has long been in the quality improvement business. Donald M. Berwick, one of the authors of this book, is the former vice president for quality-of-care measurement at HCHP and helped to introduce quality improvement principles into the organization in the mid-1980s. Since then, interest in quality has continued to be strong, with a great deal of emphasis on development of guide- lines and algorithms. Moreover, HCHP was an early participant in—and one of the leaders of—the development of the Health Plan and Employer Data and Information Set (HEDIS) at the National Committee for Quality Assurance (NCQA).[7]

The Brigham and Women's Hospital is the result of the merger of several hospitals in the late 1970s, including Boston Lying-In Hospital and the Peter Bent Brigham Hospital. In 1994, it had 720 beds and more than 350,000 ambulatory visits per year. In the late 1980s, Brigham and Women's became the main hospital for HCHP patients. Like many teaching institutions, especially on the east coast, Brigham and Women's had long resisted any form of vertical or horizontal integration. The deal with HCHP broke this mold. Moreover, in the spring of 1994, Brigham and Women's announced its affiliation with the Massachusetts General Hospital, and the two institutions—together known as Partners Health Care—began to create their own network of physicians.

Brigham and Women's has been somewhat slow to adopt quality improvement efforts. But its associations with HCHP and Massachusetts General, together with advocacy of Continuous Quality Improvement by a number of influential voices, especially the former CEO H. Richard Nesson, have led both the medical staff and the administration to see the promise of such efforts. In 1993–1994, twenty clinical care improvement teams were launched, and the new chief executive officer, Jeffrey Otten, made quality improvement a high-profile activity.

The Medical Center of Vermont is another large teaching institution that became engaged in quality improvement several years ago. In 1993, the hospital had 452 beds and absorbed 35 percent of the hospital expenditures in Vermont. The practice of medicine in Vermont is quite conservative, with per capita hospitalization costs being the lowest of the fifty states. There has been relatively low penetration of managed care in the state—somewhat less than 15 percent as of 1994. The hospital is a private not-for-profit entity that has a strong relationship with the University of Vermont Medical School.

The Medical Center of Vermont has always had dynamic leadership and so has not been complacent, even in the absence of a predatory competitive environment in the state. But Community Health Plan of Latham, New York, and the Dartmouth Hitchcock Medical Center in New Hampshire do provide some competition, and as a result, the hospital was trying in 1993 to develop a physician-hospital organization (PHO) and was also considering a merger with another, smaller hospital in Burlington. Moreover, the medical center worked closely with the Vermont Health Care Authority as health care reform bounced in and out of the Vermont legislature between 1991 and 1994.

The medical center's interest in quality improvement dates from the late 1980s. At that time, seeking strategic advantages, the hospital changed its organizational structure and created "service lines" leadership. A simultaneous quality improvement push led by Dean Lea, a vice president for clinical services, began to infiltrate strategic planning, leading to the development of quality teams. In addition, training for opinion leaders and middle management became the rule. Today, the Medical Center of Vermont has a maturing quality improvement effort, almost unique among major academic medical centers.

The other two institutions we visited also illustrate the breadth of organizational types in health care in the United States. The Henry Ford Health System, centered on the Henry Ford Hospital, is one of the dominant providers of care in southeastern Michigan. The hospital itself is a nine-hundred-bed tertiary institution. It is closely affiliated with the Henry Ford Medical Group, which consists of eight hundred physicians at twenty-six sites. The medical group and the hospital have a number of ties to community hospitals, including Cottage Hospital, Grosse Pointe Farms Hospital, and Wyandotte Hospital Medical Center. Health Alliance Plan, a mixed-model, not-for-profit HMO that serves three thousand employers and has 480,000 members is also associated with Henry Ford Health System. The total budget for the health system is $1.7 billion per year.

When Gail Warden arrived as chief executive officer from Group Health Cooperative of Puget Sound in Seattle in 1988, it was clear to him that the Ford system needed a quality initiative. He wanted to create a culture that emphasized Total Quality Management. Working closely with his senior vice president, Vinod Sahney, they selected Paul Batalden as the architect for their quality program. Their initial efforts were designed to suffuse an improvement mentality throughout the organization, the primary vehicle being the Quality Technology Council, which consisted of the top executives of each major operating unit, including the parent corporation, the tertiary hospital, the medical groups, the community hospitals, and the HMOs. A group of physician managers were trained as opinion leaders. The Quality Technology Council also identified coaches and set up a series of improvement teams. Over time, this approach has created several centers of excellence throughout the institution.

Finally, in Twin Falls, Idaho, the Magic Valley Regional Hospital, which has 160 beds—only 60 of which are occupied on most nights—has for some time been applying quality improvement techniques to care. The area of Twin Falls and its surrounding communities contains fewer than 100,000 people, but the problems confronting Magic Valley are similar to problems elsewhere in the country. The hospital faces competition from the Twin Valley Clinic, a private hospital located in Twin Falls, as well as from hospitals opening in nearby towns. As a result, Magic Valley is attempting to set up a PHO in order to create a more cohesive, vertically integrated system. It has also begun educating its governance structure about community health improvement, consisting of a board and three county commissioners (the hospital itself being a public hospital owned by the county).

The Magic Valley Regional Hospital has now undertaken an important effort to reach out and improve public health in the community at large. John Bingham, the chief executive officer, and his senior managers have designed a series of projects concentrating on pediatric injuries, motor vehicle accidents—especially among teenagers—and emergency medical systems' handling of myocardial infarctions. Under Bingham's leadership, the hospital has adopted a new goal: "To make Magic Valley the healthiest community in America." The community interventions are prompted by Bingham's belief that with capitation will come a new focus on public health and prevention. The hospital's efforts express a community interest that was certainly part of the traditional hospital role but that has been largely neglected over the past twenty years. The hospital's initiatives are therefore an exciting complement to other quality improvement efforts we have studied.

The Quality Improvement Undertaking

On our visits to institutions committed to Continuous Quality Improvement, we found a surprising number of common themes. Many institutions committed to understanding and improving the care they deliver follow a similar path. The catalyst is often the recognition by a senior member of the leadership team—often the chief executive officer—of the possibility and strategic value of continuous efforts to improve. Indeed, presidents and chief executive officers often see their personal conversion to Continuous Quality Improvement as the first step in their own institution's efforts. Often, this conversion is the result of contact with a leading proponent of improvement outside the institution. For instance, when Gail Warden arrived at Henry Ford Hospital from Group Health in Washington State, he believed it was important to craft a strategic focus on quality. Working with Vinod Sahney, he formulated a general plan and brought in Paul Batalden from HCA as a consultant. Much the same story was played out with Bill Corley at Community Hospital East, including the selection of Batalden as leading consultant.[8]

In many instances, the Total Quality Management commitment is made at a time of some flux or reengineering. Hospitals often accept Continuous Quality Improvement techniques when they perceive a need for a competitive advantage, or as they realize that they must change to meet future demands. Modern improvement techniques are based on notions of dynamic change; it follows that Continuous Quality Improvement can be especially valuable when restructuring is under way. It should come as no surprise, then, that a number of the institutions we visited began to integrate improvement techniques into their work just as significant changes were being made in the structure of their administration or after several years of financial stability had been followed by shrinking fund balances.[9]

Once top leadership is convinced that improvement must be a consistent goal, the next move is frequently to form a quality council of clinical and administrative leadership, including the key opinion leaders within an institution. This is what was done, for example, both at the Henry Ford Health System and at Sharp Health Care.

Although the quality council is typically led by the CEO, many institutions seem to have a quality champion who makes the improvement effort a full-time job. For instance, Jan Cetti at Sharp Health Care and Dean Lea at the Medical Center of Vermont help coordinate their quality councils and act as the agent of the CEO in planning and training.

Most hospitals endorsing Continuous Quality Improvement have chosen to emphasize staff training in early stages. Characteristic of this phenomenon is the training program conducted by Jeanne Mullen at Community Hospital East. Any interested employee can sign up for the five-day course. Mullen teaches much of the curriculum, assisted by CEO Corley, other quality coaches, and leaders of teams. By the summer of 1993, three hundred of the five thousand employees at Community Hospital East had gone through the full three-day program.[10] In some institutions, training involves an extraordinary investment. For instance, at Medical Center of Vermont, more than six hundred employees have gone through a two-day training seminar. Other institutions have foregone such extensive training and instead prefer to disseminate concepts of improvement throughout the institution using consultants and teams. Notably, some hospitals have segregated the quality training function from the quality improvement projects; in these institutions, the chief trainer acts more like a full-time consultant to the organization. For instance, at West Paces Ferry Hospital, Victoria Davis, head of quality resources, did the lion's share of training, while Lorraine Schiff in quality management supervised the improvement teams.

Teams are a common element of Continuous Quality Improvement efforts across the range of institutions we studied. From the smallest rural hospital to the largest metropolitan network, the vigor of an institution's effort is reflected in part in the intensity of its team activity. As an organization cultivates a new attitude toward continuous improvement, a prevalent strategy is to encourage employees to form teams to work on significant problems in particular departments.

Teams come in two generic, sometimes complementary forms. As we have discussed, the creation of a small team drawn from participants in a specific process can lead to new solutions and to employee invigoration. Such small teams can proliferate rapidly, as they did at Parkview and also at the Medical Center of Vermont, where 120 pop-up teams were operating in the summer of 1993.

The far more prevalent strategy is to have far fewer teams and to evaluate and monitor their progress carefully. In many institutions, such guided teams have been concentrated on the service side of the hospital or health care institution. Projects involving dietary services, laundry, and the physical plant are ubiquitous in the initial stages of a quality effort. Less frequently, teams form on the financial side of the institution. For example, at Parkview, one of the initial teams focused on increasing the collectability of bills.

Over time, most institutions realize that they must use the same methods to improve clinical care. Initiating clinical teams is often inhibited by the unavailability of leading physicians as participants. Many institutions told us that involving physicians in improvement was their greatest challenge. Physicians were often too busy, did not believe in the technology of improvement, or were unwilling to accept the notion of total commitment as necessary to success.

Despite these obstacles, nearly every hospital and health care organization we visited had put into place a number of clinical teams. Most common among these were teams concerned with episodes of care involving routine or repetitive use of technology and similar clinical diagnoses. For example, we often found teams in place to address improvement in cesarean sections, total hip replacements, vaginal delivery, evaluation of breast mass, and care of deep venous thromboses. Typically, these teams were trying to find new ways to reduce the cost of care, often focusing on length of stay while seeking to maintain or improve health outcomes and patient satisfaction.

To follow the progress of these larger teams, many sites identified a set of critical organizational measures that apply generically to a variety of teams. West Paces Ferry, for example, concentrated its measurement efforts on forty-five key variables. Many quality champions find it important for a health care center to create a set of measures that will fit its own environment and that clinicians and others will view with a sense of ownership.[11] A representative sample of measures would include many of the indicators promoted by the Maryland Hospital Association, some of the IMSystem indicators of the Joint Commission for the Accreditation of Health Care Organizations (JCAHO), customized satisfaction measures, and functional status tools. Some hospitals seem to have a head start in team development because their information systems allow them easy access to data that can be used to guide and evaluate improvement efforts.[12]

Guidelines and critical paths play into team functions in different ways. Guidelines help determine team selection. Especially when guidelines are promoted by payers or allied purchasers of care, a strong message is sent to the hospital that certain kinds of improvement are expected. For example, in Minnesota, the Business Health Care Action Group has asked Park Nicollet and several other organizations to develop a series of cost-effectiveness guidelines. Given the power of the purchasers' group, it can be assumed that Park Nicollet will create teams in the various clinical areas touched on by the guidelines.

Critical paths, which are specifications for routine care, are often the institution's answer to pressure for improvement in a particular area. Though the critical path methodology is strongly rooted in the nursing discipline, it is now endorsed by multidisciplinary clinical teams at a variety of institutions.[13] The paths are the more specifically tailored cousin of practice guidelines. As is the case with quality measures, critical paths are often customized for individual institutions. Indeed, many institutions are very reluctant to reveal any details of the paths their teams have constructed—a position that, of course, seriously inhibits the process of emulation.

Students of improvement emphasize that when critical paths are used, there is a risk of stabilizing care at the wrong level. Critical pathways often simply standardize the care that is presently being delivered, with little attention paid to creatively improving the care process. Path designers must be prepared to reformulate a process if they seek to achieve performance breakthroughs.

Just as quality improvement campaigns show similarities between one institution and another, so do the problems they encounter. First, nearly every hospital has difficulty getting busy physicians to participate as team members. Those that have met with some success have done so only after years of struggle. Chip Caldwell at West Paces Ferry Hospital, for example, estimated that it took five years to develop doctors into team leaders.[14] Moreover, though many physicians may receive an initial training, only a few maintain an interest in quality innovations. At the Park Nicollet Medical Center, Rodney Dueck noted that sixty physicians were initially selected for training, and forty to fifty finished the training program. However, a year and a half later, only ten to fifteen were still involved in teams. Most characteristic of our interviews was the word *skeptical* when referring to physician attitudes toward involvement.[15]

Solutions to this problem have begun to crystallize. Many hospitals have found it necessary to bring a single leading clinician into the administration on essentially a full-time basis. This individual then acts as a champion for clinical quality improvement. At Parkview, for example, a respected pulmonologist and intensive care specialist, Keith Wilson, has been drawn into the administration. Other hospitals have formalized this role. At the Brigham and Women's Hospital, Tom Lee, a leading clinical epidemiologist and cardiologist, was appointed quality chief as part of a new emphasis on quality improvement.

Alternatively, physicians can be recruited into improvement efforts through PHOs. As hospitals face capitation, high priority must be given to establishing cohesion between inpatient and outpatient settings, as well as between the administrative functions of the hospital and physician-dominated care. As has been noted, the PHO can be the vehicle for the intertwining of clinical care and administration.

Sound critical paths can be constructed only with the help of leading clinicians. Fortunately, the concrete nature and clinical content of critical paths may make them inherently appealing to physicians and nurses. Therefore, hospitals that opt for this methodology may find that they are building a strong foundation for clinicians' participation in improvement.[16]

Another consistent theme is that medical malpractice fails to rise to the attention of quality improvers. The risk-management function of hospitals is relegated to the sidelines of continuous improvement struggles. In some hospitals and health care institutions, it seems that the quality management teams are barely aware of malpractice litigation.[17] Others assert flatly that there is no conceptual relationship between quality improvement and medical malpractice litigation. As Michael Massanari at Henry Ford Hospital points out, litigation does not provide systematic data; hence even those committed to examining medical malpractice through the prism of Continuous Quality Improvement have great difficulty doing so.[18]

Some insurers have transmitted information to quality improvement teams in hospitals, attempting to build a foundation for systematic analysis of risk for medical malpractice. PHICO, the insurer for Community Hospital East, is one example.[19] The results of these collaborations are not yet available. The attitude of physicians involved in quality improvement toward malpractice and medical injuries is quite similar to that of physicians generally: most understand accidents as random events that cannot be prevented. Thus risk management tends to lead a quiet, somewhat isolated life in institutions that have tried to incorporate modern methods of quality improvement into their work.

We found quality assurance activities also to be somewhat segregated from quality improvement efforts. The office of quality assurance is frequently treated as an anachronism left in place to satisfy equally anachronistic regulations. Health care organizations we visited tended to keep assurance efforts in place mainly to satisfy the JCAHO requirement that there be a pharmacy and therapeutics committee, a tissues committee, morbidity and mortality rounds, and the like.[20] The segregation of quality assurance is also motivated by the fear that improvement efforts will be impeded by traditional methods. Therefore hospitals continue to commit resources to old systems while new systems of improvement proceed independently. This superfluous use of quality assurance is expensive, but fear of regulation is strong.

The other administrative area that tends to be isolated is utilization review. As noted in Chapter Three, utilization management grew tremendously in the mid- to late 1980s, but today its prominence in hospitals is beginning to fade. Especially in those institutions that face high proportions of capitated care, extensive utilization management becomes irrelevant.[21] Although it is important to ensure that every patient's length of stay is as short as possible, traditional utilization management may not have much more to offer in this regard. An increasing number of hospitals have come to understand that appropriate admissions, specific care pathways, and rapid discharges to well-supervised settings (all forms of "internal" utilization management) are critical. These issues are the concern of teams, and thus the role of the conventional external utilization reviewer is less and less important.

In summary, institutions that have endorsed quality improvement and have committed significant human capital and other resources to that end often follow similar routes. The appointment of a quality council, the training of large numbers of employees, the use of small clinical improvement teams, and careful management based on a carefully chosen set of parameters are the hallmarks of these efforts. Institutions that share this commitment also face similar problems, including physician indifference, structural estrangement from risk management and medical malpractice, and the perceived need to run outmoded quality assurance programs in parallel with quality improvement efforts.

Perhaps the most interesting aspect of the quality initiatives at the institutions we visited is that they were not prompted by traditional regulation. They are based, rather, on an increasingly widespread set of beliefs: that quality of care can be improved through concerted attention to care processes, that data analysis is critical to this effort, and that better quality is something the market will expect. The pressure of rules set by the JCAHO, the Peer Review Organizations, and malpractice litigation had little or nothing to do with the push for quality. Indeed, the increasing responsiveness of regulatory agencies probably results from the efforts of the health care organizations to adopt modern quality methods.

Coping with Regulation

Our critical question for providers engaged in quality improvement was this: does regulation obstruct your efforts, and if so, how? Among the institutions we studied, it was difficult to perceive a consensus regarding the interaction between quality improvement and regulation. Many observers were quite negative, readily criticizing regulatory interference, demands for meaningless additional work, and rigidity. Others were more supportive of the regulators' goals, treating their measures and efforts as appropriate to a context for quality improvement. These individuals saw regulators as one important group of external "customers" of the organization, with legitimate needs to be met. Very few of those we interviewed were openly antagonistic to the regulatory agenda, but many felt that its value was greatly exceeded by the costs of compliance. None were willing to characterize regulators as collaborators, or regulation as responsive.

CEOs rarely articulated specific concerns about the regulatory environment in health care. Some perceived very little regulatory pressure—although in the case of Charles Jacobson at Park Nicollet, this may be due to the fact that group practices are not highly regulated. Others, such as Jeffrey Otten at the Brigham and Women's Hospital, acknowledged that there was significant regulation but nonetheless maintained that the efforts of those who oversee hospitals rarely impinged on his immediate responsibilities. At Henry Ford Hospital, Gail Warden's comments were similar. He noted that the regulatory vigor in Michigan, though hardly negligible, did not compare with that in Washington State. (The critical distinction was that Washington regulated rates whereas Michigan did not.)

Assuring regulatory compliance was a job usually assigned to the first tier of management. Those in charge of relationships with regulators were well versed in the range of potential government influences. For example, Darlene Burgess, vice president for corporate government relations at Henry Ford Hospital, readily ran down the list of regulators with whom she had contact; they included the Michigan Department of Health, the Clinical Laboratory Improvement Act enforcers from the Food and Drug Administration, the state officials in charge of certificate of need (CON), the Internal Revenue Service overseers of the for-profit areas of the health system, the plaintiffs' attorneys bringing medical malpractice litigation, and the HMO regulators at the Department of Public Health.

She also noted how important antitrust litigation and disciplinary boards were as influences on the health care institution. But Burgess was an exception in the range of her regulatory duties. Most managers had frequent contact with only a few regulators.

The only ubiquitous regulator among all the hospitals we visited was the JCAHO. Very few hospital leaders criticized the commission's motives or historical contribution, yet many questioned the need for its role in an era of quality improvement. Chip Caldwell at West Paces Ferry, for example, perceived the JCAHO as an obstacle to better care; he maintained that its inspection-based oversight was incapable of promoting process improvement. Caldwell asked, why should there be a mandated tissues committee? It was far preferable, in his estimation, for individual administrators to define outcome that should occur at hospitals and provide the JCAHO with outcomes measures. Similar views were expressed by many others. Michael Massanari at the Henry Ford Hospital believed that hospitals were greatly injured by the JCAHO's agenda setting and cited surgical case review as an example. He was not at all sure that case review contributed to better care; more important, it tended to tie up key personnel in tasks that might not contribute to the health care organization's quality goals. This theme of the commission adding to costs but not to value dominated discussions of the JCAHO. There was general agreement that the diversion of energy into JCAHO compliance efforts retarded quality improvement.

But hostility to the JCAHO extended beyond the accusation that it was simply a waste of resources. At some institutions, leaders expressed a fear that JCAHO visits could lead to the undermining of dynamic quality improvement. They were specifically apprehensive that the JCAHO's surveillance mentality could threaten the carefully cultivated, but nonetheless fragile, perception among clinicians that change was desirable.[22] At the Brigham and Women's Hospital, Sheridan Kassirer, vice president for clinical services, made a point of assigning the task of preparation for a JCAHO visit to analysts associated with the old quality management department. The hospital's quality improvement effort, run by the Clinical Initiatives Development Program, was thus allowed to proceed without disruption. Similar attempts to segregate quality improvement efforts from the inspection of the JCAHO were apparent in other institutions.

The most bitter complaints about the JCAHO visits were from physicians who had been selected to be managers or quality champions. James Schibanoff, a pulmonologist who had become chief executive officer of Sharp Memorial Hospital, had recently prepared for an accreditation survey when we interviewed him in June 1994. At that time, Schibanoff oversaw both Sharp Memorial and the Cabrillo Hospital. Sharp had a positive attitude toward the JCAHO; the institution had participated as a beta site for data collection under the IMSystem and had been very supportive of the commission's Agenda for Change. However, the particular survey team that arrived at Sharp Memorial and Cabrillo did not know how to evaluate quality improvement efforts. Schibanoff often found their standards to be archaic and irrelevant.

He gave us a telling example, partially recounted at the beginning of this book. Sharp had decided to participate in the National Nosocomial Infection System (NNIS) program run by the Centers for Disease Control (CDC). The program allowed the hospital to track its experience with infection in urine, blood, wounds, and pneumonias and to compare this experience with CDC norms. The JCAHO was uninterested in any NNIS data and instead wanted to find documentation of the number of hours infection-control nurses spent on surveillance. The JCAHO surveyors' dependence on structural measures and their concomitant refusal to learn about process improvement efforts appeared to be characteristic of the commission's visits to many hospitals emphasizing quality improvement.[23]

This is not to say that negative views of the JCAHO were unanimous. For example, Ernest Lemoi, manager of internal medicine at Henry Ford Hospital, found that the JCAHO's surveyors were impressed with his quality improvement efforts, and he came out of their 1994 visit believing that the commission was on the correct track for evaluating Total Quality Management. Regina McFarland at Parkview perceptively noted that it was possible to treat the JCAHO and other outside regulators as customers. Others reiterated this view, finding some encouraging signs that the JCAHO surveyors could approve of and even praise quality improvement. However, these encouraging views fell far short of identifying a responsive approach by the JCAHO, and even failed to live up to the commission's own reform agenda.

An unbiased observer will find in our interviews a glimmer of hope for the JCAHO among advocates of quality improvement. However, this must be set against the distance still to be covered by the commission if it is to catch up with health care organizations in its approach to quality. Many hospital leaders believe that structure-focused JCAHO surveyors undermine the Continuous Quality Improvement vision. No matter what the view, however, the JCAHO still emerged in our surveys as the dominant regulatory force in the eyes of hospitals.

Indeed, by comparison, other efforts at regulation by state and federal government tend to be minor distractions. A number of our interviewees mentioned the record reviews done by Peer Review Organizations (PROs) as a tolerable nuisance that did not affect the strategy of the hospital. Others were more positive in their assessments. For example, James Taylor, chief executive officer of the Medical Center of Vermont, saw some effectiveness in PRO programs. However, the overwhelming majority of interviewees, though they may not have seen the PROs as troublesome, did not consider them to be serving any useful purpose.

Slightly more problematic, but a major influence only in a very tiny proportion of hospitals, is the federal commitment to antitrust in the health care area. Even though many of the health care institutions we interviewed were working toward vertical or horizontal integration, the antitrust issue rarely entered the conversation. In part, this is due to the fact that few health care organizations engaged in mergers or acquisitions reach the threshold of concern about market dominance. The exceptions are among hospitals in small urban areas. At the time of our interview, Parkview was attempting to merge with its cross-town competitor, Corwin-St.Mary's. Each hospital was operating at 30 to 40 percent capacity. However, in mid-1994, the Federal Trade Commission ruled any potential merger illegal, creating great dislocation at both institutions and what many in Pueblo portrayed as a perpetuation of waste in a strapped community.

State regulation garnered slightly more attention. As might be expected, its influence varied according to the state's commitment to regulation. Many states do very little to regulate hospitals, at least as far as the leaders of those institutions are concerned. Most states delegate their accreditation process to the JCAHO. Among those that do not, a number perform unannounced inspection visits at hospitals. Yet hospitals located in, for example, Colorado, Michigan, and Indiana seem to have little fear of the regulators' arrival. They find that the inspectors are often poorly trained and that their interests tend to be quite narrow; their visits are not especially disruptive. Most of the inspectors have never heard of Continuous Quality Improvement—and do not care about it.

An important exception to the pattern of innocuous state regulation is New York, where the regulatory apparatus grew significantly under the former commissioner of the Department of Health, David Axelrod. As of 1994, hospitals were dealing with four types of state regulation: mandatory reporting of certain kinds of clinical incidents, hospital surveys, oversight of physicians by the Office of Professional Medical Conduct (OPMC), and complaints investigation.[24] The most prominent regulation for the hospital appears to be the first, the reportable incidents program. Before 1993, the nature of reportable incidents had been poorly defined by the state, and the official expectations regarding the depth of the reports were not carefully delineated. As a result, the program ballooned. Strong Memorial, for example, sent out 268 reports in 1992, each of them five to seven pages long. Understandably, compliance required a tremendous commitment of resources on the part of the hospitals.

Perhaps in light of this, New York State shifted to a patient event tracking system (PETS) in 1993. Hospitals are now allowed to report events on specific, relatively brief forms. Institutions must aggregate information on incidents and can then analyze it using their own statistical processes. In some ways, the new approach is attractive for Continuous Quality Improvement. Unfortunately, it will take some time before New York's reputation as an overbearing regulator will fade.

Indeed, if anything, New York's survey program appears to be more threatening and irritating than the JCAHO's. At one week's notice, the state survey team can arrive for a two-to-four-week period. The team consists of a physician surveyor, a nursing surveyor, and others. They review policies, inspect files, and interview patients. Most of their measures are narrowly structural: the surveyors pour over minutes, policies, medical staff reports, and the like. A month and a half after such a visit, the state sends a report card noting deficiencies. The hospital then has thirty days to respond. The entire process is an archetypal inspection, with no thought given to sharing of ideas, copying, or mutual learning.

The third aspect of New York's regulatory strategy, oversight of physician licensure, is undertaken by the Office of Professional Medical Conduct. Any reportable events that would lead to questions about a physician's competence can give rise to an OPMC analysis of hospital records.

The fourth aspect is evaluation of every complaint submitted against hospitals. The extent of follow-up is significant; at a hospital like Strong Memorial, up to five to ten complaints per year must be assessed and discussed with the state.

Like others in New York, Aileen Shinaman in the general counsel's office at Strong Memorial finds state officials and inspectors to be overly interested in details, and at times quite punitive. Hospital officials seek to build a reasonable relationship with regulators and to work toward a common goal, but they believe that the regulators are less helpful than they might be. Shinaman's view is seconded by Leo Brideau, who at the time of our interviews was chief executive officer at Strong Memorial. He characterizes the state as at times adversarial and interested in micromanagement. He also cites the inordinate costs of compliance.[25] It should not be surprising, then, that the New Yorkers we interviewed find the JCAHO a welcome alternative. For example, Irwin Frank, medical director of Strong Memorial, had been through three visits from the JCAHO and characterizes its surveyors as helpful and informed. He and other members of the staff at Strong Memorial are hopeful that the JCAHO will develop some synergy between regulation and improvement efforts.

The New York Department of Health is also very rigid (and even adversarial) in its application of more traditional regulatory methods. Brideau raised significant questions about the certificate-of-need process in New York. To build certain types of facilities, Strong Memorial must gain approval from regional boards, which are dominated by consumers of medical care. Before any significant construction can occur, a variety of contingencies set forth by the boards must be met. Brideau believed this burdensome process could have a notable chilling effect on the development of new programs at Strong Memorial. He estimated that delays caused by CON requirements tend to inflate costs of new construction by as much as $100,000 per month for some projects. Leaders at hospitals in New York will no doubt be interested in the call for hospital regulatory relief put forth by the administration of Governor Pataki in 1995.[26]

Institutional leaders in other states tended to be more sanguine about certificate of need, either because the threshold for application of the laws was higher (the ceiling is $900,000 for new construction in Georgia, for example, as opposed to $400,000 in New York) or because the influence of certificate of need was receding, even collapsing, in quite a few states. In Colorado and Indiana, the

CON sun had set and was but a mildly unpleasant memory. However, a few health care leaders, like James Taylor at the Medical Center of Vermont, accepted the importance of certificate of need specifically and technology assessment generally, as part of a rational health care system. (These comments notwithstanding, the Vermont hospital's administrators were shocked by the adversarial vigor they encountered in New York regulators when New York State residents were cared for in Burlington.)

A central theme in our discussions with health care leaders and quality advocates was the claim that regulation inhibited innovation. Institutions that wished to address their customers' needs and wanted to provide the highest-quality and most cost-effective care found themselves frustrated by structure-based, safety-centered rules. One oft-recited example was the set of rules found in many states that specify the personnel required to undertake certain functions within health care institutions. As Chip Caldwell notes, hospital licensing rules in Georgia require that respiratory therapists and pharmacists, for example, perform certain functions, yet these tasks could at times be undertaken by less highly skilled—and highly paid—employees. Caldwell, though not unsympathetic to the state's concerns, asserted that the requirements simply add costs. As he and others noted, if safety is the major issue, then regulators should be satisfied with outcomes data collected by the hospitals, documenting that safety has been preserved. Another example of the same phenomenon was provided by Rick Hahn, director of the pharmacy at Parkview.[27] The state of Colorado's new uniform pharmacy code brings into the hospital setting a great deal of regulation that was originally intended only for retail pharmacies. The extension of the code to hospital pharmacies has created quite burdensome record keeping that is out of place in a hospital context. For the state, it was simply a matter of convenience to adopt a uniform code; for health care institutions, it has added expensive tasks that do not contribute to better care.

Similar concerns were voiced about federal and state oversight of clinical labs. Mark Janos, administrator of laboratory medicine at Parkview, argued that compliance with the Clinical Laboratory Improvement Act of 1988 (CLIA) has added very little quality but has created a large documentation burden. This is another example of regulation intended for one purpose having unintended negative side effects. The additions to CLIA in 1988 had been meant to modify processes in physician-owned laboratories, but because the act was applied across the board, hospital laboratories found themselves contributing more and more resources to compliance.

The solution offered by administrators interested in quality improvement was for regulators to specify certain kinds of outcomes that the institutions would then pursue. This is the sort of cooperation that is the hallmark of new rules. Our discussions with administrators in laboratories and pharmacies focused on the distinction between quality control and quality improvement. In most clinical laboratories and pharmacies, the rationale for quality control—defined as the monitoring of certain measurements on a routine basis—is quite clear. These efforts seem to interfere with quality improvement only insofar as they compete for limited resources. All interviewees agreed that quality improvement could not replace quality control. Furthermore, reducing variation in quality control measures could be understood as a quality improvement effort.

The regulatory burden is not small. Throughout health care institutions, individuals are affected in subtle and not so subtle ways by a formidable array of regulation. Engineering administrators complain about federal and state pollution standards and building codes. Those in the planning office are troubled by the potential for antitrust scrutiny. Human resources personnel note the influence of the Occupational Safety and Health Administration's rules on bloodborne pathogens. For-profit institutions, and especially the administrators of their emergency departments, are affected by the provisions of the Emergency Medical Transfer and Active Labor Act. Records administrators must accommodate the PROs and the equivalent reviewers for Medicaid and other insurance programs. In each case, the question remains: are the benefits of regulation out-weighed by the costs associated with compliance? The answer is a persistent, if at times muted, yes. On the spectrum from obstructive to responsive, the overall score is well toward the obstructive end.

Outside the hospital, it appears that regulation is even less effec-tive at promoting good care. As we have noted, managed care orga-nizations must produce a massive amount of information for insurance commissioners and other overseers regarding the nature of their networks, the kinds of incentives they offer providers, and the data they transmit to beneficiaries. However, on the clinical side and in top management, this activity is little noticed, and regula-tion of quality appears much less burdensome. J. D. Turner, an attor-ney and compliance officer at Sharp Health Care, can discuss at great length the required reporting under the Knox-Keene Act, the vehicle for regulation of managed care organizations in California. But those near the top of managed care organizations are relatively unengaged in questions of compliance with such regulatory efforts.

Most leaders at managed care organizations are aware and sup-portive of the accreditation process offered by the National Com-mittee for Quality Assurance. In fact, their views are remarkably different from those of hospital administrators who have recently faced JCAHO accreditation. NCQA strives to accommodate qual-ity improvement efforts. Though critics might suggest that this is simply a matter of regulatory capture, it would appear from discus-sions in managed care organizations that the NCQA evaluation is very thorough. Every effort is made to comply with NCQA sugges-tions, not because of fear but because the suggestions have merit and contribute to quality. Here there was a sense of responsiveness.

In what is today a minority view, the NCQA may be provider-dominated in the way the JCAHO used to be. In this light, the NCQA's HEDIS criteria, rather than reflecting the aspirations of managed care for improved quality, look like a negotiated, safe, and traditional set of parameters. Institutions generally have more dif-ficulty with self-criticism and honest assessment than is healthy.

HEDIS in its early forms can be seen here as a way of ensuring that most managed care organizations appear sound.

There will be changes in managed care accreditation over the next decade. Both the NCQA and the JCAHO, if not other regulators, will compete to oversee quality in the managed care systems and physician-hospital organizations of the future. The outcome of this competition will be telling for quality and its regulation. For now, the regulators of NCQA are quite different from their counterparts at the JCAHO and in state agencies. The NCQA strives to be supportive of efforts to improve and sees its oversight as collaborative. Traditional regulators, in contrast, often behave as though they cannot afford this luxury.

New York State regulators provide an example. In our discussions with the office of Thomas Hartman, director of health care standards and surveillance at the Department of Health in New York, top regulators asserted that they see very little nontraditional quality improvement.[28] They think there has been little success with Total Quality Management in medical areas, but they still encourage fledgling efforts. They note that the state wishes to move toward outcome measurements, along the lines of its evaluation of coronary artery bypass graft surgery, but there is a persisting sense that hospitals must be directly overseen. Although neither the hospital industry nor the regulators have data on the effect of regulation, regulators like Hartman seem convinced that without their surveillance, hospital commitment to quality and safety might fade. Nonetheless, their open attitude toward outcome measurement suggests a pathway for the future in which the state might specify outcomes that institutions would strive to meet, and regulators would step back in only when there was persistent failure to meet acceptable standards.

The Future: Purchasers, Outcomes, and Guidelines

We found hints of an outcome-based regulatory future throughout our discussions with hospital administrators. As noted in Chapter

Five, a number of states have begun building comprehensive clinical data bases. The institutions we studied, all committed to Total Quality Management, welcome these efforts, as they would like to be able to demonstrate the efficacy of their improvement programs. Moreover, benchmarking is crucial to Continuous Quality Improvement, and large clinical data bases are essential to benchmarking information.

The open attitude toward data bases is reflected in Leo Brideau's comments. New York State has successfully integrated a data base on clinical outcomes of coronary artery bypass surgery into its regulatory structure. Brideau is quite reasonably concerned about a system based on self-reporting. If the clinical data bases are to rely on reports by the institutions themselves, the rules of reporting must be carefully specified, and the inherent opportunity to "cook" the numbers—for example, by changing severity coding—must be addressed. Nonetheless, Brideau sees this strategy as a welcome change from traditional state initiatives.

Institutions in other states relate a similar story. Colorado, for example, is in the process of starting up a system in which a set of parameters based on MedisGroups will be published on each hospital. This information will be co-owned by the state and the Colorado Hospital Association. An institution like Parkview, according to Carol Guinane, is poised to demonstrate its successes in quality improvement.

The move to state-mandated benchmarking is most readily accomplished in states that already have had some sort of voluntary system in place. In Vermont, for example, hospitals have for years voluntarily put together information on length of stay and costs and shipped it to the Data Council of the Hospital Association. This fairly sophisticated system, based on McGraw-Hill's DRI methodology, has wide support within the state.[29]

The main concern about data reporting is cost. Ann Mican at Strong Memorial Hospital estimates that it may cost the hospital $200,000 to $300,000 to report on the coronary artery bypass graft program alone. If data reporting is expanded to other outcomes, its costs could become quite burdensome. Fears about costs lead inevitably to scrutiny of benefits. The utility of the benchmark measures will be based on the uniformity with which institutions report and the resulting integrity of the data. If the reporting is idiosyncratic and the measures are not comparable, the benefits will rapidly be outweighed by the costs. Equally important is the clinical integrity of the measures. Are they important to patient care? Can institutions change processes to improve performance? And does better performance mean better care?

An extension of state-based data bases is uniform guidelines for care. Very few states have guidelines in place at the present time, but they are certainly on the horizon. In Minnesota, the Business Health Care Action Group is encouraging the development of guidelines for common clinical problems. The action group has created the Institute for Clinical Systems Integration, which is to specify sixteen guidelines for cost-effective care. These rules will probably be applied across the state, although not by the state itself but by purchasers. In Massachusetts, the Department of Industrial Accidents has formulated a series of treatment guidelines for common occupational disorders. The guidelines are mandated for insurers' utilization reviews and therefore for providers. These efforts will not be the last of their kind. Movement from outcomes to guidelines is a natural one and will probably be seen in many states in the future.

It is an open question whether the use of guidelines will be promoted primarily by purchasers, as in Minnesota, or by regulators, as in Massachusetts. The former state, it should be noted, is acknowledged to be an "advanced" health care market and is the site of greatest pressure by purchasers for the extension of outcomes to guidelines. Similar efforts are already coming to life throughout managed care. A number of chief executive officers in our interviews identified aggressive sets of guidelines put into place by a large commercial payer in a particular metropolitan area.

There may be a significant drawback to some uses of guidelines.

One chief executive officer and members of his staff had misgivings about the quality of care that might be rendered under a guideline that led to an expedited schedule for treatment and discharge. There were significant negotiations with the insurer (the issuer of the guidelines) about these clinical concerns, leading to some amelioration and loosening of the guideline. No one involved in the negotiations, however, was comfortable with the real issue—the trade-off between cost-effectiveness and quality.

Providers approach this issue with a certain amount of trepidation as market incentives are magnified in health care. As discussed earlier, health care institutions were long able to ignore traditional supply-and-demand rules of the market. Consequently, true costs were often buried in somewhat inflated charges, and cross-subsidy between various payers was used to balance the books. Provider isolation from the market is no longer possible as insurers look for greater and greater economies, creating not only new pressures on the hospital's bottom line but also the need to develop methodologies for analyzing hospital costs.

The pressures of cost on health care are especially keen as capitation becomes a dominant mode of payment. California, as is well known, has led the country in development of aggressive payment structures based on covered lives. At Sharp Health Care, for example, the Rees-Stealy group is reimbursed for approximately 90 percent of its work through capitated payment. In most metropolitan areas, capitated payment has first been applied to physicians and then to hospital beds. Only when there are small numbers of covered lives does it seem that institutions will resist capitation. For example, at Parkview, where the payer mix is 70 percent Medicare and Medicaid, Bill Patterson, the chief financial officer, cannot afford to make a mistake with capitation because of the instability of the small numbers of commercially insured patients.[30] But situations like that at Parkview in turn create pressure for horizontal integration so that any one institution can compete for capitated lives.

Aggressive purchasers can affect quality improvement in a

number of ways. Most important, when bidding for services, each purchaser/employer might expect and demand different measures of quality. Individual purchasers were characterized by health care institutions as having a poor understanding of quality, yet each insisted on certain specific measures. This multitrack system induces great inefficiencies and frustrates quality improvement efforts by those on the delivery side. In effect, multiple guidelines and multiple data base criteria lead to inefficient use of resources—resources that could otherwise be used for improvement.

Beyond hampering efficiency, economic competition and the ongoing changes in health care markets pose two separate and very significant risks to Continuous Quality Improvement. First, many institutions are headed in the direction of horizontal mergers with competitors or vertical integration with physician-hospital organizations. They are also considering managed care options, and even risk holding (insuring). The ten institutions that make up our survey graphically illustrate the trend. Sharp Health Care and Henry Ford Hospital System are already vertically integrated. Harvard Community Health Plan is expanding through horizontal integration with other HMOs, most recently merging with the Pilgrim HMO in Massachusetts. The group practice Park Nicollet has recently affiliated with a hospital. Medical Center of Vermont combined with the University of Vermont's College of Medicine physicians to form the Fletcher Allen Health Care System. Three other hospitals, Community Hospital East, Parkview Episcopal Medical Center, and Brigham and Women's Hospital, have recently consummated or are pursuing affiliation with other hospitals. In this changing environment, the culture that gives rise to quality improvement efforts at one institution might not obtain at another. Attempts to transfer quality improvement are often frustrated; it appears that commitment to Total Quality Management must grow organically and cannot readily be grafted. Dedication to quality risks being left behind in what are often rough marriages.

The second risk posed by economic competition arises from the fact that when institutions combine, they usually choose to down-size (or "rightsize" or "delayer") the administration. As part of this process, quality champions may have their job descriptions rewritten or eliminated. In several institutions we visited, as consolidation occurred, there was a reduction in the overall quality management budget. These moves can devastate the sense of commitment that is so essential to quality improvement. Yet as one chief executive officer pointed out, "As belts tighten, we have to get back to our main business, which is taking care of patients." Although vertical integration creates an environment for thinking about extended processes of care, cash-strapped institutions that have recently merged might not have sufficient resources to maintain quality improvement efforts. This leaves one with the sense that the market's exaggerated concern about cost could lead to real defects in quality.

In the rush toward capitated payment and the integration it requires, some see opportunities for more effective care. At Magic Valley Regional Hospital, John Bingham believes that capitation will create incentives for better public health.[31] If under capitation, a system has to bear the costs of all health care for an individual patient, and if the health of that patient can be affected by outreach into the community, then it behooves the hospital to become more aggressive in its efforts to prevent disease and promote health. The example Bingham uses is a critical path for angina pectoris. If patients can be given thrombolytic agents faster, their survival will be higher and their complications may be less severe. Therefore the hospital should be looking into ways to provide better service from emergency medical technicians. But it should also be trying to increase public knowledge about warning signs for angina and, moving beyond prevention to promotion, encouraging changes in dietary and smoking habits. In this way, capitation aligns itself with better care and an emphasis on quality that travels outside the institution. Recently, the forty-seven-member Magic Valley Health Network, the physician organization, signed a contract with the hospital to promote preventive care in the community.

Bingham is, at least in our interviews, an outlier in his optimism. We found a considerable wearing down of commitment to quality improvement in a number of institutions. Budgets were being cut for improvement efforts and CEOs were showing less and less interest in quality management methodology. At least five of the ten institutions we visited had reduced the quality budget in the previous twelve months. Moreover, many regretted the heavy outlays on what they felt to be "tools" for "training programs." What was clear is that the push for greater quality will probably require a boost as the market develops.

If anything, then, our concerns about regulation and quality have been redoubled by our interviews. Regulation of various sorts, though not providing the massive impediments that we had hypothesized, do nonetheless frustrate certain kinds of improvement efforts. More important, regulation seldom acts in a fashion synergistic with quality improvement. There is little responsive regulation. Finally, market incentives are not appropriately engendering quality, and to date little has been done to address cost/quality trade-offs in a systematic way. Given the changes likely to be produced by a more competitive and cost-conscious environment, health care needs a framework for regulation that actively promotes quality improvement rather than simply protecting improvement from the impediments that regulation can create.

Notes

1. Interview with Jan Cetti, director, quality improvement, Sharp Health Care, June 13, 1994.

2. Interview with Carol Guinane, vice president, medical staff resources, Parkview Episcopal Medical Center, June 24, 1993.

3. Interview with Leo P. Brideau, general director and chief executive officer, Strong Memorial Hospital, September 23, 1993.

4. Interview with Glenn Bingle, vice president for medical affairs, Community Hospital East, July 6, 1993.

5. Interview with Rodney Dueck, medical director, Park Nicollet Medical Center, August 24, 1993.

6. Interview with Chip Caldwell, chief executive officer, HCA West Paces Ferry, June 2, 1993.

7. Interview with Manuel Ferris, chief executive officer, and John Ludden, medical director, Harvard Community Health Plan, February 2, 1994.

8. Interviews with Gail Warden, president and chief executive officer, Henry Ford Health Systems, July 21, 1993, and with William Corley, chief executive officer, Community Hospital East, July 6, 1993. Chip Caldwell also was impressed by Paul Batalden when Batalden was working at HCA. In fact, Batalden was important in diffusing Continuous Quality Improvement methodology throughout the HCA network. However, following the merger of Columbia Health Care and HCA, the commitment to Total Quality Management at HCA may have waned. Batalden has now left to become a professor at Dartmouth Medical School.

9. Interviews with Jim Taylor, president, Medical Center of Vermont, July 29, 1993, and with Sheridan Kassirer, vice president for clinical services, Brigham and Women's Hospital, April 12, 1994.

10. Interview with Victoria Davis, chief of quality resources, and Lorraine Schiff, chief of quality management, West Paces Ferry Hospital, June 2, 1993.

11. Some institutions have insisted on parsimony in the adoption of measures. For example, at Sharp Medical Center, twenty-four measures are used. Interview with Marie Glancy, chief of quality measurement, Sharp Health Care System, June 1994.

12. Kassirer interview.

13. Kassirer interview.

14. Caldwell interview.

15. Bingle interview; also, interview with Ernie Lemoi, administrator manager, general internal medicine, Henry Ford Hospital, July 21, 1993.

16. Interview with Judy Eastly, Community Hospital East, July 6, 1993; Kassirer interview.

17. Interview with Cynthia Miller, Park Nicollet Medical Center, August 24, 1993.

18. Interview with Michael Massanari, associate medical director, Professional Practice Review Group, Henry Ford Hospital, July 21, 1993.

19. Eastly interview.

20. For example, Davis/Schiff interview.

21. Cetti interview.

22. Davis/Schiff interview.

23. Interview with Keith Wilson, director of clinical quality improvement, Parkview Episcopal Medical Center, June 24, 1993.

24. Interview with Aileen Shinaman, associate counsel, Strong Memorial Hospital, September 23, 1993.

25. Brideau interview.

26. I. Fisher, "Pataki Will Lift Some Regulations for Health Care," *New York Times*, April 5, 1995, 1.

27. Interview with Rick Hahn, director of pharmacy, Parkview Episcopal Medical Center, June 24, 1993.

28. Phone interview with Thomas Hartman, director of health care standards and surveillance, Department of Health, New York, May 21, 1993.

29. Interview with Dave Simmons, director, accounting and budget, Medical Center of Vermont, July 29, 1993.

30. Interview with Bill Patterson, chief financial officer, Parkview Episcopal Medical Center, June 24, 1993.

31. Interview with John Bingham, chief executive officer, Magic Valley Regional Hospital, July 10, 1993.

7

Regulation for Improvement

A Prescription

Health care needs regulation. In an industry as complex and tentacular as health care, certain important social aims can be plausibly accomplished in no other way. The public's need for safety, for example, is at least as urgent in health care as it is in air travel, bridge construction, and automobile emission control, and in each such case, society has discovered no adequate private sector substitute for governmental action through standard setting and regulation. In theory, no reason exists why a private market could not itself establish an adequate mechanism for assuring that airplanes are airworthy, bridges do not often collapse, and car exhausts are clean; but actual experience indicates that private self-control does not suffice in those important fields. Nor should we expect it to in medical care.

Why self-control fails is a topic worth exploring, but it goes beyond the boundaries of this book. Garrett Harden, in his perceptive analysis of "The Tragedy of the Commons," has offered the economists' view: that the micromotives of individuals, each acting in rational self-interest, do not always sum to a sustainable social aggregate.[1] Each townsperson will rationally add one more cow or sheep to graze the common land, and at no number of beasts—even when overgrazing will kill the commons—would it be wise or logical for any individual *not* to add "one more cow." It takes a collective—a government—to stay the hand of each individual from acting on rational self-interest so that the whole can survive. Howard Hiatt has developed the medical analogy to "The Tragedy of the Commons," and the logic almost proves the need for government to regulate care.[2] "Without a certificate-of-need process," the logic claims, "each facility will rationally add its own increment of expansion to the bloated, irrational whole." The evidence bears this out. A health care system whose capital formation and growth are largely unregulated has produced an excess supply that society cannot now afford. Wennberg has shown how closely the supply of health care services tracks and predicts costs to society and how it is independent of the actual need and demand for services.[3] Government initially reacted with the certificate-of-need (CON) process and rate regulation, and later with market simulations such as prospective payment.

Few, even among those who oppose a strong governmental hand in health care, argue for the resurrection of the professionally dominated pseudoregulation of the mid-century that was documented in Chapter Two. It is hard, of course, not to be impressed by the courage of Codman and by the seriousness with which leading American surgeons in particular took on the task of self-scrutiny in the 1920s and 1930s. However, we are also haunted by the scene in the boiler room of the Waldorf Astoria Hotel in 1919, as the deans of American surgery hurled into the furnace their data on hospital adherence to the simplest rules of quality in surgical oversight. The smoke rising from the chimney of the Waldorf Astoria carried with it the basis for unquestioning trust in the capacity even of a noble profession to regulate itself.

The longer, more complex story of self-regulation, progressing to the work of the Joint Commission for Accreditation of Hospitals (JCAHO) and professional registration procedures, is less dramatic but not much more reassuring. Throughout the era of professional hegemony over the setting of standards and the inspection of performance, there is too little evidence that the safety of the public and improvement of work were indeed the highest priorities of those who claimed to hold themselves accountable for care. The standards were too lax, the tolerance of error was far too great, and the procedures for remedy—procedures protected most of all by the allegedly "self-regulating professionals"—were too cumbersome for the claim to survive that the public was fully and adequately protected by the medical profession.

This is not to oversimplify, nor to devalue, the frequent successes that did appear in professional self-regulation between the time of Flexner (when scientific practice began to be possible) and the advent of Medicare (when the public's interest became irrevocably attached to the financing of health care). The perceptiveness, courage, and innovativeness of the Lee-Jones Report and of the conferences on hospital standardization organized by the American College of Surgeons are impressive even today, many decades later. From the profession emerged John Bowman, I. S. Falk, Paul Lembcke, Beverly Payne, Kerr White, Mildred Morehead, Avedis Donabedian, and scores of other vocal and visible leaders for whom improvement was a driving aim and to whom defects in care were evident, measurable, and not to be tolerated. The Joint Commission itself became, in its own way, a conscience within the profession, and though its methods can easily be faulted, its intent must be admired: to make care safe for the public.

Yet the defects persisted, and persist today. Variation in practice runs rampant—beyond the bounds of common sense. Hospitals and doctors continue to perpetrate harms in their work, albeit unintended ones. And it is no easier now to cause an alcoholic surgeon to stop operating than it was forty years ago.

It is difficult to find even a few striking examples in which a "self-regulating" profession has, through its own initiative in public action, taken steps to fundamentally improve the safety of the public at the risk of its own economic security or collegial unity. Within medicine today, it still takes immense courage to insist that fundamental improvement is achievable, to demand it, and to accept the consequent changes. To a far greater degree than is conscionable, the fires in the furnace of the Waldorf Astoria still blaze, feeding on fear.

But regulation has not helped, either. Our review of the twentieth-century history of governmental actions taken to remedy the deficiencies of professional self-regulation is not at all reassuring. Regulatory action may have legitimate social goals that self-regulation cannot achieve, but in numerous ways, external regulation also has failed. It has emphasized only the notions of culling, inspection, and sometimes repair, to the detriment of other forms of improvement.

Even within the inspection mode, regulation has been a failure. One of its principal failings is that it costs too much for the value it provides. Among the most crucial obligations of culling or inspection is efficiency. In economic terms, inspection adds no value to a product or service; it merely seeks to minimize the *loss* of value that has occurred earlier in the process of production. Inspection is a "cost of poor quality" not a cause of good quality. For this reason, alert industries have tried continuously to make end-result inspection either unnecessary (because quality is so reliable) or, if that is not attainable, as efficient as possible. Such industries make constant attempts to reduce the burdensomeness of inspection—by using intelligent forms of sampling, by sequencing filters rationally, by smoothing and speeding the processes of inspection themselves, and by equipping and authorizing local units to respond to local deficiencies whenever possible, so as to avoid costly loops of managerial tampering.

Health care regulation has done almost the opposite. Year after year, inspection procedures by regulators have multiplied, expanded, and become more and more universal. Sampling occurs, but often it is neither technically rational nor correctly interpreted in statistical terms. Health care inspectors are still often bound to case-by-case examinations and documentation procedures that were outdated in most other industries by the 1940s. Few regulators (and as we have found in our surveys, few of the regulated entities) appear to understand or to measure the total systems costs of the inspections they introduce (costs accrued both in the inspection process itself and in the systemic response *to* inspection). We find no agreed agenda in place for continuously reducing the total cost of inspection while maintaining its accuracy, reliability, and output. For the JCAHO, the National Committee for Quality Assurance (NCQA), the Peer Review Organizations (PROs), the State Board of Registration, and all other inspectors, a key strategic issue in a resource-starved health care world should be how to reduce the total burden of inspection while improving its desired effects. The issue is rarely raised.

Beyond the question of cost, we find that the producers of care almost never regard existing regulatory procedures as adding value. Time after time, our interviewees told us that outside regulators add only to costs. We might perhaps have expected this sour claim. Inspectors are rarely welcome, and in fact, the more an individual or organization is committed to growth and learning, the less value does an unsolicited "report card" have.

But at a deeper level, the universality of the negative response to outside regulation uncovered in our interviews should make us curious. Recall first that our interviewees are not likely to be among the intended "targets" of harsh regulations. They do not run hack hospitals that should be shut down; their medical staffs are not among the loosest in self-management or the most timid in discipline. Their outcomes are not poor, and their processes are not shabby. The hospitals they represent are good hospitals—not only among the best but also seeking to improve.

For them, arguably, sound regulation might be more of a help than a threat. As devotees of quality improvement, each has learned and teaches the Japanese quality maxim that "every defect is a treasure." Each knows the value that comes even from *approximately* correct data, such as that collected by the PRO or the state public health agency. Each *could* have told us that the inspectors, though not totally welcome, did bring into the organization helpful perspectives and interesting data on the basis of which improvements could be accelerated.

None did. None told us that the outside inspectors' core product—information—was a valuable resource for the inspected organization. Why not?

At least two explanations are plausible. One is that the institutions, despite their claims to the contrary, are not in fact interested in improvement at all—that for them, "every defect is a headache," and they simply do not want to learn what the regulators have to teach.

A second hypothesis is simpler and may seem naive: that the inspector-regulators have very little to teach, that they are delivering messages either already known (and therefore wasteful) or obviously wrong (and therefore wasteful). This hypothesis suggests, to put it bluntly, that the regulators are rejected because their work is silly from the viewpoint of the well-intentioned caregiver. To use Braithwaite's term, regulation is not "responsive" to the regulated industry's needs.

It would be quite a serious matter if regulators were to judge their own performance according to the degree to which inspected parties who do not merit discipline regard the regulators as *otherwise helpful to improvement*. Yet this is precisely what we propose as one of the guiding principles for productive health care regulation in the future.

The regulation we have studied is further flawed by its wasteful and unnecessary disconnection from the best available scientific knowledge about quality and its sources. We do not know exactly when this disconnection occurred, but it became particularly evident in the mid-1960s, during the early days of regulation in Medicare. By then, Lembcke had completed his most important work, Morehead's was well under way, and a young John Williamson was writing forcefully about sophisticated models linking improvement to adult learning principles. But as the Experimental Medical Care Review Organizations (EMCROs) became the Professional

Standards Review Organizations (PSROs) and the PSROs became the PROs, no strong thread of theory became evident in the actual work of regulatory care at the federal level. Compared with Williamson's insights, Barbara Hulka's data, Donabedian's interpretive models, and (ultimately) Robert Brook's sweeping synthesis of methods, the regulatory work of those agencies pursuing the federal government's legitimate aims in health care regulation and improvement were blunt, simplistic, naive, and even technically wrong. What was already known scientifically in the mid-1970s about the value of quality and the causes of improvement gave scant grounds for predicting that the core procedures of PROs would help anyone very much. And indeed, they did not. For the most part, regulation became unscientific.

It also became fragmented. Regulation as we know it today began, so far as we can tell, in the 1930s, in two quite different areas: the profession of medicine (for example, in the committees of the American College of Surgeons) and the field of philanthropic initiative (culminating in the Committee on the Costs of Medical Care). But as we have seen, an enormous variety of agencies and regulators became involved in medical care over the next fifty years.

The complexity today is daunting. Even a small hospital must concern itself with the regulatory activities of the JCAHO, the PRO, the state professional licensure authorities, the state public health authorities, the Federal Trade Commission (FTC), the Justice Department (state and federal), environmental protection authorities (state and federal), Medicaid officials, and community health authorities. Beyond that, a new and disturbing trend has emerged of competition *among* quasi-public regulators for the right to judge. Most significantly, the NCQA and the JCAHO have elected to compete for what amounts to regulator "market share" by developing performance measures and certification procedures that many organizations must now deal with in addition to JCAHO accreditation processes. Meanwhile, private payers and large corporations have begun to engage in forms of inspection, reporting, and demands for compliance that they call *supplier management* and that feel for all the world to health care providers like another form of regulation, nearly indistinguishable in its urgency, costs, and consequences from regulation by government. Regulation has been privatized.

The momentum behind this complex, fragmented regulatory apparatus seems unrelenting. It has become implausible for most health care leaders to do much else than comply with these numerous inspections and demands for information. Like health care itself, the regulation of health care has split into isolated pieces, and there is little opportunity to fit those pieces back together. The costs of fragmentation therefore grow, seemingly without limit.

Meanwhile, of course, the health care industry has changed. Especially in the 1990s, large shifts have occurred in the structures of both health care markets and health care systems. Many communities, for example, are witnessing the formation of three major systems of care provision; one may be centered on a local managed care system, a second on an ambitious alliance of hospitals with physician-hospital organizations, and a third on the migration of indemnity insurers into physician networks or independent practice associations. The emergent vertically integrated systems offer opportunities to consolidate services, to reduce the total supply of hospital beds, to smooth patient flow among facilities, and to unify information systems.

An alert, productive, socially sensible system of regulation would respond well to (and even anticipate) such shifts in the industry. Regulations would change readily to seize new opportunities and to address new hazards in reconfigured systems. Whereas it might earlier have been important for regulators to ask, for example, How can we prevent an overbedded hospital industry from building unnecessary beds? it might now be more useful and pertinent to ask, How can we help an integrated system formed of three hospitals to close unneeded beds as promptly and safely as possible?

Some such shifts have occurred. In 1994, as noted earlier, the Justice Department issued new antitrust guidelines specifically addressing nine key strategic questions that integrated system leaders might have about safe boundaries within which to shape new collaborations. In 1992, 1993, and 1994, the JCAHO carried out major studies and changes so as to assure a better fit between its surveying standards and the needed characteristics of managed care systems.

On the whole, however, we cannot say that regulation has evolved at the same rate as the system it regulates, at least not so as to accelerate systemic changes in health care. Nor has it addressed the ever sharper cost competition that the market produces. Professional licensure procedures remain relatively unchanged, and PRO reviews have been slow to adapt to new patterns of patient management. The Health Care Financing Administration (HCFA), however, has adopted more "responsive" strategies. Though the JCAHO is struggling to change, its standards and survey methods, as we heard in our on-site surveys, often enforce old norms instead of encourage innovative designs. Professional registration procedures maintain old job boundaries when new professional roles could be far more creative.

In fact, regulation as a whole has tended to undervalue one of the most essential features of a modern health care system: innovativeness. To achieve the reductions in cost, improvement in outcome, and greater ease of access that society requires, there will need to be fundamental—and sometimes painful—redesign of care processes, products, and services. The most crucial questions may become, Why do we do it that way? and, Can we invent a way that's cheaper and better for patients?

It is unlikely that any hospital, no matter how promising a pioneer, would safely respond to a JCAHO survey or to a PRO by saying, "We rejected your standard because we have found a newer and far more powerful way to achieve the underlying aim implied by that standard." Even less can one imagine a plea from a rational organization stating, "We did indeed fail to comply with the demanded performance level because we believe it to be unimportant compared to other opportunities we have seized. These have produced gains that, in total systems terms, far outweigh the gains we would have achieved in the areas you specify. Yes, indeed, we are below your standard in immunizations, but look how we used the same resources to benefit the same children ten times as much!"

Yet this is exactly what a model of responsive regulation implies. Innovation requires risk taking; it implies some necessary failures on the road to learning. It takes energy, aspiration, and ambition, and cannot be carried through in all areas at once. These subtle but powerful characteristics of innovation and fundamental progress are hard to quantify and inspect, and may be fragile in the face of standard setting and pass-fail inspections. Indeed, we find innovation to be little valued and often discouraged in standard regulatory practice. We suggest that in a responsive regulatory environment, innovation would be nurtured, and successful innovations rewarded.

In this book, we do not shy away from recommending new approaches to the regulation of care—changes we refer to as "new rules"—but we must admit that these recommendations are based on much theory and little experience. An empirical, scientific foundation for the improvement of regulation does not yet exist. The reason is that on the whole, government *purveys* regulation but does not *test* it. Regulators know little about the effects of inspection on care because they have tried to find out very little.

We believe that regulation of health care should be treated as a domain of technology, and that regulators would be far better equipped to make recommendations for the future if they recognized the crucial importance of small-scale, short-cycle tests in learning. It would be possible to manipulate JCAHO procedures in small-scale experiments that were designed to find ways to reduce costs and improve effects. The FTC or the Justice Department could mount local and regional tests of variation in antitrust enforcement guidelines in health care, examining effects on price, outcomes, and service over relatively short time frames. Regulation is not too complex to study; it is too complex *not* to study.

We do not wish to be harsh, but we conclude overall that the regulation of American health care has fallen far short of the effects it should have on outcomes, costs, and safety in the system it regulates. Let us accept two premises. First, that the *"quality" of regulation ought to be defined as the degree to which regulation accomplishes its social aims without compromising other important aims and without creating waste*. Regulation, like health care, should be judged according to its outcomes. Second, that *regulation should be responsive and collaborative for the good of patients*. The current adversarial relationships do not permit this.

What are the desired outcomes of regulation? At some level of abstraction, they must be the same as those of the system regulated: improved health status, greater ease of use and satisfaction among users, reduction of cost and waste, and maintenance and improvement of social justice and equity.

We propose a framework to guide our scrutiny of the quality of regulation. Such a framework begins with an understanding of how performance (efficiency, safety, outcomes, minimal waste, justice) is protected and improved in any complex system. The premise for this analysis is actually quite demanding—namely, that regulation by outsiders (those who do *not* produce care) exerts an effect on care only through the behaviors and actions of insiders (those who do produce care). If we want to predict how regulation may affect quality, we must begin by asking how those who are regulated may affect quality. There are no other "responsive" routes to improvement.

The Five Approaches to Maintaining and Improving Quality

Mature organizational approaches to the maintenance and improvement of quality involve five basic categories of effort. These categories provide a framework for exploring and improving the effects of regulation on quality, and thus for designing new rules.

Repairing

No system is perfect in its effects, and all systems committed to quality must maintain and improve their ability to repair and redress defects when they occur. Consumers of products and services experience this commitment as a guarantee. The excellence of Lands' End or L. L. Bean as catalogue merchants lies not just in their capacity to provide a good product quickly and cheaply but also in their unconditional guarantees and the ability to act swiftly and pleasingly to stand behind their promise when a customer complains or returns a product. When a good hotel cannot provide a promised nonsmoking room, it upgrades the client to the concierge floor at no charge.

Health care providers have been generally uncomfortable with promises and guarantees and have lacked motivation for some types of repair. Nonetheless, it remains important for organizations to redress quickly and willingly the harms they cause. We are unable to explain why the market has not created incentives for providers to perform repair, as has occurred in some retail businesses. But the rule of regulation is to develop socially optimal strategies that the market has failed to cultivate. Regulation today may support or impede redress, as will shortly be seen. Responsive regulation should encourage it. In some ways, the compensation function of medical malpractice can be seen as a form of repair, albeit one based on adversity.

Culling (Sorting)

Repair occurs after harm is done. The same may sometimes be true of culling, but the major aim of culling is to prevent further harm. By *culling* we mean activities that assess results, performance, or quality, and seek to remove from further circulation products or services that fall below acceptable standards.

All capable quality management systems engage in culling when necessary. In manufacturing, it is the last opportunity to protect the customer. Among the great achievements of industrial quality management in this century has been the marriage of sound statistics and economic theory to systems that inspect and remove defects. The aim is to minimize the total economic loss from defective products, which arises from both the costs of inspection and the costs of the defects themselves. Attention to these statistical and technical issues makes modern inspection in most industries ever cheaper and ever more rational in economic terms.

As we have repeatedly suggested, culling is the mainstay process of American health care regulation. This is what licensure boards do when they give or take away licenses to practice. This is what CON processes do when they issue or withhold permission to build. Culling is the central job of the JCAHO, which labels its outputs "accreditation" and "citation." Malpractice prosecutions combine repair and culling in their effects. PROs cull cases for action. The main problem with processes for culling in American health care today is not in their intent but in their efficiency. Culling is necessary in any important, imperfect enterprise; but its costs and value can always be improved. This has not occurred in health care.

Copying

Culling is the outsider's best way to protect the patient in the short term. For insiders, better options exist. The simplest is *copying*, or *copying and adapting*. In this method of improvement, the core effort is not selection but learning. Copying is the mechanism through which much simple improvement, and a good deal of teaching, occur. It is the way a child first learns script. The teacher shows an example, and the learner tries to reproduce it. Why reproduce it? Because it is "correct" or "better." (It is both amusing and sad that in certain contexts we call copying from the teacher "learning" but copying from each other, "cheating." This misconception, a product perhaps of a misguided version of American individualism, robs our society of many of the benefits of cooperation.)

An enormous amount of improvement occurs by copying, and

the process can be extremely efficient. In most industries, in fact, the piracy of competitors' winning methods is a primary strategy for success. When the transistor was invented, it was smarter to copy it than either to ignore it or to try to invent a comparable device.

Actually, copying in the real world is rarely pure and faithful, but that does not diminish its value. On the contrary, the real power lies in the capability to replicate the successful method of another and then to adapt it to fit one's own local systems and circumstances. Thirty children will learn script from the same teacher, but the handwriting of each will be unique, because each is a unique "writing system."

In health care, an important example of copying as a means of improvement takes the form of investments in protocols, guidelines, and algorithms for care. No matter what the term, these mechanisms share the common underlying notion that someone knows or can discover the "best way" to carry out a task or reach a decision, and that improvement can come from standardizing processes and behaviors to conform to this ideal model. The method of improvement is *replication*—copying.

The use of guidelines is offensive to many health care professionals. For reasons unclear to us, medical organizations and clinicians seem to shift, at some point in their development, from an avid search for models (as when a student doctor asks the chief resident how to manage a patient in diabetic ketoacidosis) to an adamant rejection of them (as when a doctor dismisses a guideline as "cookbook medicine"). Whatever the explanation, medicine today stands nearly alone among complex industries in its ineptitude at copying good ideas and in its suspiciousness about replication as a legitimate route to improvement. Responsive regulation should help overcome this suspicion.

Learning in Cycles (Plan-Do-Check-Act)

A fourth common mechanism of improvement is the use of small-scale experiments in work settings. This approach to improvement is most familiar in personal growth and development. Ask a child how she is learning (improving) bicycle riding, and she will tell you, "I practice." The simple reply summarizes a complex and constant series of local experiments. From friends, parents, books, or her own digested experience ("I fell last time"), she constantly draws new ideas on how to ride—where to place her weight, her feet, her hands, how hard to push the pedals, how quickly to turn the handle bar. And she puts these ideas into direct action, learning not from the idea but from the action itself. She uses the world as a teacher, and she makes changes so that the world can teach her. This is the continuous cycle of theory and experience that John Dewey wrote about as the fundamental process of learning.[4]

This same process is codified in the lexicon of quality improvement as the Shewhart Cycle (for Walter Shewhart, who first expressed it this way), or the Plan-Do-Check-Act (PDCA) Cycle.[5] But the terms belie the absolute familiarity of the process: in order to improve, find a good idea and test it. This differs from copying, where one learns from others. In PDCA, one learns from changes that one makes oneself. PDCA is a powerful mode of improvement in most industries. When used by everyone in an organization, at all levels—each person learning from small-scale trials in his or her own work—PDCA can produce breathtaking rates of improvement and unprecedented results.

As much as medicine espouses continuous learning as a core value, in practice, PDCA cycles are rather rare in health care organizations. The evidence lies in the stability of work processes over decades. In an organization engaged in continuous cycles of improvement, people are constantly testing new ways to perform their work and retaining those that prove effective. In most hospitals, by contrast, even relatively routine procedures such as medication dispensing, physician rounds, record keeping, patient discharge, and nursing signout remain unchanged for decades.

This conservatism is easy to understand in a professional climate where the dominant rule is "First of all, do no harm." Medicine eschews changes that may introduce risks. Old practices remain in place until proof exists that new ones are better. The very idea of making changes in care "to see what happens" violates an ethical duty. As quality management, with its PDCA cycles and intentional tests of change, has made its way into health care organizations, this learned resistance to change has acted as an immune response, rejecting quality improvement as a form of irresponsible tampering, and failing to recognize that it can also be a route to responsible learning.

Nor has regulation changed this culture. In our review of regulatory initiatives, we found no significant examples of regulations encouraging learning, although recent JCAHO and PRO initiatives have the right rhetoric. Learning must be learned, especially when it is to be done by groups or in complex systems, and regulations could create a better environment for this process.

Creativity

PDCA works within the existing system. Creativity invents a new one. Whereas PDCA tends to make gains in small steps, creativity makes leaps. We call such leaps "inventions," and they demand processes and structures to support them. Characteristics of environments able to support creativity include a high tolerance for risk taking, an investment in long-term aims, and a sheltered setting where people have an opportunity to think in fresh ways. (The Greeks, interested in creativity as a social good, had in their cities a facility called *temenos*, "a garden where adults can play like children.") Most crucially, inventions may require a suspension of current rules and procedures, at least long enough for inventors to develop and test prototypes.

In health care systems, creativity may be applied in areas quite unrelated to the development of new technologies. Inventions that serve the need for care at lower cost and with better results might include new job categories, new types of interorganizational collaboration, or services delivered in novel locations.

Ideally, "regulating for improvement" should support and encourage organizational activity of all five sorts: repair, culling, copying, learning, and innovation. At the very least, regulators who choose to focus their energies exclusively on a subset of these activities should minimize toxic side effects on forms of improvement that they choose not to address directly. This is especially important in regard to the developmentally "higher" forms of improvement (learning and innovation); though these are less often the direct targets of regulatory activity, they can too easily be impaired by unwise actions in the more familiar regulatory terrain of culling.

Let us now examine how regulation can be made more responsive in regard to each of the five approaches to maintaining and improving quality.

Regulation and Repair

The willingness and ability to make promises is a strong sign of commitment by any producer. A guarantee conveys two messages: 1) "We *can* do this"; and 2) "You have a right to expect this from us." Dysfunctional producers, entitled producers, and unambitious producers make few promises to those they serve.

How does a modern organization, committed to high quality, choose the content of its guarantees? The answer in at least some commercial areas is clear: the organization guarantees what its customers have learned to expect. Bold companies, confident in their capacity to improve, guarantee more. Among the better-known recent examples is the promise made by the Lands' End mail-order company: "Guaranteed. Period." The intention is to leave the judgment of what promise *should* be made entirely in the hands of the customer. Pursuing this strategy requires more than a little faith in the rationality of customers and in their general fairness in dealing with Lands' End.

A guarantee of a different sort stands behind most airline tickets, promising carriage within several hours of a scheduled flight, failing which the airline must provide alternative service free of charge. The promise, like that of Lands' End, derives from customer needs but rests on a firmer foundation of "legitimate expectation." One reads the airline guarantee and thinks, "Darn right! Of course they should!" The Lands' End guarantee, by contrast, elicits, "How nice! They really mean to stand behind their work!" Progressive guarantees are the hallmark of an increasingly capable industry. Guarantees can motivate high quality as well as indicate it.

The two examples suggest plausible areas for regulation. First, and most important, health care regulators should encourage and reward guarantees of increasing ambition. Second, it is reasonable for regulatory policy to require that, as in the case of an airline ticket, each provider promise what every user of care has an unquestioned right to expect, and to provide prompt, easily claimed redress when that promise is broken. Such promises may apply to timely access, information exchange, modernity of therapy, and outcomes that are well within the reach of all providers of care.

Two crucial aspects of effective guarantees of this type are *ease of invocation* and *individualization of response*. A guarantee is of limited use if redress is hard to obtain. Further, guarantees at this level apply not to populations but to individuals. The main object in organizational action is prompt, individualized recovery. Great companies are not invariably right, but they are exceptional in the ways they recover when they are wrong. Specifying the requirements of recovery may be as important as specifying the guarantee itself.

Guarantees are uncommon in health care, and regulation that encourages them is nearly nonexistent. Several states require hospitals to post a patients' "Bill of Rights," dealing with such matters as the right of access to a physician, the right to review one's medical record, and the right to explanations of treatment options. But we know no examples of health care regulation that take notice of or reward more expansive statements of rights or that speak to excellence in recovery strategies when such rights are violated.

We urge experiments that positively encourage expansive guarantees, through regulatory rewards to those who offer and stand behind them. Patients might be given a promise that they will be discharged from the hospital within five days of having coronary artery bypass grafting, that medications will be given correctly and on time, that waiting times will not exceed some published maximum, or that appropriate home health services will arrive in a timely fashion. Health care is not, of course, a simple retail business. Providers of health care face enormous, uncontrollable biological diversity in its beneficiaries. But the effects of a guarantee remain the same even in the face of such diversity: a guarantee stretches the institution and encourages ambition. Responsive regulation need not always specify the content of guarantees, but it can encourage a culture of ambition by ensuring that some guarantees exist and can be invoked easily when violated.

Lands' End, of course, does not need regulators to encourage its broad guarantee policy. The market is its regulator. Good promises backed by good recovery attract customers. The guarantee is smart business. It remains to be seen if the newly emerging marketplace for health care can elicit the same level of ambition from providers of care without the goad of regulation. For the moment, we suspect not, and we therefore suggest that regulators ought at least to ask what it is that the public ought to be promised.

One final note on guarantees. Superb companies, like Lands' End, repair defects quickly, but they also capture information on warrantee invocations for the additional purpose of pattern recognition, on the basis of which products, services, and processes can be improved. If customers demand immediate refunds on the teal overcoat because of "bad fit," the company can convert this into an improvement in the product. Guarantee invocation is a signal. The same should be true in medical care. For this reason, public policies that, in effect, create guarantees but then offer opportunities to hide information on violations (or even require such secrecy) may weaken the important linkages between failures and improvement. It is important that not every failure lead to a revision of a system (that is "tampering," and wasteful), but it is equally important that data on patterns of defect be accumulated and studied, providing a foundation for systematic improvements. For this reason, the National Aeronautics and Space Administration maintained in its heyday an elaborate centralized system of "trouble reporting," not to nail inadequate employees but rather to highlight the link between, say, a weak weld that appeared in Pasadena and a pattern of welding failures in several otherwise disconnected sites. For the same reason, the Food and Drug Administration maintains reporting systems for adverse drug events, and the Centers for Disease Control ask doctors everywhere to report unusual occurrences of disease. Properly reported, failures of guarantee can guide improvement work.

Regulation and Culling

Health care regulators are at home in the neighborhood of culling. It is the mainstay of their current processes. Examples abound: professional licensure, certificates of need, public release of hospital mortality data, report cards (Health Plan and Employer Data and Information Set [HEDIS] and others), JCAHO accreditation, public health department inspections, clinic licensures, and punitive and deterrent aspects of malpractice law—all these and more rest on foundational logic involving measurement and selection. It does not matter if the selection itself is done by a state agency, a quasi-public board, a jury of peers, or a consumer of care. For each, the method is the same: assess the population and classify the object of study as acceptable or unacceptable; if unacceptable, take appropriate action for removal or change.

No quality management system is complete without culling as a process. It becomes more and more crucial as the stakes for failure rise, and as the trustworthiness of the underlying systems of design and production decays. Culling is the final sentinel guarding the customer. (Only repair comes later, and sometimes repair is impossible.) Travelers want airplanes to be carefully inspected every time they fly.

Excellent health care providers do their own culling. They have no less interest than do external regulators in protecting customers. Indeed, the inspection and culling processes within health care, most conducted voluntarily by managers and clinicians, are at least as pervasive and rigorous as those imposed from outside health care. Morbidity and mortality conferences, tumor boards, student examinations, supervision of junior staff, cosigning of orders, duplicate narcotic signouts, and incident reports all represent forms of culling. In their daily work, health care managers call it "fire fighting" or "crisis management"; they watch events and intervene when necessary.

Sound culling rests on two foundations: efficient management of the inspection process and adjustment of action thresholds to the best economic levels. These are the hallmarks of responsive regulation, and in both respects, health care regulation could be performing much better than it is.

Our interviews, along with widely publicized criticisms of government, suggest that culling today is not managed well. The symptoms are everywhere. First, much inspection is needlessly universal. A rational inspector would design JCAHO surveys, for example, to vary widely from hospital to hospital, so that energy was focused where the yield would be greatest. This would reduce the time and energy required in each facility both for preparation and for the actual survey.

Second, inspection and culling in health care take too long. Among the key quality characteristics of a JCAHO survey or a HEDIS report are cycle times—the duration of a survey, the time between measurement and report, the speed with which criteria and standards are improved. The JCAHO has recently reduced the time between its surveys and reports, but on the whole, cycle times in health care inspection processes remain extremely long and are not improving.

Third, sound inspection makes good use of historical trends in making predictions about the future. The best example outside health care is the use of control charts (graphical portrayal of statistical information), which can give an early warning signal when an otherwise stable process is becoming unstable. Health care regulators, by contrast, rarely make sophisticated use of trends over time. Instead, certification, accreditation, and other culling practices rely on current measurements and snapshots and therefore have trouble making sound predictions.

Most important, those who manage inspection and culling practices in health care seem only rarely to evaluate the extent to which those practices are indeed making care safer and better. The few evaluations that have been performed in the past few years are not at all reassuring. PRO activities, for example, often look wasteful and ineffective under the lens of health services research. Many Boards of Registration in Medicine require evidence of continuing medical education (CME) from doctors seeking renewal of their licenses, despite research that shows CME to be of little or no value. Even after decades of JCAHO surveys, there is not even one major research study, by the JCAHO or anyone else, of the actual impact of those surveys on the quality of care; the few studies that do exist are descriptive, not experimental.

Briefly put, we have no systematic answers to the two most important questions about the performance of systems of culling in health care: 1) Do they achieve their aims? and 2) What do they cost? An entire industry of inspection in health care is built on the sands of assumption.

It is time for a change. Those who argue, with good reason, that we must preserve inspection and culling as key processes for maintaining and improving health care quality must also recognize the need for improving these processes. Future regulation of this type should

1. Take account of, and continuously reduce, its costs and the costs to the inspected system

2. Take account of, and continuously reduce, its cycle times

3. Adjust inspection processes according to their predicted yield, rather than use universal and standard inspection procedures for all

4. Make greater use of control charts and other means of evaluating trends over time, for the purposes of minimizing the burden of inspection and permitting better predictions

5. Link inspection to aims, so that culling occurs with respect to dimensions of performance known to be valued by customers and required by society

In short, like the most advanced of those they inspect, inspectors must demonstrate a commitment to modern notions of quality improvement.

Regulation and Copying

Sound responsive regulation would encourage the prompt diffusion of improved processes and services throughout the health care industry. When copying holds the seeds of rapid improvement, secrecy is an enemy.

Government can be an active participant in the enterprise of learning from others. For example, it can aggregate information when others cannot, as is done for purposes of airline safety at the National Transportation Safety Board and the Federal Aviation Administration. It can also act as a distribution system for sound information, as it does in the Agricultural Extension Service or the National Library of Medicine. It can facilitate copying by promoting uniformity of practice or manufacture, as it does in establishing standards for weights and measures, enforcing certain accounting principles, mandating gauges in transportation systems, and setting communication rules for the airwaves.

We recognize that a conflict may develop between a regulator's role in inspection, which may require the prying of information from the regulated entities, and his or her role as a facilitator of copying. The problem arises because extracting information for the purposes of evaluation may require guarantees of confidentiality that inhibit the exchange of ideas.

One unfortunate example of this conflict has occurred in the administration of the Malcolm Baldrige National Quality Award by the National Institute of Standards and Technology (NIST).[6] The Baldrige Award is a form of positive culling—inspection followed by judgment. NIST felt—and may have been right—that a guarantee of confidentiality was necessary in order to encourage companies to apply honestly for the award; they might not do so if they felt they were giving away their trade secrets. As a result, the entire award process is conducted behind a veil of secrecy, and thousands of pages of applications, examiner reports, site visit reports, and records of deliberation by the judges are all locked away or destroyed instead of being studied and used for national learning. The award system (culling) confounds the system of learning from the examinations (copying).

As a whole, health care regulation is profoundly overinvested in culling at the expense of copying. Improved regulation would specifically design and test methods through which lessons from one health care system or organization could easily and openly be made known to others. If health care competition is to be the rule of the day, it ought not to occur at the expense of the spread of sound improvements in care that can save social resources or patients' lives. We could make good use of an "extension service" for health care improvement.

One form of encouragement of copying that has dressed itself in regulatory clothing is the movement toward guidelines for care. Such guidelines reflect, to some extent, a well-reasoned effort to put the best available knowledge into a form that has immediate practical application. Guidelines can be helpful, but they can also be counterproductive if they ignore the need for copying to be adapted to local circumstances if real improvement is to result. Thus regulators who purvey guidelines must recognize that they will and must vary in actual use.

Regulation and PDCA Cycles

"New rules" should encourage local learning in the form of trials of change, or PDCA cycles. A hospital or managed care system that is rapidly improving must necessarily be testing new ways to do its work. Change may be triggered by a minor suggestion from a single employee that is rapidly tested and deployed throughout the organization, or it may follow an enormous redesign of major services. In the quality management movement, PDCA cycles can take the shape of quality improvement teams, or improvement projects, or pilot tests.

Regulation can slow this work of improvement if it insists, directly or indirectly, that boundaries between functions be kept high. This is the case when regulations specify job boundaries (what registered nurses or clerks can or cannot do, for example) or when they require that certain procedures (such as record keeping, attestation, drug dispensing, registration, transport, or diagnosis) be conducted in traditional, classical ways, even when better ways may be found that achieve higher performance or lower cost. Less directly, regulation can quench the impulse toward improvement when the consequences of failure in a trial are too onerous. Legitimate learning involves taking some risks. Regulators must be able to distinguish between the responsible try that marks real improvement efforts and irresponsible guesswork that runs too high a risk for too slight a potential payoff.

We encourage regulators, especially those who certify or accredit organizations, to give high value to well-managed improvement trials. Requirements that processes be conducted "by the book" may be less useful for improvement than requirements that welcome *either* performance by the book *or* a conscientious search for even better ways to accomplish the same aims. The JCAHO, for example, has attempted to train its surveyors to recognize quality improvement efforts as an appropriate response to a performance standard.

We believe that regulations can be designed to *encourage* the breaking down of barriers between professions and between organizations. Accreditors can seek evidence of cooperative behaviors, collaborations, shared aims, and more integrated work flow. A standard that requires each job position to work within precise parameters may be less valuable than one that promotes continuous reductions in overall cycle times—a development requiring more cooperation and flexibility among job positions. The former approach might require that perfusion pump technicians complete so many hours of instruction per year; the latter might inquire about safe and continuous reductions in elapsed pump time in cardiac surgery.

An example of regulation that is potentially toxic to improvement cycles emerged when an educational institution seeking the right to award physicians CME credits was visited by surveyors from the accrediting body, the American College for Continuing Medical Education (ACCME). Among the qualifying questions asked was the degree to which the educational experience was "specifically aimed at doctors, and not others." ACCME criteria make it difficult to give accreditation for courses taught to, say, both doctors and nurses, with the aim of improving cooperative relationships between them. To this extent, at least, the accreditation procedure impedes the breaking down of barriers between professions, even if outcomes of care are thereby improved.

Regulators seeking to support continuous improvement should avoid such myopia and make sure that their procedures encourage cooperation at a system level. When the system involved is a community or a group of organizations, this principle, of course, easily runs afoul of antitrust regulation. The core question is one of aim. If the key value to be pursued in antitrust enforcement is preservation of an active, competitive market, then antitrust regulators must avidly block cooperation on too large a scale. The price, however, will be suboptimization of the system, as a more rational use of resources can almost always be achieved by enlarging the boundaries of a system. It follows that if the key aim is rational optimization of the system as a whole, more cooperation should be encouraged.

Take the example of specialization of function on a regional scale. Respectable health services research shows that for many technical procedures in health care, higher volume is associated with better outcomes. A single cardiac surgical unit doing five hundred procedures a year will generally have better outcomes than five units each doing one hundred a year. In addition, economies of scale and learning should operate, making the larger unit less expensive per unit of service. Not many American cities need more than a single cardiac surgery unit, and most would have better outcomes if units now operating separately were combined. In the service of improvement of the system as a whole, consolidation of high technology units is desirable. From antitrust perspectives, it may not be. With the antitrust enforcement, employers in a medium-sized city may not be able to find full-service managed care systems each of which performs cardiac surgery at a volume high enough to support excellent outcomes. The choice will be difficult: competitive systems, or cooperative ones with better outcomes and lower costs. Responsive antitrust might allow combination of high-technology efforts yet maintain competition in primary care.

Regulation of health care has been responsible for a great deal of waste in the form of failed cooperation. We wish to see a new generation of regulation emerge that permits and encourages a great deal of cooperative exchange in the oversupplied medical marketplace. If, in a small city, two hospitals can make a deal whereby one closes its duplicative neurosurgery service while the other closes its duplicative cardiac surgery suite, perhaps holding each other harmless economically, we believe this should be not only permitted by the regulatory framework but encouraged. American medicine is too large, but survival of the fittest is among the silliest ways to shrink it. In actual fact, this will result in "survival of the middle-sized," and the benefits of full cooperation will be lost.

We wish there were a way to make the dissemination of good news about better methods of care mandatory. Among physicians, hiding a safer surgical approach from one's colleagues would be regarded as childish and unethical. The same should be true of the improvement work of health care organizations. Perhaps responsive regulators can find a productive role in ensuring that a hospital in possession of a better way to administer analgesia tells others as soon as possible. Improvement knowledge in health care, perhaps more than in other industries, should be treated by regulation as a public good.

Regulation and Innovation

Improvement can take place in two ways: gradually over time or suddenly, in a quantum jump. These two modes are represented, respectively, by PDCA and innovation, and effective organizations can use both to their advantage—that is, they can change incrementally *and* they can innovate from the ground up. A bicycle rider can discover how to ride a bicycle faster or switch to a motorcycle.

Regulation is relatively silent about fundamental innovation. True invention occurs in a minority of organizations and when effective, usually builds on a level of general competence that would put most health care organizations well outside the perimeter of concern of safety-minded regulators.

Probably the main assignment for health care regulators who wish to facilitate innovation is simply not to slow it down. As for specific tasks, these would probably involve—as in the encouragement of PDCA cycles—supports for collaboration. We believe that the most promising arena for innovation in health system design (as opposed to new health technologies) is at the community level, where the sources of ill health often lie, and where the redesign of organizational roles can be groundbreaking. In the field of children's health, we have seen innovation in the form of new partnerships between schools and hospitals for the extension of outreach services and prevention counseling. Perinatal morbidity and mortality, injury prevention, and control of violence are all health-related agendas that must involve non-health-care organizations. This has special implications for financing, since money spent in injury prevention may save many multiples of the cost in health care needs averted, but injury prevention budgets are only rarely tied in with health care dollars, making transfers difficult.

Regulators who wish to encourage innovation at the community level will have to value and reward cooperation. Where innovative regulation is required, we suspect that ERISA constitutes a major impediment. We can think of few regulatory reform agendas more crucial to real redesign of health care than the rewriting of ERISA to allow innovative state-based regulators to move "upstream" to the causes of disease, in the search for better outcomes at lower cost.

We also assume that among the most promising innovations in the future of health care will be the redesign of professional roles, especially in primary care. Regulations whose underlying motive is to preserve current professional boundaries will be hindrances to innovation in meeting the social need for primary care and health information. We feel similarly about record-keeping requirements that are based on fossilized systems of documentation. Medical records and communication systems are in need of fundamental redesign, and we believe that regulators should give a great deal of leeway to those who believe they can accomplish the aims of record keeping and communication with totally new approaches.

Improving Regulation

Our objective is to suggest changes in today's prevailing regulatory practices that will create a climate more nurturant of rapid and continuous improvement in the costs and outcomes of health care. We believe that a modicum of effort is needed in the traditional regulatory activities of surveillance and culling, but we also believe that the public would be better served if future regulatory activities could also nurture other elements of a total system of quality management—especially copying, organizational learning, and innovation. The emerging competitive markets in health care will increase the energy of the search for more effective and efficient practices. Regulation has a double-edged potential both to slow and to speed this search. Responsive regulation will speed it.

Some things should not be changed. There are babies in the bathwater of contemporary regulation, and we might best begin by specifying those activities worth preserving more or less intact. First and most important, governmental regulators have an ongoing obligation to assure public safety. This applies no less to health care than it does to other industries in which error can have consequences that echo far beyond a local commercial relationship. The public has an interest in assurance that minimal standards exist and are enforced, and that any person or organization operating below those standards forfeits the right to continue in business. For this reason, governments perform or arrange for inspections and licensure of aircraft and pilots, building plans and elevators, restaurants and chefs, and—for exactly the same reasons—hospitals and doctors. We will argue later for improving the activities of inspection so that this public obligation can be discharged with a minimal burden on all and without harm to other important aims. However, nothing we write here or elsewhere should be construed as denying that health care regulation should include surveillance to assure public safety. Braithwaite's analysis of coal mining arrives at much the same conclusion—some background surveillance provides a context for responsive regulation.

Second, we are in general sympathy with the current and expanding movement to obtain and release to the customer accurate information on the performance of health care systems and providers. The public pays those providers nearly a trillion dollars a year and has a right to make informed choices. We find no justification for denying respectful disclosure, and following Codman, we believe such disclosure can inform not only choices but also learning and exchange in the service of improvement. Equally, we are aware of the hazards of disclosure, which include costly gaming, silly debates, and even dishonesty.

We will ask later not for an end to public reports of performance, but for the improvement of the systems of reporting. Among the crucial steps to refining "report cards" are commitments to link reports to carefully developed aims (so that they are reporting on whether those aims have been achieved), to adjust and change reports in response to variations in aims over time and among populations, to assure technical excellence in the measurements that underlie the reports, and to continuously reduce the total costs of the measurement and reporting systems themselves.

We believe strongly that there must be continuing efforts to detect and punish fraud and abuse in health care provision, whether it be misuse of public funds or exposure of individual consumers to harm. Though the increasing influence of managed care systems will create internal dynamics in health care organizations to prevent fraud, we believe that governmental policing functions will continue to be needed as well.

Finally, we would do nothing to impede the extension of accreditation activities beyond their traditional focus (hospitals) into the more contemporary and salient arena of managed care and integrated health systems. Accreditation agencies that remain concerned with hospitals alone will rapidly become anachronisms. This applies particularly, of course, to the Joint Commission for Accreditation of Health Care Organizations, whose new name ought accurately to describe its activities. But the emergence of integrated systems of care as dominant models does not mean that accreditation should end, only that it should be refocused.

Thus we believe that many current inspection-oriented regulatory activities are well worth retaining and improving. Overall, however, the system of health care regulation in the United States does not need stabilization; it needs change. It is too expensive, too grounded in the past, too concerned with old forms, and too little addressed to new ones. It is too much a creature of its own old habits, and if it is to accelerate improvement in health care, it must itself change and improve a great deal.

We offer our prescription in parts, each concerned with the changes needed in a specific arena of regulation.

Rx 1: Reduce the Costs of Inspection

We have argued for the need to retain inspection as part of responsive regulation, specifically to ensure that minimal standards of safety are met. Governments should continue to ensure, for example, that people who call themselves "Medical Doctors" have in fact completed formal training, that hospitals dispose properly of their hazardous wastes, that narcotic medications are securely stored and accurately accounted for, that highly technical and dangerous equipment is properly maintained, and that hospital elevators, like elevators in all buildings, will not harm their occupants. We believe that routine relicensure and accreditation procedures are wise, and we even believe that relicensure of physicians, especially those who perform dangerous procedures, should be extended beyond current practice. If airline pilots must regularly demonstrate their competence to fly familiar planes, it is inexplicable to us that surgeons, once licensed, are never again required to show that they can perform risky or unfamiliar procedures. The rationale that makes initial licensure a necessity applies with equal force to relicensure.

But even as we argue strongly for retaining inspection, licensure, and accreditation procedures, we wish to argue even more strongly that these procedures badly need improvement. There are better ways and worse ways to inspect, and many of the inspections that now characterize the surveillance of medical care are among the worst known in any industry. Bad inspection is wasteful, misdirected, inaccurate, and unimaginative. It is the opposite of real vigilance.

Inspection practices such as licensure, accreditation, reaccreditation, and reviews for fraud could be improved by application of the following basic principles, among others:

Avoid universal inspection. Substitute rational sampling. One example of universal inspection is the routine three-year cycle of JCAHO surveying. Such standard patterns simplify decision making for the regulator, but they probably bear little relationship to the underlying aims of inspection or to a rational view of the important defects and risks found in health care. If the inspection system were being created from scratch today, would we subject all hospitals to the same review schedule? Or might we look more frequently at hazardous services and less frequently at those of lower inherent risk? Would full reviews be given to all institutions, or would we look most intensively at organizations for which there is reason to predict a higher yield of findings requiring action? What is the minimum number of medical records that must be audited to obtain a reliable profile of activities?

Accredit modern management and quality assurance processes and structures. At a deeper level, in attempting to assure safety, it may sometimes be better to examine the systems and competence of an organization or individual than to inspect results further "downstream." Modern manufacturers, for example, are more interested in understanding their suppliers' procedures for assuring the quality of supplies prior to shipping than they are in expanding their own processes for "receiving inspection" at their own plants. This notion is consistent with many longstanding JCAHO survey practices that study procedures for quality assurance within hospitals. The JCAHO, for example, studies *whether hospitals have procedures for reviewing unexpected deaths* as carefully as it studies *rates of unexpected deaths.*

What has not yet occurred, however, is an integration of modern understandings of ideal management practices into inspection systems. The ISO9000 standards for quality assurance processes formulated by and now widely adopted in non-health-care industries are far more sophisticated than the conventional criteria applied today in hospitals. Even more, the ambitious management standards required by the Malcolm Baldrige National Quality Award offer a model of modern management for quality that few regulators, accreditors, or licensing agencies in health care would recognize.

Minimize internal costs of response to inspection. Preparing for a JCAHO survey is expensive—far more expensive than it needs to be. It would be productive for all inspectors and accreditors to inquire into the kinds and amounts of cost incurred by producers of care as a consequence of inspection activities, and then to work collaboratively with institutions to progressively reduce those costs while maintaining or improving inspection quality. Cost reduction could come from many types of change, including the following:

Minimize preparation of materials never actually used in the inspection

Increase flexibility in use of existing internal documents, instead of requiring transcriptions or duplication

Minimize the number of copies of documents requested

Minimize the number of people required at inspection events

Increase intervals between inspections

Reorder events to conform with internal needs and constraints.

Schedule inspections during periods of low service demand, to permit reallocation of idle capacity

Avoid unexpected changes that require additional work

Smooth scheduling processes

Decrease cycle times. Time lags throughout inspection processes tend to cost money without adding value. An accreditor who manages to issue a final report immediately on completing a survey visit has saved everyone time and money. Instead, current habits and processes of accreditation and licensure often contain months-long delays during which little or nothing of value is happening. People are simply waiting for some next meeting to occur or for a decision to be made. Speed in every phase is probably a key characteristic of quality in most inspection processes, and it calls for continual improvement.

Make fuller use of tiered inspection. One way to avoid universal inspection is to create (or improve) efficient decision rules for movement from one "tier" of the subject population to another. One generally efficient rule is: "Get to an 'exit' as quickly as possible." Imagine, for example, that one were deciding whether or not to perform a mammogram on a patient. One excellent question to ask first is, "Are you a woman?" The reason this is such a good first question is that so many people can answer no and thus exit the system immediately. (Imagine an alternative proposal that one first ask people about age, family history, and presence or absence of a palpable lump in the breast, and only afterward find out their gender; the inefficiency is obvious.)

Our impression is that accreditors and inspectors tend to establish too few tiers of examination (often, there is only a single tier, which is, by definition, universal inspection) and frequently do not sequence their inquiry in the most efficient order. One useful question to ask in designing inspection sequences is, "How can we quickly exempt as many as possible from further inspection?" This reserves inspection energies for application where they can do the most good and saves time and money for providers as well.

Rx 2: Link Regulation Explicitly to Shared Aims

A broad defect in today's approach to health care regulation is the absence of explicit and widely shared aims as the touchstone. By *aims*, we mean goals for the system of care itself. More specifically, we mean goals that might be measured, rather than vague— albeit important—concepts like "safety," "access," and "fair pricing." We believe that regulation would be better designed if all involved had a common set of measurable objectives. Suppose, for example, that it were possible to state that the goals of regulation included the following:

Narrowing of the racial gap in infant mortality

Reduction in the number of medication errors

Reduction in the number of inappropriate and unnecessary surgical operations

Reduction in the costs of intensive care units by 20 percent while improving functional outcomes

If such specific priorities could be set, it would become possible to study and measure the extent to which any particular regulatory activity was supporting progress in the desired direction. Without explicit goals, it becomes much more difficult to judge regulation itself.

It is easy to see why setting explicit systemic goals is so difficult and rare. A list of goals must be finite, and constructing it therefore requires choices about what will and will not be attempted (for now). Such choices are politically provocative. Systemic goals (such as reducing infant mortality) require negotiation and cooperation among elements of the system that may not be used to cooperating.

It is also hard to imagine who would be able credibly to set goals for health care. Would it be professional societies? Governmental agencies? Citizens' groups? Legislatures? Any one of these acting alone risks threatening others. Furthermore, each lacks leverage to induce the needed changes and cooperative behaviors.

However, American regulation is not unfamiliar with such goal-directed behavior. A prime example is the Clean Air Act, which explicitly defines environmental targets for pollution levels and creates both directives and flexibility for government regulation of industry through which these targets may be achieved. We would like to see health care regulation similarly guided by a Healthy Public Act, setting out ambitious but achievable targets that would inspire specific regulatory activities.

In health care, it may be especially important that shared aims be customized to populations and regions. Aims (and therefore regulatory priorities) in rural Utah should logically be different from those in Harlem, simply because the burdens of disease and the configurations of resources differ so greatly in the two locations. Efforts to achieve equity in health status require not identical aims in all areas but locally responsive aims. This implies flexibility in adapting regulations to local community needs. The same applies to accreditation practices and priorities. It may be important to focus on accrediting geriatric care in Fort Lauderdale and trauma care in Aspen, not vice versa.

Rx 3: Focus Regulation and Accreditation on Managed Care and Integrated Systems Wherever These Are Prevalent

It is an anachronism to regulate fragments in an era when the primary goal is to reconnect the parts into a whole. As of this writing, the JCAHO and federal regulators are only beginning to tackle the job of designing surveillance activities to fit the new market of integrated delivery systems (IDSs). NCQA has been somewhat more in the forefront of this effort, but it should not stand alone. The challenge for regulators in this new environment is the same as for the newly aligned caregivers: to understand, measure, and improve care from the viewpoints of the patient and the community, rather than from those of the old categories of service, whose boundaries must now be broken down.

It will now become more important for both providers and regulators to ask how diabetic patients are cared for through time than to ask whether lengths of stay for diabetes are appropriate. It will become more important to assess cardiac disease prevention than cholesterol screening rates. Students of the field might give their attention to continuity of care between hospitals and nursing homes instead of focusing on each site separately. They might become more interested in what doctors and nurses do cooperatively together and less interested in what each professional group does separately.

The new, integrated aims require new tools of measurement and inspection, just as they do new processes of care. This represents a major transition for regulators, who are less well equipped to inspect care on a population basis than on an institutional or professional basis. In regulating an integrated care system, the Board of Registration in Medicine and the Board of Registration in Nursing now have new reasons to coordinate and link their regulatory work. If they do not, they will both be out of step with care. Regulatory agencies that have heretofore seen themselves as quite separate and independent must recognize their interdependencies and learn to cooperate with each other far more than ever before. In fact, they should not just recognize interdependency, they should create it—and require those they regulate to do the same.

Rx 4: Reduce Competition and Duplication Among Regulators

Whereas a competitive marketplace for health care may be good for care, a competitive marketplace for regulation is, in our opinion, bad for care. We have lately seen the emergence of strong competitive postures among quasi-public regulatory bodies; the JCAHO and NCQA, for example, have each tried to gain "market share" in accrediting elements of integrated care systems. In some regions, private groups such as business coalitions and major corporations have added their voices, which are indistinguishable from those of governmental regulators in their demands for data, for compliance with standards of care, and for performance targets. As a result of this fragmentation and competition among regulators, providers of care—even those most willing to cooperate with regulators—are forced into wasteful and needlessly complex efforts of internal measurement, report preparation, and record keeping.

A pure-market enthusiast might claim that a market among regulators will improve regulation. Though plausible, this argument finds little support in experience; the evidence of excessive costs introduced by heterogeneous regulation is strong. If NCQA and the JCAHO both lay claim to accrediting managed care organizations, and if they fail to cooperate in doing so, most organizations will be forced to maintain expensive, duplicative systems of reporting and response. State and federal law has preemption rules to avoid contradictions and silliness of this type; private accreditors and regulators do not. They must rely on self-restraint and voluntary cooperation with each other.

Rx 5: Establish Safe Havens for Major Innovation

To realize the full potential for improvement in health care delivery will require major reengineering of many processes, roles, and structures, including some not often challenged in the long history of medical care delivery. Consider the resistance of the banking industry twenty years ago to the idea that banking transactions might be accomplished faster and less expensively by machines operated by customers in shopping malls, without the involvement of tellers or any bank employee. The ATM machines we now take for granted represented at first a major threat to an entrenched system of beliefs and habits within the industry. It is hard enough to accomplish such innovations within organizational cultures without the drag of inhibitory regulation. A regulatory climate that discourages bold experiments may kill such changes completely.

No one can know for sure what changes in health care systems today might become the dominant breakthroughs of tomorrow. Some promising leads exist, however. More and more, for example, it seems possible for patients to give themselves care that formerly was thought to be the preserve of professionals. Renal dialysis patients can operate dialysis machines themselves, inserting their own IV needles and managing their own drugs and electrolytes. A hospital in New York operates several floors essentially without nurses, where family members and patients perform highly technical nursing tasks at levels of reliability equal to or greater than those in units with classical staffing. Several organizations are experimenting with technicians trained to perform diagnostic and therapeutic procedures formerly done only by doctors, including sigmoidoscopy and colonoscopy.

The need for innovation goes far beyond the research conventionally performed in laboratory and academic settings. In other industries, major innovation comes from active research and development in real-world settings and in nonacademic organizations. The same will occur in health care, but at a pace strongly influenced by the burdens and risks that regulators place on innovation. Licensing bodies must create room for explorations of new job descriptions and new roles for existing professionals. Facilities inspection and JCAHO accreditation must leave room for reengineering of physical space, equipment, and flow of material and people. Since no genuine developmental effort can have absolute assurance of success, the regulatory climate must be tolerant of failures incurred in the authentic search for better approaches providing safe havens for innovation. Tests of innovations should be as safe as is feasible, but they cannot be completely without risk.

We suggest that regulators engage in a diagnostic self-study to learn where and how their activities impede brave and constructive innovation in the design and provision of health care services. By staying focused on the aims of regulation, not its processes, they may be able to decrease the drag. Some will fear that forces of irresponsibility might be unleashed, but to them we reply that risks can come from two types of imbalance: too much innovation and too little. When it comes to the redesign of the actual processes of care, we observe today little sign of the first type of imbalance—and a virtual addiction to the second.

Rx 6: Encourage the Progression of Managed Care

State insurance commissioners and other regulatory authorities simply have not been able to keep pace with the changes in the health care industry as it moves into integrated delivery systems that manage care, usually under capitated fees. At the present time, there is relatively little external oversight of managed care, and that which is accomplished—primarily through NCQA—may be a weak form of self-regulation, highly dependent on voluntarism and consensus among the regulated entities. In most states, the notable exception being California, state insurance and public health officials have simply not penetrated the managed care environment.

The greatest concerns about quality under integrated managed care funded through capitation are the cost/quality trade-offs that will be made by individual practitioners. As noted earlier, unlike the previous financing structure of the health care system in which physicians were not required to bear the costs of additional resources for diagnosis and treatment, the modern system of capitation puts the physician's economic interest in conflict with some patients' needs for such resources. The threat of implicit rationing is real, and this raises new and acute concerns about quality. How is managed care, whether in traditional managed care organizations or integrated delivery systems, to be regulated?

Providers have seized on "any-willing-provider" laws, which reduce the ability of managed care systems to specifically select physicians with whom they will contract to provide care. Some aspects of any-willing-provider laws might be helpful, especially insofar as they require additional information for consumers on the nature of utilization review. These laws should, however, be fine-tuned. Consumers need to know, in simple terms, the amount of risk that physicians are assuming on capitated or prepaid contracts. The average consumer should understand that if the economic risk to the physicians is high, the incentives for rationing and the risk of compromised quality may also be high. Thus we applaud the "sunshine act" aspects of managed care regulation. We know, however, that any effort to force public disclosure will mean radical change for the managed care industry, because health care organizations have not traditionally made public the exact nature of internal physician incentives.

The more important aspect of any-willing-provider laws from the viewpoint of physicians is the central requirement that all managed care networks be opened to any provider who wishes to join. We doubt the wisdom of this requirement. If responsible cost consciousness is to be integrated into health care, managed care will have to do much of the heavy lifting. The discounts available through capitated payment are critical in a cost-conscious environment. We must emphasize a culture of parsimony in day-to-day medical practice, and managed care does this. It is rational and responsible to develop a counterweight to the excesses of resource use that have grown habitual in the fee-for-service medical care world. More is not necessarily better. If an organization is to be held responsible for the quality and costs of the care it delivers, then it must be able to exercise responsibility for the choice of physicians on whom it will rely to deliver that care. Networks should not be opened. If they are, quality is just as likely to deteriorate as to improve.

Nor do we find any compelling arguments in favor of encouraging physician-dominated managed care programs to the exclusion of other forms of management. Organized medicine would like to raise the limit on the proportion of specialists in a given geographical area who can participate in a managed care plan (currently 20 percent). While one could argue that physicians in management might be more attuned to patient needs, it seems equally probable that physicians would respond to profits just as much as would other health care managers. The argument for physician-dominated networks is simply not compelling, but the antitrust concerns it raises are.

How, then, can managed care organizations be responsively regulated? We believe the model should be based on large doses of self-policing. NCQA may in the future become a more demanding regulator and more ambitious in the aims it sets for the industry, but in our view, the initial set of HEDIS measures shows many of the characteristics of a negotiated settlement for managed care organizations. Rather than relying on NCQA alone, we would strongly encourage HMOs to specify the quality standards that they will meet, and would expect them to be tough. Compliance by practitioners with specified processes of care and publication of patient satisfaction data are the foundations on which we would build this self-regulation. Moreover, managed care organizations and burgeoning networks must be able to demonstrate good outcomes in the areas of care that are most vulnerable in managed care settings. The public should be especially interested in the care provided for patients requiring significant resources and should be able to evaluate critical incentive structures. Profiles of patients who are referred for hospitalization with certain diagnoses should be made available by those delivery systems that place the hospitals at risk for care. Regulators could help by standardizing certain processes of care—for example, by requesting clinical information on and outcomes for patients with unstable angina. Publication of this information, and discussion of outcomes between regulators and managed care organizations, are important elements of a responsive approach to regulation.

The regulators themselves must be prepared to identify superior methods within managed care organizations. Though competition is appropriate in a health care scheme, those innovations that appear to improve quality at no additional cost should be shared among organizations. Regulators can help in such networking and exchange. The regulatory model should not be one of biannual or unannounced visits to survey particular organizations. Rather, every major alternative delivery system should have regulatory teams assigned to it. This will be made easier as health care competition becomes increasingly oligopolistic. The teams and the organizations should consult with one another, and the regulators should encourage learning. When and if outcomes begin to deteriorate in specific care processes, regulators should confer and help managed care organizations understand why this is the case long before sanctions are visited.

Perhaps the best place for this point of regulatory contact is a quality oversight board. We envision that state-based regulation of alternative delivery systems and managed care organizations would require that health care organizations create such quality boards to exercise oversight of care. These quality boards could be made up of leading providers and selected patients, following the model of institutional review boards that oversee biomedical research.

The quality boards should have some independence and should constantly be reviewing quality information from within the organization. They would examine all new critical pathways, short-stay mechanisms, and case management concerns. They would report to top management. The quality board would play an ombudsperson role within the organization, advocating quality of care. For example, the board might limit the amount of risk that could be devolved to the practitioner, so as to decrease the likelihood of inappropriate trade-offs between cost and quality. It might prohibit use of a new care pathway if that pathway seemed to be too stringent in reducing the hospital stay. Or it might insist on careful outcome measures when a specific program is initiated.

In some ways, the boards would provide an organizational pathway for the altruistic commitment of provider to patient. Their goal would be to oversee the effectiveness of systems for quality improvement and to ensure that economic incentives were not adversely affecting the quality of care.

Working with quality boards, the regulators would become less surveyors and more quality consultants. Of course, regulators would be empowered to enforce fallback standards should the accountable health plan fail to promote a sturdy quality council or fail to demonstrate its compliance with the self-set quality measures. As Braithwaite has suggested, there would be a strong regulatory stick held in the background that would help promote the more cooperative relationship between plan and regulators.

The oversight of alternative delivery systems will probably be the dominant regulatory mode of the future. The transformation of the health care system makes a great deal of traditional regulation appear anachronistic. The notion of independent hospitals and independent physicians will fade as health care becomes more corporate. In the meantime, however, modifications in existing regulatory structures can speed the creation of a culture of responsive regulation.

The regulation of physicians will probably continue to fade into the background as health care integrates. Though hiding problems may be emotionally easier in the short run, it is in almost no one's long-term interest to protect deficient physicians within an organization. The culling function performed by medical boards can probably be replaced by increased attention on the part of accountable health plans to the quality of care provided by individual practitioners.

Rx 7: Build on Traditional Provider Oversight Mechanisms

As noted earlier, it is sensible to continue to license physicians. The licensing authority can play some coordinating role as the health care system moves further toward complete integration. Physicians who are the subject of numerous complaints, who have been disciplined by organizations, or who perhaps are strong outliers for malpractice claims should be scrutinized by medical boards. As the role of these boards is reconceived, they should be viewed as sturdy agents of oversight that lie in the background of self-regulation. For example, medical boards, along with other authorities, can investigate claims that physicians inappropriately ration care under pressure from capitation. So long as the thresholds are fairly high, and the oversight once called into action is rational, there is no reason why medical boards should pollute responsive regulation.

The role of hospital regulation is more complex. As hospitals are absorbed into integrated delivery systems, regulation of the single institution runs the risk of creating uncoordinated signals. A regulatory focus on the IDS offers the prospect of cohesion. Yet for the foreseeable future, hospital regulation through the JCAHO will persist. The JCAHO is slowly restructuring, as surveyors learn to teach rather than to survey. The emphasis on benchmarking and measurement is appropriate. The JCAHO is at this point groping toward models of responsive regulation.

Two important caveats attend our analysis of hospital regulation. First, the JCAHO would really begin to improve the quality of care if its ongoing organizational liaisons were invigorated. The commission should be encouraged to disseminate information about interesting new forms of quality improvement. The lessons learned in one hospital should be part of the communication between the JCAHO and other hospitals. If copying were promoted, and if lessons were applied with the help of PDCA methods, the efficacy of JCAHO oversight would be greatly increased.

Second, the JCAHO should allow much more flexibility in meeting standards. It could provide a valuable model for future regulation if it were willing to negotiate with hospitals to create institutional self-regulation for compliance with customized outcome measures. The JCAHO's Indicator Measurement System has been widely criticized, for good reason. Many providers and critical decision makers find its measures unhelpful. Instead of insisting on a single track, the JCAHO should be willing to promote innovation in measures and then hold institutions to their word.

This new attitude would go some way toward removing the sustained reputation of the JCAHO as a punitive overseer. Today's perception of the JCAHO as simply a culler and remover of defects is very strong. Continuing the Agenda for Change on a more radical trajectory might lead to even more impressive accomplishments by the JCAHO, and might successfully catapult the organization into a position of regulating IDSs.

However, without a much greater commitment on the part of the JCAHO to responsive regulation, we would be hesitant about endorsing the commission as the regulatory locus for accountable health plans of the future. The next five years are critical. As the new competitive health plan system emerges, so too might a JCAHO willing to play a more insightful and thoughtful regulatory role. If this is the case, and if the commission can metamorphose sufficiently to shake its reputation as a hostile surveyor, it may emerge as the vehicle for regulating for improvement.

The future of the Peer Review Organizations is somewhat cloudier. Like the JCAHO and NCQA, the PROs would like to be the arbiter of quality measurement and the consultant of choice regarding quality improvement. However, the PROs' responsibility is limited to Medicare. Given the emphasis on fiscal responsibility in Washington in the mid-1990s, it seems unlikely that Medicare revenues will increase greatly in the near future. Therefore the PROs will remain somewhat shackled to care for the elderly and disabled.

The new health care system needs coordinated regulation. It is difficult to see how a prominent role for the PROs could be a part of such regulation. Should another overarching regulator of accountable health plans emerge, such as the JCAHO, what further important role could the Peer Review Organizations take on, especially as Medicare increasingly utilizes capitation-based risk contracts? Of course, HCFA oversight will not fade away, particularly while the elderly constitute a strong lobby. Yet is it really necessary? Will not PRO requirements, insofar as they differ from those of other regulators, simply create additional work and inefficiencies? Although the Peer Review Organizations, to their credit, are less easily captured than other regulators, the question still remains whether additional signals do not simply add dissonance. Copying and learning can be promoted by others, to whom oversight of Medicare should perhaps be shifted.

Public data reporting should become more prominent in a responsive regulatory environment. We do not advocate that all health care institutions be required to meet the same outcome measures. Rather, we suggest that individual institutions provide their own data on quality, with a fallback position set by regulators. As long as a health care institution can appropriately justify a set of standards to consumers and regulators, it seems that the public will be able to judge the institution's ability to meet those standards.

Higher-quality performers will set higher standards for themselves, and consumers should be able to recognize this.

We would also suggest that health care institutions be required to make public their leading quality interventions. We want to promote copying and learning and believe public sharing of new insights is desirable. Although, as we have mentioned, this may be somewhat at odds with the notion of competition in health care, it is very much in keeping with the collaborative, honest, and open sharing of care improvements seen in the past. As new and exciting technologies were integrated into health care—for example, coronary artery bypass grafting—the innovators acted like any other scientists and shared their techniques and efforts in the scientific literature. Our insistence that quality innovation methods be shared with the public and with other health care institutions is merely an outgrowth of this sense of collaboration that has been so important to patient care. To use the analogy of report cards, it is important to share not only one's test scores or final marks but also one's study techniques. As the system relies increasingly on competition, it must also be prepared to nurture collaboration.

Rx 8: Change Malpractice Liability Law to Incorporate No-Fault Provisions and Enterprise Liability

Medical injury compensation demands reform. Two critical insights drive our negative assessment of the efficacy of malpractice as a quality promoter. First, identifying negligent care has always been extraordinarily difficult. Because case reviewers disagree on whether negligence occurred, the administrative costs of the medical malpractice system are very high. Many potential suits are not brought, yet at the same time, a large amount of litigation concerns cases in which there was no negligence. Patients are not compensated, and the deterrence signal is difficult for providers to understand.

The situation is likely to become worse as capitated care brings some rationing to the bedside. In the past, the negligence determination was simplified somewhat by the cost-blind nature of medical care. In the future, it will not be possible to assume that the physician's standard of care is founded on the deployment of all available resources on behalf of patients. Although some commentators have suggested that cost considerations will readily be integrated into the medical malpractice standards, others are not so sanguine.[7] It seems likely that attempts to understand the standard of care will become ever more difficult as physicians weigh the costs of every test and procedure.[8]

The second major difficulty with medical malpractice is the way in which the legal issues are presently evolving. Greater amounts of care are being rendered through organizations. Medical malpractice, however, is based primarily on the responsibility of the individual practitioner. Insofar as litigation is unable to reach the accountable health plan, either because it is ERISA-qualified or because organizational liability simply does not exist in the state where the suit would be filed, attempts to obtain redress may be thwarted. Although integrated delivery systems are the appropriate targets for litigation, current law makes it very difficult to reach them, and physicians pay the price. Medical malpractice must be reformed if it is to play any sort of definable role in contributing to quality of care.

Medical malpractice does have some positive attributes. First, it is not prone to capture, thanks to the independence of the trial bar. Second, its deterrence signal, though based on a deficient system of identifying defects, is nonetheless registered by institutions. Empirical research on deterrence suggests that the deterrent effect is noted primarily at the level of the organization.[9] Therefore, as the organizational structure of medicine becomes ever more important, malpractice litigation should play a proportionately significant role.

In light of these facts, we would recommend two significant changes in malpractice regulation. First, we suggest dropping the requirement of a demonstration of negligence and moving to a strict liability/no-fault approach. One of us has advocated this in other contexts in the past,[10] but here it is intended to bolster quality of care. Most medical injuries are preventable, and thus can be the targets of quality improvement efforts on the part of the system as a whole. Focusing on the medical injury rather than on the difficult-to-define negligence that may have caused it creates the context for appropriate efforts toward improvement.

Second, we favor an enterprise liability focus and therefore hope for reforms in ERISA that will allow this to occur. No-fault provides a much clearer signal, and insofar as it is supported by risk-adjusted premiums paid by an enterprise, it brings about deterrence. Malpractice litigation based on an enterprise liability/no-fault model would increase incentives to identify process defects that are associated with medical injuries.[11]

We realize that any medical injury compensation scheme will provide an uncoordinated series of deterrence signals. However, it may make good sense to have a system for addressing quality that is completely free of any possibility of capture, especially as the prevalence of self-regulation increases. No-fault compensation for injuries serves an important social process in itself (providing compensation for uninsured costs of accidents). But more important, it can provide a source of clear and uncaptured signals for safety.

Rx 9: Revise ERISA to Permit Adequate State Regulation of New Health Care Structures

The most appropriate locus for reasonably responsive regulation is at the level of the state (which encompasses state designates such as the JCAHO). Some regulatory power must be brought to bear on institutions when self-regulation is not functioning smoothly. We believe that the states are better positioned to set up the appropriate liaisons and consulting relationships with health care organizations. The federal government is too distant and the task too massive for it. The federal government cannot possibly consider creating the bureaucracy needed to oversee all institutions in all fifty states. A prominent state role is appropriate.

This regulatory oversight will have to be protected from ERISA preemption. There is no doubt that, given the advantages, employers will continue to self-insure and will increasingly contract directly with integrated delivery systems. This means that a good portion of the operation of IDSs will fall under the preemptive umbrella of ERISA. There is a need for state oversight—and the hovering threat of the state's fist—if the regulated industry is to have incentives to improve quickly. But if ERISA's immunities continue to expand despite the *Travelers* decision (see Chapter Five), the reach of these incentives will steadily decline.

Rx 10: Encourage Antitrust Enforcement to Promote Cooperative Behaviors That Reduce Cost While Improving Outcomes

Antitrust litigation emphasizes containment of cost much more than improvement of quality. Given the complex series of new configurations in integrated care, the antitrust regulators' concentration on horizontal arrangements between providers is somewhat outdated. It makes little sense for physicians or others to fix prices at artificially high levels when there is competition between integrated systems. If price-fixing occurs, capitated payment will simply go elsewhere—assuming, of course, that there are competing groups of physicians in the marketplace. The physicians are no longer the dominant economic player.

Nevertheless, many of the impulses of federal authorities are reasonable. They have sought to clarify the complex rules guiding enforcement and to provide safe harbors. In the case of mergers, they have moved in the direction of reasonable settlements, allowing partial mergers. But in Pueblo, Colorado, for instance, they appear to have failed (see Chapter Five). Two struggling hospitals in a single small city do not provide care of as high a quality as one robust center. In many such circumstances in our bloated health care industry, consolidation of services, even at the expense of competition, is the wiser choice.

In their oversight of physician-hospital organizations and networks, federal officials have been willing to accommodate new organizations as long as the risk of horizontal price fixing is minimized. The courts have now indicated that they will review cases of monopolization of physician services by managed care organizations; this is the next major step in the evolution of antitrust regulation—one that is quite important for quality competition.

We do not see a need to remake antitrust law from the ground up. It is important for IDSs to compete appropriately with one another. We are supportive of the Justice Department's insistence that no one delivery system dominate care within particular specialties. Such domination would undermine the effect of capitation by creating an imbalance in negotiations on capitation fees and the cost-saving benefits that should come from managed care. We do, however, encourage serious reconsideration of enforcement behaviors when they stand in the way of rational system development, especially when they impede consolidation of high-technology services in areas of oversupply or underuse. We would, at a minimum, expect antitrust enforcement policies to be flexible enough to allow sharing and copying of interventions that improve quality (a policy the federal authorities have followed).

Rx 11: Rethink the Role of Fraud and Abuse Regulation

We believe that fraud and abuse litigation is misguided. The regulatory basis for litigation against fraud and abuse is culling. Such litigation is intended to protect patients from illegitimate profit making, especially through overuse of procedures. But again, with strong capitation, what motivation would physicians have to overuse resources? The major problem will be with underuse, and the trade-offs between cost and quality that occur as a result. The purpose of deploying fraud and abuse litigation in a health care system dominated by IDSs is difficult to discern.

Perhaps more important, the attempt to rein in provider profit making is being made in a health care system whose evolution is driven by the pursuit of profit (or in the case of not-for-profit entities, growth in fund balances). It is imperative that these prohibitions of such kickbacks be reconsidered. The definition of kickbacks have fallen behind the actual and justifiable trends in relationships between managed care systems and the clinicians they rely on.

There will, of course, be moral hazard within organizations, and a strong desire to profit by reducing resources for patients. However, the regulatory apparatus described earlier for oversight of IDSs should identify areas in which this might occur and should establish appropriate quality measures for them. Federal fraud and abuse regulation seems only to hamper the further coordination of health care oversight and has almost nothing additional to contribute.

Current tax laws are somewhat more valid than fraud and abuse regulations. They are intended to protect the public's interest in the gain reaped by benefits organizations from tax-exempt status. Nonprofit hospitals that do not pay taxes and that can accept tax-deductible contributions cannot allow these benefits to inure to profit-making entities. Of course, the regulations (IRS rulings) that result from the government's well-founded intentions do complicate integration, but these complications should be acceptable to organizations interested in retaining its nonprofit status, and are to some extent inevitable.

Both fraud and abuse litigation and tax law raise the major question with which we have been wrestling in our consideration of quality incentives in an integrating health care system. Market incentives are clearly driving the effort to reduce costs, and that effort is dependent on managed care and integration. A similar dependency may develop where competitive efforts are directed toward quality improvement. However, trade-offs between cost and quality are cause for concern. Fraud and abuse regulation and the tax laws only tangentially address this issue, to the extent that they seek to reinstate a less competitive, less profit-driven environment. It is better, in our view, to let state regulators take up this issue as the health care system evolves.

Rx 12: Monitor Quality for the Impoverished

At this point, it appears that the Health Care Financing Administration will engage in less and less oversight of changes in Medicaid. This is worrisome, because the Medicaid population may be especially vulnerable in an immature capitated market. Medicaid patients may often be "money losers" for organizations in a capitated arrangement with poor adjustment for risks. Moreover, many Medicaid recipients will be less able to understand information available to consumers and will be in a weaker political position to retain and exercise choice. For this vulnerable group, the trade-offs between cost and quality may be damaging ones.

Given these circumstances, it may make sense to have specific oversight for state Medicaid plans. The task might be handled by IDS regulators, but we suggest that this is one area in which additional governmental oversight may be more important than complete coordination of regulation. We favor safeguards for Medicaid patients that may go beyond those for other consumers.

To provide such safeguards is probably going to require changes in the legal process through which states obtain Medicaid waivers. Waivers have so far been intended to allow states to experiment with alternative mechanisms for delivering care. Yet many states would like to make permanent changes—for example, to move Medicaid into managed care. How should the federal government oversee this process? In particular, how should it oversee quality of care?

We favor an explicit recognition, in the form of new federal statutory law, that states are able to move Medicaid from fee-for-service to managed care mechanisms. The waiver process must be modified to allow for oversight of such shifts. We also favor a federal requirement that states submit Medicaid care to quality measures of outcomes and process. HCFA could specify rules on data gathering, processing, and reporting. This would provide the agency with information necessary to regulate for improvement and would provide the nation with comparative data on the performance of different types of Medicaid programs. HCFA should be empowered to discipline those programs that do poorly on such measures. Such a system provides an opportunity for HCFA and states to engage in responsive regulation.

Finally, it goes without saying that the uninsured do not receive the same standard of care as that received by the insured. Lack of access to care remains a salient problem for the quality of the American health care system. States should have the opportunity to address this issue—if necessary, through Medicaid and ERISA waivers.

Rx 13: Establish Public Processes for Exchange of Information on Improvements and Innovations

Secrecy about improvement impedes improvement. According to medical tradition, it is also unethical. A surgeon who invents a better approach to the pancreas is expected to publish it. The daylight of open dissemination of good ideas subjects those ideas to review and critique and allows benefit to accrue to many. If the surgeon replied, "I wish to keep this a secret so that I can use my knowledge for my economic benefit and compete more effectively against my colleague surgeons," there would be an outcry of criticism couched in the language of professional duty and ethical responsibility. In effect, clinical ethics (at least as espoused) treat knowledge as a public good.

The norm has its limits. Most physicians would probably not view it as unethical for a surgeon who invents a new device to patent it and to derive economic benefit from its sale. A hospital that created a new computerized patient registration system that smoothed flow and offered local market advantages would probably escape criticism for keeping it secret, even if an argument could be made that its wider use would save medical resources in the community as a whole.

The newly energized competitive health care market will put pressure on the distinction between improvement knowledge that is a public good and improvement knowledge that is a property useful for competitive gain. If "immunization rate" is measured in the HEDIS report card, should a managed care organization able to improve that rate through a clever new approach to high-risk patients keep that approach to itself? Or should it make it widely known so that larger numbers of high-risk children can be immunized everywhere? If better pain control earns a hospital a larger share of the surgical market, should its approach to pain management be a secret? What about an innovation that reduces operative death rates in a marketplace where death rates are published to support consumer choice?

Advocates of market forces as a key to improvement may regard such questions as coming from a self-important "medical model" or worse, naïveté. But they must nonetheless face them. Who will be the stewards of knowledge that can benefit the public's health and conserve strained medical resources? Is the market steward enough?

We think not. There is some force that moves government to spread knowledge. Why else would we have an Agricultural Extension Service to spread awareness of good farming practices, even among competing farmers? Why would we have a National Transportation Safety Board that investigates accidents so that all travelers may be safer? Who would not find it abhorrent and seek legal sanctions if an airline discovered a consequential problem in its Boeing 747s, kept it a secret, fixed it in its own planes, then waited for others, unaware of the problem, to crash, thereby giving the airline a competitive advantage in the marketplace?

The fragmented, local, and increasingly competitive and fearful medical market holds insufficient promise for sustaining rapid, open exchange of great ideas for improvement. The skills, systems, and habits of exchange are underdeveloped. Innovations in processes of care spread too slowly already, and we believe that the pace may even slacken for a while. We favor the development, as a matter of public policy, of governmentally supported mechanisms to collect and disseminate good ideas for change. President Clinton's ill-fated Health Security Act contemplated such a vehicle in the form of "regional professional foundations," whose purpose was to support data collection, exchange, and open study of good practices among professionals and organizations. The model built on the great success of the Maine Medical Assessment Project and other examples of voluntary collaboration among clinicians searching for improved processes and outcomes. Without governmental action, we fear that such collaborations will not build or spread. The time may come when the health care market will have matured enough to support collaborative learning in the private sector, but that time is not yet in sight.

We suggest that regional professional foundations, or perhaps some medical analogue to Agricultural Extension Services, be developed and supported. This would best be done at the federal level, where economies of scale may be found. However, we also recognize that sometimes local innovation and local networks—exploiting similarities and common understandings—can better support rapid exchange of ideas. Some states have already taken steps of this type. The state of Washington, for example, has lately supported collaborative work on improvements in obstetrical practice.

Although we advocate governmental stewardship of mechanisms for exchange of improvement ideas, we are equally concerned that professional groups support and insist on such exchange. Professional self-regulation should include strong stands by the professions themselves on the need to preserve scientific publication and professional collaboration in learning as important norms of behavior. We recently learned of a hospital that refused to share information on how it achieved significant improvements in out-comes for pneumonia patients, lest that information find its way into the hands of its competitors. Neither professions nor govern-ments should be tolerant of such behavior, and both should be active in efforts to prevent it and to encourage openness.

Rx 14: Maintain Governmental Support for Community-Based Health Improvement Initiatives

Most ill health is engendered far from the world of medical care, and most basic prevention has little to do with the technologies of care. A hospital admission is "rework." The real failure often lies upstream. McGinnis and Foege, in a landmark essay,[12] analyzed the pattern of mortality in the United States and determined that about half of all deaths in 1990 could be attributed to tobacco, diet and activity patterns, alcohol, firearms, risky sexual behaviors, motor vehicle accidents, and illicit drug use. The greatest opportunities to improve health in the nation lie in the control and reduction of these everyday causes of mortality and morbidity.

Will the developing medical marketplace respond? Perhaps in the long run, it will. Progressive employers and the HEDIS score-card, for example, treat certain prevention activities as an index of quality in provider organizations. Some, for example, examine smok-ing rates among enrollees, or rates of mammographic screening.

But it is a long jump—a chasm, actually—between care designs that assure mammograms and effective actions that reduce avoidable injuries, motor vehicle crashes, and risky sexual behaviors. One key maneuver for the reduction of tobacco use, for example, is to enforce age restrictions on the purchase of cigarettes from vending machines. How, exactly, is an HMO to achieve that? What if reducing motor vehicle injuries requires innovations in teenage driver education?

One real hospital, the Magic Valley Regional Hospital in Twin Falls, Idaho, undertook the role of leading a citywide campaign to reduce bicycle injuries in children. It worked. The program achieved a 40 percent reduction in emergency room visits for head injuries in bicycle accidents within a few months. It also "achieved" a major financial headache for the hospital, whose emergency room revenues fell by several hundred thousand dollars. This hospital had the ethical stamina to maintain the preventive activity nevertheless. But how many would?

Nor will capitation solve the problem. If a competitive market in capitated managed care were to develop in a small city, how could one hospital find advantage in supporting community efforts to prevent bicycle injuries? The resulting cost savings would be spread among competitors as well as in the initiating organization. This is often the nature of community-based health improvements.

The market may suffice to induce improvements in care within organizations; we doubt that it will also achieve improvements that require community-level action and high degrees of coordination among agencies and organizations. For this reason, pursuit of the health of the public must fall to governments and others able to act across institutional and economic boundaries. We have heard a good deal of optimistic talk about how managed care competition will support prevention of disease, but we believe that many causes of death and disease will yield more readily to collaborations supported and organized by government. The need for strong federal support of such institutions as the Centers for Disease Control, the U.S. Office of Disease Prevention and Health Promotion, and the National Center for Health Statistics will remain, even in the Darwinian era of health care provision. Similar needs exist for state-level epidemiology, public health services, and bridge-building programs of prevention and outreach.

Summary and Conclusion

Health care markets and providers are moving into a new era. Regulation must follow. As systems of care replace divided and fragmented individual providers, the eyes of the regulator must adjust their focus, lest regulation become the oversight of fossils. As the need for improvement of care becomes more and more evident, and as methods for the measurement of progress become more and more available, regulators must be able to master new means in the service of new ends.

We find much worth preserving in the current regulatory apparatus but even more that needs to change. Slowly but inexorably, the regulatory mechanisms that were birthed to keep health care both honest and safe may, without change, become serious impediments to the best efforts of health care to evolve and improve. Like health care providers, regulators who cling too tightly to their own past will find themselves less and less able to serve those who depend on them.

We have made recommendations for change, but in the final analysis, the system has become too complex for reliable predictions. For the regulator of the future seeking to make sound changes, there can be little certainty about what is right. However, what is *wrong* is to stay still. The best alternative—the only responsible alternative, in fact—is to agree to change, and then to test promising approaches under circumstances in which all can learn by reflecting together. Regulation is a technology. It must evolve, be tested, and always bear the burden of proving its worth.

We suggest that regulators become responsive in the manner outlined by Braithwaite. They should attempt to cooperate with health care providers, to specify outcomes, and to cultivate innovation. They should adopt many of the modern methods of improving the quality of their work that providers are now adopting for theirs. We believe that if they do so, they will cultivate quality *and* avoid capture.

We propose the move to responsive regulation because we believe the market alone cannot produce incentives for high-quality care. One of our greatest concerns is indeed that the market may overemphasize costs to the detriment of quality. If anything, regulation has a larger role as the market evolves, not a smaller one.

Notes

1. G. Hardin, "The Tragedy of the Commons," *Science* 162 (1968): 1243–48.

2. H. H. Hiatt, "Protecting the Medical Commons: Who Is Responsible?" *New England Journal of Medicine* 293 (1975): 235–241.

3. See J. E. Wennberg, J. L. Freeman, and W. J. Culp, "Are Hospital Services Rationed in New Haven or Over-Utilized in Boston?" *Lancet* 1 (1987): 1185–89; see W. P. Welch, M. E. Miller, H. G. Welch, E. S. Fisher, and J. E. Wennberg, "Geographic Variation in Expenditures for Physicians' Services in the United States," *New England Journal of Medicine* 328 (1993): 621–627.

4. A. F. Bentley and J. Dewey, *Knowing and the Known* (Boston: Beacon Press, 1949).

5. W. Shewhart, *Economic Control of Quality of Manufactured Product* (New York: Van Nostrand Reinhold, 1931).

6. National Institute of Standards and Technology, *Malcolm Baldrige National Quality Award Application Criteria* (Gaithersburg, Md.: National Institute of Standards and Technology, 1995).

7. M. A. Hall, "Institutional Control of Physician Behavior: Legal Barriers to Health Care Cost Containment," *University of Pennsylvania Law Review* 137 (1988): 431–536; E. H. Morreim, "Cost Containment and the Standard of Medical Care," *California Law Review* 75 (1987): 1719–1763.

8. For a different solution to this problem, see E. H. Morreim, "Redefining Quality by Reassigning Responsibility," *American Journal of Law and Medicine* 20 (1994): 79–104.

9. See T. A. Brennan, "Letter: Questioning the Value of Liability in Medical Malpractice," *Health Affairs* 14 (1985): 320–321.

10. T. A. Brennan and M. Rosenthal, "Medical Malpractice Reform: The Current Proposals," *Journal of General Internal Medicine* 10 (1995): 211–218.

11. See L. A. Petersen, T. A. Brennan, A. C. O'Neil, E. F. Cook, and T. H. Lee, "Does Housestaff Discontinuity of Care Increase the Risk

for Preventable Adverse Events?" *Annals of Internal Medicine*
121(11) (1994): 866–872.

12. J. M. McGinnis and W. H. Foege, "Actual Causes of Death in the
United States," *Journal of the American Medical Association* 270
(1993): 2207–12.

Index